Psychiatric Care in
the Nursing Home

Psychiatric Care
in the
Nursing Home

Edited by

William E. Reichman, M.D.

Associate Professor of Clinical Psychiatry
Robert Wood Johnson Medical School
University of Medicine and Dentistry
of New Jersey

Paul R. Katz, M.D.

Associate Professor of Medicine
University of Rochester
School of Medicine & Dentistry

New York   Oxford
OXFORD UNIVERSITY PRESS
1996

Oxford University Press

Oxford   New York
Athens   Auckland   Bangkok   Bombay
Calcutta   Cape Town   Dar es Salaam   Delhi
Florence   Hong Kong   Istanbul   Karachi
Kuala Lumpur   Madras   Madrid   Melbourne
Mexico City   Nairobi   Paris   Singapore
Taipei   Tokyo   Toronto
and associated companies in
Berlin   Ibadan

Copyright © 1996 by Oxford University Press, Inc.

Published by Oxford University Press, Inc.,
198 Madison Avenue, New York, New York 10016

Library of Congress Cataloging-in-Publication Data
Psychiatric care in the nursing home / edited by William E. Reichman,
Paul R. Katz.
p.   cm. Includes bibliographical references and index.
ISBN 0-19-508515-9
1. Nursing home patients—Mental health.   2. Geriatric psychiatry.
I. Reichman, William E.   II. Katz, Paul R. (Paul Richard)
[DNLM: 1. Mental Disorders—in old age.   2. Nursing Homes.   WT
150 P9661   1996]
RC451.4.N87P78   1996
362.2'3—dc20
DNLM/DLC
for Library of Congress   95-36063

1 3 5 7 9 8 6 4 2
Printed in the United States of America
on acid-free paper

Foreword

Lissy F. Jarvik

For many years there were very few of us laboring to advance the field of geriatric psychiatry and to improve the delivery of mental health care to the elderly. It is most gratifying, therefore, to find that so much knowledge has been accumulated as to fill a hefty book dealing with the delimited topic of psychiatric care in nursing homes. The editors have targeted the primary care physician as the key reader for this book, and have succeeded in providing a very readable and well-illustrated volume. It is enriched with case history material and will serve well the needs of the busy practitioner. But it is also well-referenced so that anyone wishing to pursue any topic in greater depth will have the opportunity to do so.

The chapter authors include several with outstanding national and international reputations which might make us forget the caveat issued by the editors in their preface: "... Much of what we know about the treatment of mental illness in the nursing home is extrapolated from data gathered in other settings and our unreplicated clinical experiences."

We all look forward to a future when wisdom and contentment will characterize the last part of life, but as long as dementia and depression remain associated with old age, as long as the full understanding of the mental infirmities associated with old age remains elusive, this volume will continue to meet an important need.

Preface

This is among the first multiauthored texts devoted exclusively to psychiatric problems in the nursing home. The need for such a book becomes evident after a quick review of the characteristics of the population currently residing in nursing homes. Numerous studies document the very high prevalence of psychiatric-related illness in nursing facilities. Dementia, mood and anxiety disorders, psychosis, sleep disorders, and nonspecific disturbances such as restlessness or aggression all contribute significantly to morbidity and mortality in nursing home residents (Borson et al., 1987). Indeed, 70% of nursing home residents may meet diagnostic criteria for dementia (Rovner et al., 1990), while 90% of residents may have at least one form of behavioral disturbance (Tariot et al., 1993). Estimates that the total number of nursing home residents in the United States will exceed 2 million by the turn of the century and 4 million by the year 2040 (Schneider and Guralnik, 1990) indicate the need for psychiatrically oriented care in this setting. Even now it has been estimated that once one reaches the age of 65 years, the risk of a nursing home admission before death exceeds 40% (Kemper and Murtaugh, 1991).

While psychiatric problems are commonplace in the nursing home, detracting significantly from quality of life, specific psychiatric diagnoses accompanied by reasoned care plans are applied in only a small minority of cases. Zimmer and colleagues, for example, observed that serious behavioral problems were documented in less than 10% of affected cases, while psychiatric consultation was appropriately requested for only 1 of 7 residents (Zimmer et al., 1984).

Care for nursing home residents is further complicated by the presence of significant physical disability as well as a paucity of social supports (see following table). In addition, the management of psychiatric illness in very old and frail nursing home residents is often constrained by the systems of care or the "milieu" of the nursing home. Direct care in nursing facilities is provided, in large part, by unlicensed staff (i.e., nursing assistants) who generally lack the training necessary to accommodate the host of medical and psychosocial needs of the resident population. Further, professional nurses are forced to expend much energy complying with regulatory requirements, thus limiting their involvement

Selected Characteristics of Nursing Home Residents Aged 65 and Above

Subject	Percent Living in Nursing Homes, 1985 (n = 1318)	Percent Living in Community, 1984 (n = 26,343)
Age		
65 to 74	16.1	61.7
75 to 84	38.6	30.7
85+	45.3	7.6
Sex		
Men	25.4	40.8
Women	74.6	59.2
Race		
White	93.1	90.4
Black	6.2	8.3
Other	0.7	1.3
Marital status		
Widowed	67.8	34.1
Married	12.8	54.7
Never married	13.5	4.4
Divorced or separated	5.9	6.3
Requires assistance in		
Bathing	91.0	6.0
Dressing	77.6	4.3
Using toilet room	63.2	2.2
Transferring	62.6	2.8
Eating	40.3	1.1
Difficulty with bowel and/or bladder control	54.5	(NA)

Source: U.S. Senate Special Committee on Aging and the American Association of Retired Persons. *Aging America: Trends and Projections.* Washington, DC: USDHHS Pub. No. (FCOA) 91-28001, 1991.

at the bedside. Although adjusting to a "sicker" population over the past several years, nurses make up just over 10% of all nursing home employees, with a ratio of one registered nurse per 49 nursing home residents (Mezey and Knapp, 1993).

Care in nursing homes has been affected not only by levels of staffing and proficiency but also, very importantly, by legislative mandates. A number of such mandates were set forth with passage of the nursing home reform amendments contained within the Omnibus Budget Reconciliation Act of 1987 (OBRA). Stemming from a 1983 Institute of Medicine report documenting significant deficiencies in the care of nursing home residents, the recommendations embodied in OBRA sought to enhance resident rights, shift from process-based to outcome-based criteria in the assessment of quality, and guarantee the provision of standardized comprehensive assessments to all residents while clearly detailing the rationale for medications, particularly psychoactive agents (Elon and Pawlson,

1992). While nursing home practice, in many ways, has been revolutionized since OBRA, as evidenced by significant declines in the use of chemical and physical restraints, the benefits of such reform for other critical aspects of nursing home care have been more elusive. For example, the recruitment of specialists to nursing facilities who are expert in the treatment of psychiatric-related illness remains problematic.

In this context who, then, can be expected to deliver the services needed to maintain the mental health of the approximately 1.6 million individuals currently residing in this nation's 16,000 facilities? To all intents and purposes, it is the internist and family practitioner who have assumed this responsibility. These primary care physicians, who typically spend less than 20 minutes per nursing home resident per month, clearly need as much support as possible when it comes to managing the vagaries of psychiatric illness in an increasingly complex nursing home environment. It is primarily for these physicians that *Psychiatric Care in the Nursing Home* was written. While psychiatry and psychology consultants, nurse specialists, and other professionals should find valuable information in this volume, our overriding goal has been to provide clinically oriented material to assist the nursing home practitioner in addressing the main diagnostic, treatment, ethical, and social dilemmas in the care of their patients. All of the authors, recognized experts in their respective fields, have practical hands-on experience in the nursing home setting. To further assist the reader, we have attempted, whenever appropriate, to structure each chapter so as to cover a broad range of issues in epidemiology, pathophysiology, differential diagnosis, and contemporary approaches to pharmacological and nonpharmacological treatment. Despite this effort, our understanding of these issues is limited by a paucity of rigorously conducted observations of the phenomenology of mental illness in the nursing home setting.

Additionally, much of what we know about the treatment of mental illness in the nursing home is extrapolated from data gathered in other settings and from our unreplicated clinical experiences. While acknowledging the many questions that remain unanswered, we are hopeful that *Psychiatric Care in the Nursing Home* will provide some much-needed building blocks while highlighting the urgent need for more research in this area.

Over the years, our devotion to nursing home care has been fostered by many generous colleagues who have provided support and much-appreciated mentorship. We are also very grateful to the numerous contributors to this volume who worked diligently to provide insightful clinical information despite a relative paucity of research data. Last, we wish to express tremendous gratitude to Ann Rauchbach for her continuous devotion and important contribution to the project, as well as the assistance of our editor, Mr. Jeffrey House at Oxford University Press.

Piscataway, N.J.   W.E.R.
Rochester, N.Y.   P.R.K.
May 1995

References

Borson S, Liptzin B, Nininger J, et al. Psychiatry in the nursing home. *Am J Psychiatry* 144:1412–1418, 1987.

Elon R, Pawlson LG. The impact of OBRA on medical practice within nursing facilities. *J Am Geriatr Soc* 40:958–963, 1992.

Kemper P, Murtaugh CN. Lifetime use of nursing home care. *N Engl J Med* 324:595–600, 1991.

Mezey M, Knapp M. Nurse staffing in nursing facilities: Implications for achieving quality of care. In: Katz PR, Kane RL, Mezey M (eds): *Advances in Long Term Care, II.* New York: Springer, 1993.

Rovner BW, German PS, Broadhead J, et al. The prevalence and management of dementia and other psychiatric disorders in nursing homes. *Int Psychogeriatr, 2,* 13–24, 1990.

Schneider EL, Guralnik JM. The aging of America: Impact on health care costs. *JAMA* 263:2335, 1990.

Tariot PN, Podgorski CA, Blazina L, Leibovici A. Mental disorders in the nursing home: Another perspective. *Am J Psychiatry* 150:1063, 1993.

Zimmer JG, Watson N, Treat A. Behavioral problems among patients in skilled nursing facilities. *Am J Public Health* 74:1118–1121, 1984.

Contents

Contributors

DONALD BLIWISE, PH.D.
Associate Professor, Department
of Neurology
Director, Sleep Disorders Center
Emory University School of Medicine
Atlanta, Georgia

SOO BORSON, M.D.
Associate Professor
Department of Psychiatry and
Behavioral Sciences
University of Washington School
of Medicine
Seattle VAMC
Seattle, Washington

JEFFREY CUMMINGS, M.D.
Professor, Departments of Neurology
and Psychiatry
Reed Neurological Research Center
UCLA School of Medicine
Chief, Behavioral Neuroscience Section
Psychiatry Services, West Los Angeles
Veterans Affairs Medical Center
Los Angeles, California

PAGE MOSS FLETCHER, M.D.
Fellow in Geropsychiatry
Department of Psychiatry and
Behavioral Sciences
University of Washington School
of Medicine
Seattle VAMC
Seattle, Washington

MARION GOLDSTEIN, M.D.
Clinical Associate Professor
SUNY Buffalo, School of Medicine
& Biomedical Sciences
Department of Psychiatry and
Internal Medicine
Erie Country Medical Center
Buffalo, New York

HILARY T. HANCHUK, M.D.
Assistant Professor of Clinical Psychiatry
Director, Geriatric Psychiatry Training
UMDNJ—Robert Wood Johnson Medical
School
Piscataway, New Jersey

GREGORY A. HINRICHSEN, PH.D.
Assistant Professor of Psychiatry
Albert Einstein College of Medicine
Acting Director of Internship Training
Director, Fellowship Program
Clinical Geropsychiatry
Hillside Hospital
Glen Oaks, New York

TIMOTHY HOWELL, M.D., M.A.
Director, Mental Health Clinic
Associate Professor (CHS)
Co-Director, Geriatric Psychiatry
Fellowship Program
Departments of Psychiatry and Medicine
University of Wisconsin School of Medicine
Department of Veterans Affairs
William S. Middleton Memorial
Veterans Hospital
Madison, Wisconsin

MARY HOWELL-RAUGUST, M.D.,
PH.D., J.D.
57 Russell Avenue
Watertown, Massachusetts

SANDRA A. JACOBSEN, M.D.
Assistant Professor
Department of Psychiatry
Tufts/New England Medical Center
Boston, Massachusetts

LISSY F. JARVIK, M.D., PH.D.
Professor of Psychiatry
University of California, Los Angeles
Distinguished Physician
West Los Angeles VA Medical Center
Los Angeles, California

MARSHALL B. KAPP, J.D., M.P.H.
Professor, Department of Community
  Health
Director, Office of Geriatric Medicine
  & Gerontology
Wright State University School of Medicine
Dayton, Ohio

JURGIS KARUZA, PH.D.
Visiting Professor
Department of Medicine
University of Rochester School of
  Medicine & Dentistry
Co-Director
Western New York Geriatric Education
  Center
State University of New York at Buffalo
Professor of Psychology
State University College at Buffalo
Buffalo, New York

PAUL R. KATZ, M.D.
Associate Professor of Medicine
University of Rochester School of
  Medicine & Dentistry
Medical Director
Monroe Community Hospital
Rochester, New York

EDWARD KIM, M.D.
Instructor, Department of Psychiatry
  and Human Behavior
Jefferson Medical College
Geriatric Psychiatry Program
Wills Eye Hospital
Thomas Jefferson University
Philadelphia, Pennsylvania

SANDRA R. LEIBLUM, PH.D.
Professor of Clinical Psychiatry
Department of Psychiatry
Associate Professor of Clinical
  Obstetrics & Gynecology
UMDNJ—Robert Wood Johnson
  Medical School
Piscataway, New Jersey

ADRIAN LEIBOVICI, M.D.
Clinical Assistant Professor of
  Psychiatry
University of Rochester School
  of Medicine & Dentistry
Associate Chief, Department
  of Psychiatry
Rochester General Hospital
Director, Geriatric Psychiatry
Rochester Mental Health Center
Rochester, New York

ANDREW F. LEUCHTER, M.D.
Associate Professor of Psychiatry
  & Biobehavioral Sciences
UCLA School of Medicine
Los Angeles, California

MICHAEL MEGA, M.D.
Clinical Instructor
Department of Neurology
Reed Neurological Research Center
UCLA School of Medicine
Los Angeles, California

DEBORAH J. OSSIP-KLEIN, PH.D.
Senior Scientist
Departments of Community and Preventive
*   Medicine and Psychology*
University of Rochester School of
*   Medicine & Dentistry*
Monroe Community Hospital
Research Health Scientist
Department of Veterans Affairs Medicine
*   Center*
Canandaigua, New York

PETER RABINS, M.D.
Professor of Psychiatry
Department of Psychiatry and
*   Behavioral Sciences*
Johns Hopkins Medical Institutions
Baltimore, Maryland

WILLIAM E. REICHMAN, M.D.
Director, Division of Geriatric Psychiatry
Associate Professor of Clinical Psychiatry
Department of Psychiatry
UMDNJ—Robert Wood Johnson
*   Medical School*
Piscataway, New Jersey

RAYMOND C. ROSEN, PH.D.
Professor Psychiatry and Medicine
Department of Psychiatry
UMDNJ—Robert Wood Johnson
*   Medical School*
Piscataway, New Jersey

BARRY ROVNER, M.D.
Medical Director
Department of Geriatric Psychiatry
Wills Eye Hospital
Associate Professor
Thomas Jefferson University
Philadelphia, Pennsylvania

TERESA M. SCHAER, M.D.
Chief, Division of General Internal
*   Medicine & Geriatrics*
St. Peter's Medical Center
Clinical Assistant Professor of
*   Internal Medicine*
UMDNJ—Robert Wood Johnson
*   Medical School*
New Brunswick, New Jersey

JAMES B. SHACKSON, M.D.
Fellow, Division of Geriatric
*   Psychiatry*
Department of Psychiatry and
*   Human Behavior*
St. Louis University School
*   of Medicine*
St. Louis, Missouri

KENNETH SOLOMON, M.D.
Associate Professor
Division of Geriatric Psychiatry
Department of Psychiatry and
*   Human Behavior*
St. Louis University School of
*   Medicine*
St. Louis, Missouri

ILANA P. SPECTOR, PH.D.
Assistant Professor of Psychiatry
Douglas Hospital Center and Department
*   of Psychiatry*
McGill University
Verdun, Canada

PIERRE N. TARIOT, M.D.
Associate Professor of Psychiatry,
*   Medicine, and Neurology*
University of Rochester School of
*   Medicine & Dentistry*
Director of Psychiatry
Monroe Community Hospital
Rochester, New York

RICHARD A. ZWEIG, PH.D.
Assistant Professor of Psychiatry
Albert Einstein College of Medicine
Staff Psychologist
Geriatric Psychiatry Division
Hillside Hospital
Glen Oaks, New York

Psychiatric Care in
the Nursing Home

1

The Nursing Home as a Psychiatric Hospital

Edward Kim and Barry Rovner

The aging of the American population and the associated higher risk of developing dementia and disabling physical conditions have raised concerns about long-term institutionalization and the care that takes place in this setting. Approximately 1.5 million people, or 5% of those over age 65, currently live in nursing homes; 20 to 50% of those over age 65 will eventually live in nursing homes at some point (German et al., 1992). The prevalence of psychiatric disorders in nursing homes is estimated to be as high as 80% (Rovner et al., 1990a). Among patients with dementia, the presence of noncognitive psychiatric symptoms such as agitation, delusions, and depression can increase the likelihood of nursing home placement (Knopman et al., 1988; Morriss et al., 1990; Pruchno et al., 1990; Steele et al., 1990). Moreover, studies in medically ill populations indicate that depression can predict persistent disability in conditions as diverse as cardiac disease (Stern et al., 1975; Schleifer et al., 1989), stroke (Robinson et al., 1983), and hip fracture (Mossey et al., 1989). This chronic disability can lead to nursing home admission.

Nursing home care has traditionally emphasized the treatment and management of chronic, disabling physical disorders such as arthritis, heart disease, and cancer. Contemporary nursing homes closely resemble general hospitals in architecture, epidemiology, and models of care (Johnson and Grant, 1985, p. 38). Patients are evaluated and treated by doctors and nurses in a subacute medical setting. Given the high prevalence of psychiatric disorders such as dementia and depression in nursing homes, however, the reality of nursing homes in many cases more closely resembles that of chronic mental institutions of past generations: ''. . . the characteristic picture is that of a dozen residents arrayed in front of a television or sitting in a hall, each staring ahead. If anyone is talking, it is mostly to herself'' (Vladek, 1980, p.26).

The management of psychiatric disorders such as dementia and depression lags far behind that of physical disorders in both sophistication and optimism in many nursing home settings. Therapeutic nihilism, often based on erroneous misconceptions of the aging process and mental illness, can lead to a purely custodial approach without regard to rehabilitation or active treatment. Nursing home care models that fail to address the psychiatric needs that so often arise in this population omit a major source of disability. In addition, inappropriate management of psychiatric disorders can lead to overuse of medication and physical restraint, resulting in increased side effects and complications. Accurate psychiatric diagnosis and effective treatment is therefore a fundamental aspect of nursing home care.

Psychiatric Disorders in Nursing Homes

Until recently, no researchers have investigated the prevalence of mental disorders among the elderly in nursing homes using current diagnostic criteria (Rovner and Katz, 1994). Rovner et al. (1990a) studied 454 new admissions to eight nursing homes in the Baltimore area in an attempt to analyze psychiatric morbidity in nursing home residents and its effects on quality of life. Overall, 364 (80.2%) of the new admissions had a diagnosable psychiatric disorder, dementia being the most common ($N=306$, 67.4%). Primary dementia of the Alzheimer type accounted for 172 cases, or 37.9% of the entire sample. Multi-infarct dementia accounted for 81 cases, or 17.8%. Of the nondemented patients, 58 (12.8% of the entire sample) were depressed, and 11 (2.4%) had schizophrenia. Rovner et al. (1990a) also found that 122 (40%) of the demented patients in the Baltimore nursing home study suffered from noncognitive psychiatric symptoms such as depression or delusions that complicated their management. Indeed, behavior problems occur in up to 64% of all nursing home residents (Zimmer et al., 1993). ''Perhaps it is not unreasonable to consider nursing homes as places beset with an epidemic of dementia. This line of reasoning is useful because it leads to two relevant concepts of public health care, namely the contribution of the environment to provoking and sustaining aspects of disease, and the development of preventive procedures and practices'' (Rovner and Katz, 1994, p. 14).

The high prevalence of psychiatric disorders among nursing home residents is striking in that nursing home care typically is administered by internists or family practitioners and nurses with medical-surgical training. In the presence of significant behavioral and cognitive disturbances such as depression, hallucinations, delusions, and agitation, staff may feel overwhelmed by symptoms that they have not been trained to manage. In response, they may resort prematurely or inappropriately to physical restraints and sedating medications, resulting in limited benefits and unnecessary side effects as well as potential morbidity.

While behavioral and psychotic disturbances associated with dementia may lead to rather excessive treatment responses, depression is quite frequently undertreated. As few as 10% of nursing home residents who suffer from depression are treated with antidepressants; a larger percentage receive neuroleptics or benzodiazepines, and most receive no treatment at all (Heston et al., 1992). This has significant implications, since depression increases the risk of mortality independent of the severity of medical illness (Rovner et al., 1991). Moreover, depression can cause cognitive dysfunction above and beyond the underlying dementia. This reversible dementia syndrome of depression is often clinically indistinguishable from irreversible dementia syndromes (Mahendra, 1985). Depression tends to be manifest somewhat differently in the elderly, with more weight loss, psychomotor disturbances, and hypochondriasis rather than guilt and sadness (Caine et al., 1993). This more ''organic'' presentation, complete with associated cognitive deterioration, may convince staff members that the individual is experiencing a natural, expected progression in his or her dementia. This can lead to underdiagnosis and undertreatment of a reversible condition, resulting in further disability. Since 60% of treated cases have recovered significantly at 1 year follow-up (Katz, 1990), the failure to treat depression adequately represents neglect, which can lead to increased complications and even death. The reader is referred to Chapter 7 for a more complete discussion of depression.

Psychotropic Prescription Practices in Nursing Homes

The high incidence of behavioral disturbances among nursing home residents reflects the proportionately high prevalence of dementia and other psychiatric disturbances in this population. Accordingly, the prescription of psychotropic medications is quite frequent in nursing homes. Rovner et al. (1990a) found that 34% of nonpsychotic demented nursing home residents received neuroleptics. Restlessness and wandering were likely to result in neuroleptic use (Nygaard et al., 1990). Schneider and Sobin (1991) suggest that medications such as trazodone, anticonvulsants, and buspirone may be as effective as neuroleptics in reducing behavior disturbances associated with dementia. Neuroleptic use can increase the risk of hip fractures (Ray et al., 1987) and lead to cognitive impairment (Rovner et al., 1988). This raises concerns regarding the inappropriate or indiscriminate use of these medications. While antipsychotic medications can be effective in the short-term management of agitation and wandering in demented patients (Schneider et al., 1991), excessive and inappropriate use of these medications is common in nursing home settings. In order to curb the inappropriate and excessive use of psychotropic medications in nursing homes, the 1987 OBRA regulation restricted the use of neuroleptic and sedative-hypnotic medications in nursing homes. Federal regulations now require that nursing home residents receiving neuroleptics have a specific psychiatric diagnosis and behavioral indications documented in their charts. This has resulted in a 36% decrease in neuroleptic usage without a concomitant increase in benzodiazepine prescriptions (Rovner, et al., 1992). Moreover, neuroleptic use can be reduced in nursing homes without compromising patient care (Avorn et al., 1992). This may be due to the fact that medical staffs at nursing homes typically consist of physicians who are not psychiatrically trained. In addition, nursing staff may not be trained in behavioral and environmental interventions, which may reduce behavioral disturbances without the use of medications. (See Chapter 4 for a discussion of psychopharmacological principles and issues.)

In response to the current deficiencies in psychiatric treatment in many nursing homes, the American Association for Geriatric Psychiatry, the American Geriatrics Society, and the American Psychiatric Association (AAGP, AGS, APA, 1992) published a "position statement" on the use of psychotropic medications in nursing homes. The tenets of this statement are as follows:

1. Support for both clinical training and research is needed to optimize the use of psychotherapeutic medications in nursing homes.

2. Appropriate use of psychotherapeutic medications for the treatment of diagnosed psychiatric disorders is an important aspect of the care of nursing home residents.

3. The basic principles underlying the treatment of psychiatric disorders and behavioral problems in nursing homes are identical to those for the treatment of geriatric patients in other settings.

4. Nursing home residents with Alzheimer's disease and other dementias should be evaluated to determine whether they are experiencing secondary psychiatric symptoms. When present, such symptoms should be treated.

5. Psychiatric disorders such as depression are common in nursing homes and should be treated. These disorders frequently coexist with and complicate the disabling physical conditions that make long-term care necessary.

Psychosocial Aspects of Nursing Home Care

Nursing homes that provide therapeutic stimulation of demented patients may slow the progression of functional disability despite progression of the underlying dementing process, thereby improving patient outcomes (Rovner et al., 1990b; Spector and Takada, 1991). Comprehensive treatment of demented patients in nursing homes must first address the generally irreversible and often progressive nature of these conditions. Degenerative changes in the brain lead to a decreasing ability to adapt to environmental changes on the affective, cognitive, and behavioral levels. Neuropsychiatric responses to such situations of adaptive overload include depression, agitation, and delusions. Since it is impossible, in most cases, to restore these adaptive capacities, attention must be devoted to adjusting the environment to better fit the individual's needs, strengths, and deficiencies. This may reduce or eliminate the need for psychotropic medications in some demented individuals. What is striking is the absence of studies investigating the interaction between pharmacological and psychosocial interventions in these conditions. Often, this sort of care necessitates the development of specialized dementia care units.

In 1991, it was estimated that 10% of American nursing homes had special care units (OTA report, 1991). Rabins et al. (1987) discussed how such units could provide better care by concentrating resources and maintaining dedicated, highly trained staff. Higher levels of patient agitation can be tolerated with less staff distress in such units. Such units make less use of physical restraints and tend to utilize different criteria for the use of physical restraints and psychotropic medications (Sloane et al., 1991). This may be due to the staff's anticipation of and preparation for such behavior, which results in a larger repertoire of management strategies.

Conclusion

Nursing homes have evolved from the almshouses and mental institutions of the nineteenth century to subacute medical facilities. Unfortunately, due to lack of interest or social stigma, the treatment of age-associated mental disorders has not kept pace. The high prevalence of psychiatric disturbances and of psychotropic drug prescriptions in nursing home populations indicate that nursing homes function as long-term psychiatric hospitals for the elderly. To provide comprehensive high-quality care, nursing homes will have to develop programs designed to meet the psychiatric needs of their residents. In this way they will come to resemble psychiatric hospitals of the present rather than mental asylums of the past.

References

AAGP, AGS, APA. Position statement: Psychotherapeutic medications in the nursing home. *J Am Geriatr Soc* 40:946–949, 1992.

Avorn J, Soumerai SB, Everitt DE, et al. Psychotherapeutic medications in the nursing home. *N Engl J Med* 327:168–173, 1992.

Beers MH, Ouslander JG, Rollingher I, et al. Explicit criteria for determining inappropriate medication use in nursing homes. *Arch Intern Med* 151:1825–1837, 1991.

Caine ED, Lyness JM, King DA. Reconsidering depression in the elderly. *Am J Geriatr Psychiatry* 1:4–20, 1993.

German PS, Rovner BW, Burton LC, et al. The role of mental morbidity in the nursing home experience. *Gerontologist* 32:152–158, 1992.

Heston LL, Gerrard J, Makris L, et al. Inadequate treatment of depressed nursing home elderly. *J Am Geriatr Soc* 40:1117–1122, 1992.

Johnson CL, Grant LA. *The Nursing Home in American Society.* Baltimore: Johns Hopkins University Press, 1985.

Katz IR, Simpson GM, Curlick SM, Muhly C. Pharmacologic treatment of major depression for elderly patients in residential care settings. *J Clin Psychiatry* 51(suppl):41–48, 1990.

Knopman DS, Kitto J, Deinard S, Heirig J. Longitudinal study of death and institutionaliza-tion in patients with primary degenerative dementia. *J Am Geriatr Soc* 36:108–112, 1988.

Mahendra B. Depression and dementia: The multifaceted relationship. *Psychol Med* 15: 227–236, 1985.

Morriss RK, Rovner BW, Folstein MF, German PS. Delusions in newly admitted residents of nursing homes. *Am J Psychiatry* 147:299–302, 1990.

Mossey JM, Mutran E, Knott K, Craik R. Determinants of recovery 12 months after hip fracture: The importance of psychosocial factors. *Am J Pub Health* 79:279–286, 1989.

Nygaard HA, Bakke KJ, Breivik K, Brudvik E. Mental and physical capacity and consump-tion of neuroleptic drugs in residents of nursing homes. *Int J Geriatr Psychiatry* 5:303–308, 1990.

OTA Report. Special care units for persons with dementia. K. Maslow, *personal communi-cation,* 1991.

Parmelee P, Katz IR, Lawton MP. Depression among institutionalized aged: Assessment and prevalence estimation. *J Gerontol* 44:M22–M29, 1989.

Pruchno R, Michaels JA, Potashnik SL. Predictors of institutionalization among Alzhei-mer's disease victims with caregiving spouses. *J Gerontol* 45:S259–S266, 1990.

Rabins PV, Rovner BW, Laron DP, et al. The use of mental health measures in nursing home research. *J Am Geriatr Soc* 35:431–434, 1987.

Ray WA, Griffin MR, Schaffner W, et al. Psychotropic drug use and the risk of hip fracture. *N Engl J Med* 316:363–369, 1987.

Robinson RG, Kubos KL, Starr L, et al. Mood changes in stroke patients: Relationship to lesion location. *Comp Psychiatry* 24:555–556, 1983.

Rovner BW, David A, Lucas-Blaustein MJ, et al. Self care capacity and anticholinergic drug levels in nursing homes. *Am J Psychiatry* 145:107–109, 1988.

Rovner BW, German PS, Broadhead J, et al. The prevalence and management of de-mentia and other psychiatric disorders in nursing homes. *Int Psychogeriatr* 2:13–24, 1990a.

Rovner BW, Lucas-Blaustein J, Folstein MF, Smith SW. Stability over one year in patients admitted to a nursing home dementia unit. *Int J Geriatr Psychiatry* 5:77–82, 1990b.

Rovner BW, German PS, Brandt LJ, et al. Depression and mortality in nursing homes. *JAMA* 265:993–996, 1991.

Rovner BW, Edelman BA, Cox MP, Schmuely Y. The impact of anti-psychotic drug regulations (OBRA 1987) on psychotropic prescribing practices in nursing homes. *Am J Psychiatry* 149:1390–1392, 1992.

Rovner BW, Katz IR. Neuropsychiatry in nursing homes, In: Coffey CE, Cummings JL, eds. *Textbook of Geriatric Neuropsychiatry.* Washington, DC: American Psychiat-ric Press, 1994.

Schleifer SJ, Macari-Hinson MN, Coyle DA, et al. The nature and course of depression following myocardial infarction. *Arch Int Med* 149:1785–1789, 1989.

Schneider LS, Sobin PB. Non-neuroleptic medications in the management of agitation in Alzheimer's disease and other dementia. *Int J Geriatr Psychiatry* 6:691–708, 1991.

Sloane PG, Matthew LJ, Scarborough M, et al. Physical and pharmacological restraint of nursing home patients with dementia: Impact of specialized units. *JAMA* 265:1278–1282, 1991.

Specter WD, Takada HA. Characteristics of nursing homes that affect resident outcomes. *J Aging Health* 3:427–454, 1991.

Steele C, Rovner BW, Chase GA, Folstein MF. Psychiatric symptoms and nursing home placement in Alzheimer's disease. *Am J Psychiatry* 147:1049–1051, 1990.

Stern MJ, Pascale L, McLoone JB. Psychosocial adaptation following myocardial infarction. *J Chronic Dis* 29:513–526, 1975.

Vladek BC. *Unloving Care: The Nursing Home Tragedy.* New York: Basic Books, 1980.

Wolinsky FD, Callahan CM, Fitzgerald JF, Johnson RJ. The risk of nursing home placement and subsequent death among older adults. *J Gerontol* 47:S173–S182, 1992.

Zimmer JG, Watson NM, Levenson SA. Nursing home medical directors: Ideals and realities. *J Am Geriatr Soc* 41:127–130, 1993.

2

General Approaches to Behavioral Disturbances

Pierre N. Tariot

Careful surveys have documented that 90% or more of nursing home patients have at least one form of behavioral disturbance, with as many as half exhibiting four or more (Rovner et al., 1986; Tariot et al., 1993). In some cases, the severity of these behavioral syndromes is equivalent to that encountered among psychiatric inpatients (Tariot et al., 1993). Despite the complexity of these problems, most caregivers have little or no mental health training; indeed, most are non-professionals. The frequency and severity of behavioral disturbances, combined with the lack of preparedness in most nursing homes, are sufficient justification for devoting an entire textbook to the subject.

There are other important reasons for addressing behavioral disturbance in the nursing home. The kinds of psychological symptoms seen are undoubtedly distressing to those experiencing them, such as frightening hallucinations or delusions, abiding depression, sleeplessness, or anxiety of phobic proportions. In addition, a variety of adverse consequences can ensue from disturbed behaviors, including violent interactions with others, the appropriate use of psychotropic medications but with undesired effects, or the inappropriate use of such medications and physical restraint (Tariot and Blazina, 1993). Caregivers can suffer serious psychological and physical consequences from their attempts to deal with these behaviors (Rabins et al., 1982; Chenoweth and Spencer, 1986; Colerick and George, 1986; Deimling and Blass, 1986). Whereas relief of these symptoms can promote increased function, autonomy, and improved quality of life for the patient as well as others, unattended behavioral pathology can lead to greater distress for all concerned.

This chapter proposes a systemic general approach to the evaluation and management of behavioral disturbances in the nursing home, summarized in Table 2.1. The approach is grounded in traditional medical and psychiatric principles of diagnosis and therapy and builds on earlier proposals (Leibovici, 1988; AAGP, AGS, APA, 1992). It is easy for these traditional principles to get lost in the face of the extremely complex, atypical behavioral disturbances that are so common in the nursing home. Nonetheless, returning to basics pertains for these atypical problems as well as any other medical problem. Thoughtful application of diagnostic and therapeutic principles is, in itself, therapeutic in settings involving multiple disciplines, yet where many of the caregivers may have minimal medical or psychiatric expertise.

TABLE 2.1.　General Approach to Behavioral Disturbance

1. Define target symptoms
   Elicit data from multiple sources.
   Arrive at a consensus about target symptoms and aggravating and ameliorating factors.

2. Establish or revisit medical diagnoses
   Perform traditional evaluation.
   Rule out delirium.
   Rule out other medical diagnoses.
   Assess for associated excess disability (e.g., pain).
   Treat medical disorders specifically.
   Monitor target symptoms.

3. Establish or revisit neuropsychiatric diagnoses
   Make traditional evaluation.
   Rule out depression.
   Rule out other discrete disorders.
   Rule out organic mental disorder such as dementia.
   Watch for interacting medical/psychiatric variables.
   Treat specific syndromes when present.

4. Assess and reverse aggravating factors
   Sensory impairment.
   Environmental disturbance.

5. Adapt to specific cognitive deficits
   Is busy area vs. quiet spot better?
   Pictures or labels can help.
   Place important objects or memory book in room to help orient.
   Simplify environment.
   Provide cues for activities.
   Allow pacing, wandering.

6. Identify relevant psychosocial factors
   Allow for adjustment at admission.
   Perceived or real loss of support can lead to systematic behaviors.
   Support, validation, reminiscenses are helpful.
   Psychotherapy is sometimes indicated.
   Optimize physical and social stimulation.

(continued)

TABLE 2.1.   General Approach to Behavioral Disturbance (*continued*)

7. Educate caregivers
     Review evaluation, outline further diagnostic steps.
     Summarize functional and cognitive status.
     Redefine target symptoms.
     Support caregivers.
     Educate the system.

8. Employ behavior management principles
     Staff behavior has a major effect.

9. Use psychotropics for specific syndromes
     Treat primary syndromes specifically.
     If a sydrome is superimposed upon an organic disorder, treat the syndrome first.

10. Symptomatic pharmacotherapy
     For severe, acute problems, consider hospitalization or neuroleptics.
     For the rest, develop "psychobehavioral metaphor": fit target symptoms into a syndrome
        known to be drug-responsive, such as depressive, manic, psychotic, anxious, or vegetative.

11. The process of treatment
     Assess risk/benefit ratio.
     Start low, go slow.
     Use lowest effective dose.
     In the absence of prompt efficacy, maintain subtoxic dose for an appropriate period, then
        withdraw.
     Perform trial in reverse. Watch for flare of behavioral problems.
     Subsequent trials may be in order.
     Even effective medications should be empirically withdrawn.
     Medicatioins do not always work: go back to step 1!

A General Approach

Define Target Symptoms

The term "behavioral disturbance" refers to a behavioral or psychological syndrome or pattern associated with subjective distress, functional disability, or
impaired interactions with others or the environment (Tariot and Blazina, 1993).
An important first step is to delineate the patterns carefully; they will have
diagnostic and therapeutic implications that will help the caregiver to succinctly
summarize the "target symptoms": for instance, "bangs on table repeatedly, calls
out loudly, resists care, cries intermittently, expresses self-deprecatory ideation,
doesn't complete meals without cueing, attempts to leave with apparent purpose
in mind," and so on. Since many behaviors are ephemeral, it is helpful to elicit
observations from the multiple sources that are available in the nursing home:
aides, nursing staff, social workers, dietary staff, clergy, and physical, occupational, and recreational therapists, looking for "ground swells" of opinion that
particular patterns do or do not exist.

Establish or Revisit Medical Diagnoses

The next step is a comprehensive medical evaluation. It is not unusual for a behavioral disturbance to be the proximate cause for the first detailed medical evaluation: in many cases, preexisting neuropsychiatric diagnoses, for instance, have been undetected. A complete evaluation includes a full medical history, review of medication, physical examination, laboratory testing, and assessment of cognitive and functional performance.

Although behavioral problems can occur by themselves, they often indicate that the patient has one or more treatable medical disorders that are causing the disturbed behavior. These must be established or revisited. The most dreaded is delirium. One of the truisms of geriatrics is to presume that the new onset of disturbed behavior results from delirium until proven otherwise, since virtually any behavioral symptoms or syndrome can result from delirium. It has been observed in 6 to 7% of nursing home residents and can present as an acute, subacute, or even chronic picture (Rovner et al., 1986; Rovner et al., 1990). While psychoactive medications are the most common culprit, intercurrent infectious processes, dehydration, electrolyte disturbance, and trauma are other precipitants of delirium. (See Chapter 5 for a thorough discussion of delirium.)

Other medical disorders, by themselves, can cause behavioral symptoms in the absence of delirium. The classic examples are the ''depressive'' manifestations of thyroid disease, infections, head injury, sedating medication, and so forth. In addition, medical disorders can result in behavioral symptoms as a result of secondary disability such as pain, sensory impairment, disrupted sleep, or physical limitation.

When medical problems or metabolic abnormalities are present, treatment should be directed toward correcting them, and the patient should be monitored for his or her response. The same principle holds for associated secondary consequences of medical disorders: they should be corrected where possible or at least accommodated.

Establish or Revisit Neuropsychiatric Diagnoses

It is possible that the disturbed behavior is a consequence of a long-standing, chronic, or recurrent psychiatric disorder, or it could be the initial presentation of a new psychiatric disorder. Establishing the presence of a psychiatric diagnosis entails evaluation of current symptomatology, response to therapy, and family history. Perhaps the most important psychiatric diagnosis in the nursing home, in terms of prevalence and likelihood of therapeutic success, is depression. The prevalence of major depression among cognitively intact nursing home residents has been estimated to be as high as 25% (Parmelee et al., 1992), a figure an order of magnitude higher than that found in the community. The crucial role of drug therapy in the treatment of major depression has been emphasized in the recent practice guidelines developed by the Agency for Health Care Policy and Research and the American Psychiatric Association. The efficacy and safety of treatment of depression in the elderly is relatively well established, although there are uncertainties about the applicability of carefully done research studies in depressed subjects to frail elderly patients in the nursing home setting (Katz, et al., 1990). The evidence is substantial, however, that the value of such treatment is extremely high. (See Chapter 6 for a complete discussion of depression and Chapter 3 for psychopharmacological considerations.)

Surveys have also indicated a substantial proportion of other psychiatric disorders in the nursing home, such as schizophrenia (Chapter 8), mania (Chapter 6), anxiety disorders (Chapter 7), and substance abuse (Chapter 12) (Rovner et al., 1986; Rovner, et al., 1990; Tariot et al., 1993). In all instances where these are presumed to be the primary etiology of the disturbed behavior, specific appropriate therapy should be applied and the response monitored. Adjustment disorders are worth special mention: it should be presumed that admission to a nursing home will be a significant stressor. Recognizing this may helpfully focus attention on needs that will diminish over time.

A very large proportion of nursing home patients will suffer from dementia (Chapter 5) or some other organic mental disorder: in fact, these are the most prevalent neuropsychiatric diagnoses in the nursing home (Rovner et al., 1986; Rovner et al., 1990; Tariot et al., 1993). It is obvious that the etiology of the organic mental impairment must be established, as it may offer clues to definitive therapy for the behavioral problem. Likewise, it is also perhaps obvious that a patient with an organic mental impairment may suffer a superimposed medical illness, which, while benign in itself, produces unusual behavioral disturbance in the vulnerable patient. Patients with such organic mental disorders can also experience concomitant discrete psychiatric disorders. Since behavioral disturbances in such patients can occur for either reason, it is important to try to make the distinction. It is especially helpful to describe and categorize the target symptoms, as alluded to previously. This will facilitate monitoring and can guide symptomatic pharmacotherapy. Where a syndromal psychiatric disorder is superimposed upon an organic mental disorder, the syndrome should be treated first.

Assess and Reverse Aggravating Factors

Whether psychiatric or medical pathology is present, it is also important to bear in mind other factors that can precipitate or aggravate behavioral disturbance. First among these is sensory impairment. It is unfortunately common to observe health professionals who fail to recognize that a patient cannot see or hear well, or cannot use assistive devices properly because of cognitive impairment. For such patients, simplification and clarification of communication is essential. This includes making one's face fully visible to facilitate lipreading, experimenting with different volumes of speech, inserting or adjusting hearing aids, using amplifiers, reducing communication to simple phrases or words, communicating by writing or letter board, and so on. As a related issue, English is a second language for many, and interpreters can be very helpful.

Environmental disturbances such as excessive heat or cold during unusual climate changes, noise from construction or other disruptive residents, or altered daily routines can lead to discomfort that is expressed only by disturbed behavior such as calling out or other apparently purposeless efforts to leave or remedy the problem. Adjustments in light, noise, temperature, or change in room or roommate can sometimes be helpful. Although not strictly environmental, music may help relax certain patients.

Adapt to Specific Cognitive Deficits

In some cases, "problem" behaviors can be better understood as well-intentioned but perhaps confused or disruptive efforts to communicate or adapt (Cohen-Mansfield, 1992). For instance, pacing may reflect a need for stimulation, "wandering" may result from an incorrect belief that the patient needs to get to another place, and verbally disruptive behaviors may represent efforts to obtain assistance.

Suspiciousness may occur when impaired comprehension leads to the understandable perception that the environment or another person is threatening. A host of behaviors may be understandable as "environmentally dependent." This occurs typically in an organically impaired patient with executive control dysfunction (Lezak, 1983). It is common for such patients to react to what is in front of them: an open door prompts passage through it (perhaps into another's room); a visible overcoat is put on, triggering the desire to leave; any food item in view is eaten; and so forth.

A variety of interventions may be designed according to a patient's particular pattern of cognitive impairment. Patients with disorientation but some ability to interpret pictures or words may respond to pictures or labels identifying their room, possessions, family members, activities for the day, and so on. Some will benefit by being in a quiet location, while others may enjoy being in a busy public area. Some patients find it helpful to be "anchored," more firmly aware of their personal history, by important possessions such as pieces of furniture or art as well as family photos. A "memory book" can be considered for certain confused patients, consisting of an album of photos and phrases to help remind them of important events, places, and relationships. Patients can also be helped by reducing clutter in their environment or reducing the number of environmental cues to which they might respond inappropriately. On the other hand, those who need to be engaged in a physical activity can respond to cues from the environment (and staff) about this. These could range from simply having magazines available to providing repetitive tasks that patients are capable of completing (e.g., counting, folding, and so on). It may be valuable to create a physical environment where it is possible for patients to stimulate themselves by walking and exploring, such as circular corridors and safe outdoor walking areas, or to design visual or physical barriers to reduce the chances of unsafe egress.

Identify Relevant Psychosocial Factors

Anger, sadness, and even denial can accompany nursing home admission. Once admitted, the patient may experience loss of contact with others through death, a move, or simply a vacation taken by an important other, resulting in a temporary but frequently significant sense of loss or abandonment. A variety of other psychological themes are common and may respond to opportunities to speak of them without requiring psychotherapy. Such themes can include loss of health, function, autonomy, privacy, possessions, and intimacy. Reviewing and acknowledging these losses and stressors can help reduce feelings of sadness and anxiety. It is also important to support those patients who are striving to make healthful adaptations—to accommodate new realities without resigning themselves to despair. Encouragement and validation, and ongoing efforts to reclaim positive memories and experiences from one's prior life, are basic therapeutic tools. It is also obvious, and often overlooked, that the patient's personality plays a major role in determining adaptation to the nursing home setting. How has he or she historically coped with loss, transition, and interaction with others? A developmental history that includes this information should be part of every patient's database. In some cases, it is desirable to obtain a consultation regarding the utility of psychotherapy, although this is not a generally available option. (The reader is referred to Chapters 13 and 14 for discussions of psychotherapy in the nursing home.)

It is almost always desirable to optimize physical activity and social stimulation. This entails working collaboratively with nurses, clergy, and social workers, and physical and recreational therapists to clarify what "mix" of activities is best for a particular patient. Are there appropriate group therapeutic activities? Are religious activities important and available? Are there existing social activities that are well suited to a given patient's temperament? Is it medically safe to go on picnics, shopping trips, or overnight passes?

Educate Caregivers

Education of staff, families, and patients is essential. This typically entails a review of the medical and psychiatric evaluation as it stands and possible further diagnostic steps, a summary of functional and cognitive deficits, a concise summary of the disturbed behaviors ("target symptoms"), and consideration of possible aggravating and ameliorating factors. This first step demonstrates that the team's response to the behavior will be logical, thorough, and thoughtful. This reassuring message is initially established by the manner in which one collects information, and it is reinforced by the manner in which the case is summarized. This feedback phase provides all concerned with an improved and specific behavioral lexicon, which is also reassuring and facilitates improved communication and monitoring of the subsequent course. Clarification of the prognosis and of therapeutic options also help caregivers and patients cope. It is reassuring to know that there can be discernible and predictable patterns, that "confused" behaviors can actually have understandable origins, and that certain frightening behaviors are a manifestation of a pathological substrate rather than an emotionally laden personal attack. Such knowledge allows caregivers, some of whom have limited experience and training, to interact more helpfully and specifically with their patients. Finally, it is important to emphasize the value of the clinician's ongoing presence during efforts to manage a disruptive patient. Relatively brief visits can bolster staff and patient morale considerably, as can explicit validation of the demanding nature of caring for such patients.

Similar messages can have a great impact on family and friends.They may learn how certain of their behaviors are either provocative or helpful. They may be able to appreciate that, although the patient may be aphasic, the perceived abandonment at the time of a vacation can lead to distress that could be ameliorated by asking other friends or family members to help out temporarily by visiting more frequently. At the same time, family and friends may have valuable information and suggestions to offer the multidisciplinary care team regarding optimal care of the patient.

At a broader level, education of the larger system beyond the health care team can be considered as well. Adequate recognition of behavioral disturbances in the nursing home would lead to sensible implementation of educational programs for all caregivers, thoughtful development of appropriate policies and procedures, establishment of mental health consultation resources in the facility, and ties to the acute care system for those patients requiring inpatient management.

Employ Behavior Management Principles

The fundamental principles of behavior management are quite relevant to the nursing home without invoking rigorous behavior modification programs. It is easy for staff to underestimate the extent to which their own behavior can influence the behavior of patients, particularly those who are organically impaired. When staff behave in a calm, reassuring manner and are confident in their approach, most patients will respond with reduced fear and anxiety and improved ability to cooperate with care. Conversely, sudden or apparently aggressive approaches or obvious fearfulness are likely to provide an unsettled response. Patients who call out or grab at caregivers repeatedly may do so less often if they are approached at times when they are not calling out, eventually learning that they do not have to send out distress signals in order to have their needs adequately met. Some patients benefit considerably from brief moments (even a few seconds) of social contact offered repeatedly, as often as every few minutes. A gentle touch can also go a long way. Staff must understand that approaches such as this are very effective but require consistent application over sustained periods.

Use Psychotropics for Specific Syndromes

As in the treatment of any psychiatric disorder, psychosocial and environmental interventions such as those outlined above should be considered first and may be effective by themselves. In other cases, they serve as necessary and helpful adjuncts to psychopharmacological treatment.

For behaviors that remain disturbed despite interventions such as those identified above, there is a legitimate role for psychotropic medication. As emphasized previously, when a specific, diagnosable syndrome is present, this syndromal diagnosis should determine the treatment plan. Where the syndromal diagnosis is superimposed upon an organic mental disorder, that syndromal diagnosis should also determine the initial treatment plan. For instance, if a nursing home patient with dementia is referred for evaluation of pacing and is found to have features of a concomitant major depressive disorder, the depressive syndrome should become the focus of the treatment, even if the pacing is mild and manageable. An adequate trial of antidepressant treatment can determine the extent to which the depressive syndrome is contributing to the patient's cognitive and functional disability. Similarly, if the patient is found to have either a delusional disorder or a diagnosable anxiety disorder, treatment should be initiated with medications known to be effective for these conditions. The decision about treatment should be based on estimates of the extent to which the syndrome is associated with the behaviors in question as well as on impaired function.

Symptomatic Pharmacotherapy

It should be recognized, however, that many patients with organic mental impairment and behavioral disturbance do not have a specific diagnosable syndrome. For these patients, intervention directed toward symptom reduction is necessary. The most common set of problems is usually referred to loosely as "agitation" (Cohen-Mansfield, et al., 1992). The choice of medication in such patients may be influenced by the urgency of the situation. If rapid control of grossly disturbed or unsafe behavior is necessary, neuroleptics are frequently used first, or the patient may be admitted to an acute care hospital.

In most cases, however, the choice of drugs and optimization of therapy may involve a lengthier process of trial and error. There is remarkably little empirical evidence to guide decision making. In view of this, a rational approach has been proposed. An initial step in this process is to develop a "psychobehavioral metaphor" (Leibovici and Tariot, 1988). The term "metaphor" is used to emphasize the heuristic and tentative nature of the process. The aim is to formulate a working hypothesis regarding the nature of the patient's psychopathology that is to be tested in a carefully monitored trial of drug treatment. The clinician obtains information derived from multiple sources, emphasizes the most salient features, and attempts to define a patter (that well may be fragmented) roughly analogous to a more typical drug-responsive syndrome. Although this process is logical and valid on its face, the clinical evidence in its favor is not strong, since choice of medication is derived primarily from case reports, open studies, and extrapolations from studies in other populations. The following provide examples of some typical "psychobehavioral metaphors."

Depressive Symptoms

Patients with agitation or withdrawal may exhibit negativistic, irritable, dysphoric, or anxious symptoms even in the absence of overt syndromal depression. In such cases an empirical trial of antidepressant medication can be considered. It would be appropriate to select a medication without prominent anticholinergic or sedating properties such as nortriptyline, desipramine, trazodone, selective serotonin reuptake inhibitors, bupropion, or possibly monoamine oxidase inhibitors.

Manic Symptoms

Some patients with dementia may exhibit hyperactivity, pressured speech, overly cheerful or irritable mood, decreased sleep, and, rarely, sexual preoccupation. In such cases, therapy with carbamazepine or lithium can be considered. A preliminary report suggests that carbamazepine in low doses may show efficacy for relief of agitation in some patients, although confirmation is necessary (Tariot et al., 1994). In the absence of extensive data regarding toxicity, nursing home patients must be presumed to be especially vulnerable to the toxic effects of these drugs.

Psychotic Symptoms

At times, paranoid features or hallucinations may be readily apparent. Occasionally, however, they can be inferred only from fragmented data such as poorly articulated fears, inappropriate accusations, or agitation that occurs primarily in the presence of interpersonal interactions. In such cases, this suggestion of paranoia could provide the logical basis for initial trial of an antipsychotic agent. Once again, the anticholinergic and sedative properties of standard agents will very likely dictate the choice of agent.

Anxious Symptoms

High levels of anxiety or restlessness may respond to anxiolytic agents. This may be particularly helpful in patients with prominent insomnia, or when a reversible situational component is present. It should be emphasized that it may be difficult to distinguish between anxiety and depression in patients with organic disorders; therefore, it may be prudent to consider antidepressant medication first in such patients.

Other Behavioral Symptoms

Repeated episodes of violence might lead to consideration of the use of beta-adrenergic blockers, anticonvulsants, or antipsychotics. Affective lability, which is generally distinguishable from depression, may respond well to antidepressant therapy or anticonvulsants. If apathetic or withdrawn behaviors are prominent, the first question must be whether these are manifestations of a depressive disorder or psychosis. In such cases, specific therapy is indicated. In other cases, empirical trials of antidepressants or stimulants may also be reasonable.

Vegetative Changes

Changes in diurnal rhythm, pattern or quality of sleep, appetite, diet, weight, and sexual energy are common noncognitive aspects of behavior that may represent a therapeutic opportunity in organically impaired patients with disturbed behavior. For instance, sleep disturbance occurs in up to 47% of patients with dementia. The question naturally arises whether this is associated with a depressive disorder, and, in turn, whether that disorder causes/contributes to disturbed behavior. If so, empirical trials of psychotropics (e.g., antidepressants) are sometimes in order.

The Process of Treatment

An aphorism in the field is that every psychotropic trial in this population is an experiment with an *n* of 1. This reflects the confusing heterogeneity among patients resulting from variable etiology of behavioral disturbance, medical and psychiatric comorbidity, age, phenomenology, history of prior illnesses and treatment, vulnerability to adverse effects, and so forth. Concern about the magnitude of the danger resulting from drug therapy is well justified but based largely upon cases in which medications were used inappropriately, in large doses, and without ongoing monitoring and adjustment. The balance between risk and benefit is improved if the process for initiating treatment follows the principles outlined above and if the patient is monitored on a regular basis with honest assessment of benefit as well as toxicity. In the absence of benefit at appropriate doses, or if there are significant adverse effects, the medication should obviously be decreased or discontinued.

Another general principle is "Start low, go slow." Medications should generally be started at low doses and increased gradually, with ongoing monitoring for adverse effects as well as efficacy. Dose increases should be planned to allow for the assessment of both and should allow time for input from multiple members of the treatment team. In some cases standardized rating scales are useful for tracking behavioral change and documenting efficacy, although most have not been validated in the clinical setting. Doses should generally be titrated upward until there is evidence of either clear benefit or early toxicity. In some cases, medications permit measurements of plasma levels, which can serve to guide treatment (e.g., nortriptyline). In other cases, a "subtoxic" dose (i.e., that below which mild adversity occurs) can be maintained for a period of weeks before concluding that a trial has been ineffective.

Where a medication appears ineffective, it is reasonable to perform the empirical trial in reverse, tapering the medication and watching for problems during withdrawal, such as the unmasking of behavioral problems that were actually better during the treatment period. Assuming that symptoms are still present and that the patient does deteriorate, a trial with a second, presumably different class of medication can be undertaken. In especially difficult cases, this process is repeated several times. Although there are instances where no agent appears to be helpful, these are fortunately uncommon.

When a treatment trial is positive, it is reasonable to continue treatment for a period of weeks or months and at some point to taper the medication and reevaluate symptoms, once again performing the clinical trial in reverse. There is almost no evidence guiding decision making in this regard. The usual factors taken into account include the severity of symptoms, prior history of relapse, stability of other relevant variables, and adequacy of monitoring capability—in addition to the duration of treatment. (See Chapter 3 for additional techniques and pharmacotherapy.)

Summary

Many of the key points of this chapter were highlighted in the 1992 position statement of the American Association for Geriatric Psychiatry, American Geriatrics Society, and American Psychiatric Association, which is paraphrased here (AAGP, AGS, APA, 1992). The basic principles underlying the treatment of psychiatric disorders and behavioral problems in the nursing home are identical to those for the treatment of geriatric patients in other settings. The initial step in the evaluation of any psychiatric disorder or behavioral symptom is to establish whether the symptoms result from a medical illness, previously diagnosed or undiagnosed. The next step is to establish or revisit psychiatric disorders. Comprehensive treatment planning takes into account both pharmacological and nonpharmacological interventions. The latter may include modifications of sensory, environmental, or psychosocial variables; education and support of patients as well as families; staff support of behavioral management; or psychotherapy. Despite concerns about overuse of psychotropic medications in the nursing home, they are of value for the treatment of behavioral disturbances and should be applied specifically where possible. Empirical trials of symptomatic pharmacotherapy can be aided by the use of therapeutic metaphors—that is, subtyping behavioral syndromes according to target symptoms that might be suggestive of a good response. Whenever psychotropics are used, the patient should be monitored for reduction of target symptoms as well as undesired effects. Useless medications should be stopped and even effective medications may be successfully withdrawn after a period of treatment. This will help assure that the patient will be neither over- nor undertreated.

References

AAGP, AGS, APA. Psychotherapeutic medications in the nursing home. *J Am Geriatr Soc* 40:946, 1992.

Chenoweth B, Spencer B. Dementia: The experience of family caregivers. *J Gerontol* 26:267, 1986.

Cohen-Mansfield J, Marks M, Werner P. Agitation in elderly persons: An integrative report of findings in a nursing home. *Int Psychogeriatr.* 4(supp 2):221–240, 1992.

Colerick E, George L. Predictors of institutionalization among caregivers of patients with Alzheimer's disease. *J Am Geriatr Soc* 34:493, 1986.

Deimling G, Blass D. Symptoms of mental impairment among elderly adults and their effects on family caregivers. *J Gerontol* 41:778, 1986.

Katz IR, Simpson GM, Curlik SM, et al. Pharmacologic treatment of major depression for elderly patients in residential care settings. *J Clin Psychiatry* 51(suppl):41, 1990.

Leibovici A, Tariot PN. Agitation associated with dementia: A systematic approach to treatment. *Psychopharm Bull* 24:49, 1988.

Lezak MD. Executive functions and motor performance. In: Lezak MD, ed. *Neuropsychological Assessment,* 2nd ed. Oxford Press, New York, 1983:507.

Parmelee PA, Katz IR, Lawton MP. Depression and mortality among institutionalized aged. *J Gerontol* 47:P3, 1992.

Rabins P, Mace N, Lucas M. The impact of dementia on the family. *JAMA* 248:333, 1982.

Rovner BW, German PS, Broadhead J, et al. The prevalence and management of dementia and other psychiatric disorders in nursing homes. *Int Psychogeriatr* 2:13, 1990.

Rovner, BW, Kafonek S, Filipp L, et al. Prevalence of mental illness in a community nursing home. *Am J Psychiatry* 143:1446, 1986.

Tariot P, Blazina L: In: Morris J, ed. *Handbook of Dementing Illnesses,* New York: Marcel Dekker, 1993:461.

Tariot PN, Erb R, Leibovici A, et al. Carbamazepine treatment of agitation in nursing home patients with dementia: A preliminary study *J Am Geriatr* 42:1160–1166, 1994.

Tariot PN, Podgorski CA, Blazina L, Leibovici A. Mental disorders in the nursing home: Another perspective. *Am J Psychiatry* 150:1063, 1993.

3

Psychopharmacology

Adrian Leibovici

Psychotherapeutic drug use in long-term care facilities has received a lot of attention in the last 5 to 10 years, including public outcry and government regulation. This chapter will review the use of psychotropics for the mental health problems most commonly encountered in nursing homes, some of the specific problems associated with prescribing psychotropics in this environment, and the current status of public and scientific debate surrounding this topic.

Psychotherapeutic Medications Used in Nursing Homes

As described in Chapter 1, psychiatric morbidity is highly prevalent in long-term care facilities. For example, 94% of residents in an intermediate care facility in Maryland had a mental disorder according to DSM-III criteria (Rovner et al., 1986). Two more recent studies replicated similar prevalence figures: 94 and 91% respectively (Chandler and Chandler, 1988; Tariot et al., 1993). Dementia and related organic brain syndromes, depression, agitation, anxiety, and sleep disorders are among the most common psychiatric problems for which psycho-therapeutic drugs are sometimes useful.

Antidepressants

Depression is prevalent in the nursing home environment: one study found that 50% of the institutionalized elderly had a depressive syndrome and 12% of them met DSM-III criteria for major depression (Parmalee et al., 1989). The whole spectrum of depressive illness is present in nursing homes: adjustment reactions, major depression with melancholia or with psychotic features, and organic mood syndromes in the context of cerebrovascular or neurodegenerative processes. Severity ranges from very mild to catastrophic. Some of the most severe cases of depression can be found in nursing homes, where many residents experience multiple, major losses in a short period of time (see Chapter 6).

Along with a number of nonpharmacological interventions like individual and group supportive contact, formal psychotherapy, and environmental manipulation, antidepressant medication can play a crucial role in the successful treatment of this disabling condition (see Table 3.1).

Tricyclic antidepressants are still the most widely used, although newer and better-tolerated drugs are gradually replacing them. Efficacy is probably similar for all members of this class, but price and side effect profiles vary. These drugs are divided into the subgroup of tertiary amines (including amitriptyline, imipramine, doxepin, and clomipramine) and the subgroup of secondary amines (including nortriptyline, desipramine, protriptyline, and maprotiline).

Their mechanism of action is not well understood, but they are thought to increase the net availability of serotonin and norepinephrine in the synapse by inhibiting presynaptic uptake. Newer theories stress the modulating effect on pre- and postsynaptic receptors (Charney et al., 1981). The antidepressant effect of these agents is gradual and may be delayed for 2, 4, or even 8 weeks, which can be quite frustrating; this is why these medications are often prescribed for insufficient amounts of time before being prematurely determined "ineffective."

With the use of these medications, side effects are numerous, including anticholinergic toxicity (xerostomia, constipation, urinary retention, blurred vision, delirium of variable severity), orthostatic hypotension, sedation, quinidinelike delays in atrioventricular conduction, and mild memory impairment. In general, secondary amines are thought to be more "activating," inducing fewer side effects but sometimes being responsible for restlessness and insomnia if given at night. In most situations, they are preferable to tertiary amines, which are associated with more anticholinergic effects, cardiac toxicity, and sedation. When agitation or insomnia are prominent features, however, drugs like imipramine or doxepin can be very useful. Dosage is guided by tolerability, clinical effectiveness, and, to some extent, blood levels. The elderly are expected to require blood levels in a similar range as for younger adults or, for some patients, a lower range (Alexopoulos, 1992). In general, dosage is expected to be smaller than for a younger population due to both heightened receptor sensitivity and to age-related changes in liver metabolism and volume of distribution (Nies et al., 1977).

Nortriptyline is favored by many clinicians because the correlation between blood level and efficacy is well established and points to the existence of a "therapeutic window," an attractive feature considering the time saved in reaching optimal dosage. Doses of 25 to 50 mg daily are often sufficient in the elderly.

Not infrequently, these drugs are used for other indications than depression. Small doses are well documented to augment the action of analgesics; anxiety and especially panic anxiety respond well to imipramine and other tricyclics;

TABLE 3.1. Antidepressants for Elderly Nursing Home Residents

Class	Generic	Brand	Geriatric Dose, mg/day
Tricyclics			
Tertiary amines	Imipramine	Tofranil	50–150
	Amitriptyline	Elavil	50–150
	Doxepin	Sinequan, Adapin	50–150
	Trimipramine	Surmontil	50–150
	Clomipramine	Anafranil	50–150
Secondary amines	Nortriptyline	Aventil, Pamelor	25–75
	Desipramine	Norpramin	50–150
	Protriptyline	Vivactyl	10–25
	Maprotyline	Ludiomil	25–100
	Amoxapine	Asendin	75–200
SSRIs	Fluoxetine	Prozac	10–40
	Sertraline	Zoloft	25–100
	Paroxetine	Paxil	10–40
Atypical agents	Trazodone	Desyrel	75–200
	Bupropion	Wellbutrin	75–225
	Venlafaxin	Effexor	75–225
MAOIs	Phenelzine	Nardil	15–60
	Tranylcypromine	Parnate	10–30
	Isocarboxazide	Marplan	10–30

clomipramine is a good anticompulsive agent; doxepin, in small doses, has been used in agitated dementia (Friedman et al., 1987).

Trazodone is an antidepressant structurally unrelated to tricyclics. It is widely used in nursing home residents. Compared with tricyclics, it has less anticholinergic toxicity, although—infrequently—it can be responsible for symptomatic alpha blockade: orthostatic hypotension and dry mouth. Although less frequently than tricyclics, it has been associated with cardiac arrhythmias. In nursing homes, it is used for its "antiagitation" effect in behaviorally disturbed, demented residents, especially in those who display repetitive verbal or motor actions (Aisen et al., 1993). Trazodone is also a very good hypnotic, an effect that tends to occur faster and at lower doses than those required for the antidepressant effect.

Selective serotonin reuptake inhibitors (SSRIs: fluoxetine, sertraline, paroxetine) have become quite popular with prescribing nursing home physicians, since these medications are practically devoid of serious cardiac toxicity and might have an edge over traditional antidepressants when an "activating" or antianxiety effect is sought. Ease of administration (once a day) is another advantage. Their use in elderly nursing home residents can be limited by side effects (anorexia, nausea, hyponatremia, jitteriness, and agitation) and by their high price. Fluoxetine 10 to 20 mg daily is a commonly used dose in the elderly, but in some cases doses as low as 10 mg every other day and as high as 60 to 80 mg a day have been tried and were well tolerated. According to their manufacturers, sertraline 50 mg and paroxetine 20 mg are equivalent to fluoxetine 20 mg.

Bupropion is another "atypical" antidepressant that has been tried with some frequency in nursing home residents, who seem able to tolerate it well (Kane et al., 1983). It is described as an "activating" drug, to be avoided at bedtime. Its mechanism of action is not well understood: it blocks dopamine reuptake, but only at very high doses. The major attraction for its use in the long-term-care population is the lack of cardiac toxicity and the fact that, unlike SSRIs, it does not inhibit appetite or sexual function. With the use of high doses (over 400 mg/day), it was associated with a higher incidence of seizures than other antidepressants. Like the SSRIs, bupropion is comparatively quite expensive. In the elderly, the dose can range from 75 mg once or twice a day to 100 or 150 mg three times a day (Schatzberg and Cole, 1991).

Monoamine oxidase inhibitors (MAOIs) used in this country for depression include phenelzine, isocarboxazid, and tranylcypromine. They are as effective as tricyclics in geriatric depression (Georgotas et al., 1986). The activity of MAOI is increased in geriatric depression (especially if cognitive impairment is a feature), in patients with Alzheimer's disease, and in older individuals in general (Alexopoulos, 1987). This makes the use of MAOIs in nursing home residents theoretically attractive. The most feared and well-publicized characteristic of these drugs is their association with a hypertensive crisis caused by inadvertent ingestion of catecholamine precursors like tyramine-rich foods and phenylephrine, which is found in over-the-counter cold remedies. This complication is dramatic and can lead to stroke or death. It requires urgent treatment with strong hypotensive agents, usually in a hospital setting, but fortunately it is rare and can be virtually eliminated with a proper tyramine-free diet and exclusion of certain medications. In fact, the nursing home environment—where, in general, diet and medication dispensing are controlled—is more favorable to the use of MAOIs than the ambulatory setting.

The most common side effects of these drugs include orthostatic hypotension, weight gain, overstimulation or sedation, and an anticholinergic syndrome that, for similar doses, is weaker than for tricyclics. In younger patients, these drugs have been advocated in panic disorder, "rejection sensitivity," or "atypical depression" and in cases where other antidepressants are not effective or tolerated. They are probably not widely used in nursing homes (Leibovici et al., 1993).

Antipsychotics

Drugs in this class are also known as major tranquilizers or neuroleptics. They have been prescribed extensively in nursing homes primarily as sedatives for agitated, aggressive patients and, more than any other psychotropics, their use has drawn attention to their sometimes inappropriate use as "chemical restraints." In fact, their more specific indication is for delusions, hallucinations, illogical thinking, and fearful social withdrawal, but they are effective in the treatment of dangerous agitation whatever the context: psychosis, delirium, dementia (see Table 3.2).

TABLE 3.2.   Antipsychotics for Elderly Nursing Home Residents

Class	Generic	Brand	Geriatric Dose	Chlorpromazine Equivalents
Low potency	Chlorpromazine	Thorazine	25–200	100
	Thioridazine	Mellaril	20–200	95
	Mesoridazine	Serentil	10–100	50
Intermediate	Molindone	Moban	5–50	10
potency	Loxapine	Loxitan	5–50	10
	Perphenazine	Trilafon	4–32	8
	Thiothixene	Navane	2–20	5
	Trifluoperazine	Stelazine	2–20	5
High potency	Fluphenazine	Prolixin	0.25–6	2
	Haloperidol	Haldol	0.25–6	2
Atypical	Risperidone	Risperidal	1–3	?
	Clozapine	Clozaril	12.5–150	60

The therapeutic effects, as well as many of these drugs' side effects, are linked to their antagonism of dopamine receptors in different areas of the brain. The twenty or so antipsychotic drugs approved for use in this country form a continuum, from the ''low-potency'' end (e.g., chlorpromazine, thioridazine) to the ''high-potency'' drugs (e.g., haloperidol, fluphenazine). Sedation, orthostatic hypotension, and anticholinergic toxicity are common side effects of the low-potency drugs, while extrapyramidal syndromes (akathisia, parkinsonism, acute dystonia, dyskinesia) are more common with the use of high-potency drugs. Tardive dyskinesia is associated with prolonged use of all traditional antipsychotics, and it is commonly believed that duration of exposure, advanced age, and female gender are risk factors. Recent research confirmed only duration of exposure as having predictive value, but the data are preliminary (Sweet et al., 1994). Neuroleptic malignant syndrome is a rare but potentially lethal complication of antipsychotics, characterized by spasticity, fever, autonomic dysfunction, and delirium. Its occurrence in the elderly is not infrequent. The extent to which antipsychotics are still used in nursing homes is highly variable. Lately, the percentage of residents taking these drugs has tended to become a quality-of-care indicator, as nursing homes are encouraged to institute drug-reduction programs. From a clinical point of view, however, it is important to recognize that psychosis, a frequent occurrence in nursing homes, can be a disabling condition and is best treated with neuroleptics. Haloperidol, in doses as low as 0.25 mg once or twice a day, is a frequent starting point. Many residents will respond to very low doses (0.5 to 3 mg daily). All antipsychotics are equally effective in equivalent dosages. Elderly individuals with preexistent functional psychosis (e.g., chronic schizophrenia) and a minority of agitated demented patients will need and tolerate high doses, sometimes comparable with those used in young adults. In general, the choice of a particular drug in this class is driven by the side-effects profile. In theory, a patient with preexistent parkinsonism should receive a low-potency drug, but in practice the anticholinergic and alpha-blocking effects of these compounds are so predictably detrimental that most practitioners consider high-potency drugs to be a first choice. Intermediate-potency antipsychotics—including molindone, thiothixene, and loxapine—can offer a less extreme side-effects spectrum. Clozapine and risperidone are two newly available antipsychotic drugs. They have a different mechanism of action than typical antipsychotics and, at least in the case of clozapine, are proven to be effective in a sizable minority of schizophrenic patients resistant to traditional drugs. The geriatric use of these drugs has been only marginally researched, although some anecdotes and open-ended studies suggest that they might be effective (Heylen et al., 1988; Ball, 1992). One of the implications for nursing homes to be considered is their very high price. Clozapine is associated with a relatively high incidence of agranulocytosis, and weekly white blood cell testing is mandated by the manufacturer via a cumbersome distribution and monitoring system. Both clozapine and risperidone can cause orthostatic hypotension, thus limiting their tolerability in the elderly.

Anxiolytics-Hypnotics

Benzodiazepines are widely used in nursing homes for the treatment of anxiety, insomnia, and agitation as well as for muscle relaxation, although in some institutions small doses of antihistaminic drugs, like diphenhydramine or hydroxyzine, are preferred. By and large, older drugs like meprobamate and barbiturates have been all but abandoned because they are more difficult to tolerate and do not offer any advantages over benzodiazepines. All benzodiazepines have the same pharmacological effects and a common mechanism of action, which is believed to consist of facilitating the action of gamma-aminobutyric acid, an inhibitory neurotransmitter with receptors on a macromolecular complex containing so-called benzodiazepine receptors as well (Teicher, 1988).

The choice of a particular benzodiazepine in the elderly will be dictated by differences in pharmacokinetic properties. For instance, the rate of onset (time from administration until desired effect) is shortest with diazepam, a drug with fast and almost complete absorption, and delayed with drugs like oxazepam and temazepam. The subjective perception of benzodiazepines by residents and staff in nursing homes is probably heavily influenced by this variable: drugs that act quickly are easier to correlate with their intended effect and might be perceived as more useful or powerful.

Duration of effect, which depends on the elimination half-life of the parent drug and active metabolites, is also very important, differentiating between long-acting drugs like clonazepam, flurazepam, or diazepam and shorter-acting ones like lorazepam or alprazolam. Obviously, with repeated dosing, long-acting drugs are likely to establish "steady state" at higher levels, adding to the danger of side effects like oversedation, ataxia, confusion, tolerance, and dependence. Withdrawal symptoms, which may result from too rapid tapering of an established regimen with benzodiazepines, occur faster with short-acting drugs, which are associated with more rapid changes in blood levels.

Hepatic metabolism is another relevant variable to consider: oxazepam and lorazepam are inactivated by conjugation with glucoronic acid only (a metabolic pathway independent of age or disease), but other benzodiazepines, which are also metabolized via demethylation and hydroxylation (age- and disease-dependent processes), are expected to be slower to clear in the elderly. This is the theoretical basis for preferring oxazepam and lorazepam for use in nursing home residents.

The best use of benzodiazepines depends on a good understanding of their effects and limitations and of the patient's clinical picture. For instance, anxiety with onset late in life is many times organic in nature, and medical causes must be explored and treated before or in addition to symptomatic treatment. Intermittent use is appropriate, since standing doses for long periods of time will most often lead to habituation.

Lorazepam 0.5 to 1 mg or oxazepam 10 to 15 mg once to four times a day are commonly prescribed. When depression or panic are part of the picture, attempts should be made to gradually replace the benzodiazepine used acutely with an antidepressant that is likely to control anxiety as well. Obsessions and compulsions are best treated with SSRIs or clomipramine from the outset.

Sleep disorders are also very common in the elderly nursing home resident, but "sleeping pills" should be a last-resort solution after a thorough assessment of the problem has been undertaken and issues like "sleep hygiene," daytime naps and sedentarism, medical problems, or sleep apnea are considered (see Chapter 9). Many times the elderly nursing home resident complains bitterly of insomnia and insists on having a sleeping pill, but when staff keeps a sleep log, it becomes clear that the resident's sleep is not disturbed at all. Insomnia—associated with intercurrent problems like acute medical illness or adjustment to a new room or roommate—is most likely to respond to short-term benzodiazepines like lorazepam 0.5 mg, oxazepam 10 mg, or triazolam 0.125 mg at bedtime, as needed. Other nonbenzodiazepine hypnotics like chloral hydrate 250 to 1000 mg or zolpidem 5 to 10 mg are sometimes prescribed, but they all share the same tendency to lead to tolerance and loss of efficacy with prolonged use. The hypnotic effect of the antidepressant trazodone has already been mentioned.

Agitated dementia is sometimes treated with benzodiazepines like diazepam, lorazepam, or oxazepam. When acute control is needed, as before medical procedures or when agitation occurs as severe but infrequent outbursts, these drugs might be appropriate; but for persistent forms of agitation, benzodiazepines are better avoided (Loebel and Leibovici, 1994). A "paradoxical" increase in agitation, in response to administration of benzodiazepines, has been reported in a minority of elderly patients with preexistent brain disease.

In the last several years, the nonbenzodiazepine anxiolytic buspirone has been promoted for use in agitated, demented individuals; as such, its use in long-term-care institutions has increased (Herrman and Eryavec, 1993). Doses as high as 80 mg daily have been used safely in the elderly, but the starting dose can be as low as 5 mg twice a day. The main attraction to this drug is its relatively benign side-effects profile, although it has been associated with extrapyramidal syndromes. The major criticism is its still questionable efficacy both for anxiety and agitation. The manufacturer stresses the fact that sometimes the full therapeutic effect occurs only after weeks of treatment.

Mood Stabilizers

This class includes lithium, carbamazepine, valproic acid, and possibly clonazepam, a long-acting benzodiazepine. They are useful in the treatment of mania, prophylaxis of manic and depressive episodes, enhancement of antidepressant drugs in difficult to treat depression, and, relevant for nursing home residents, in decreasing aggression and agitation in patients with brain disease (Leibovici and Tariot, 1988). The extent of their use in long-term-care facilities is less well characterized, but in a recent survey of psychotropic utilization in a teaching nursing home, we found a frequency of 5.34% (Leibovici et al., 1993). Lithium is quite neurotoxic in the elderly, sometimes at doses otherwise within therapeutic range. Using lithium citrate, which comes as a liquid containing about 60 mg lithium/mL, allows for fine titration of dose, which is often necessary in this population. Doses as low as 60 mg twice a day might be effective. Dehydration from febrile illness, diarrhea, or perspiration during heat waves (especially in nursing homes without air conditioning) can rapidly lead to lithium toxicity. Staff must be aware of this danger in residents on lithium, and fluid intake should be increased when needed. Other lithium-induced side effects include tremor, ataxia, sedation, cardiac arrhythmias, hypothyroidism, and skin rash.

Carbamazepine is an effective antimanic agent as well, and several studies have now addressed its potential role in the treatment of agitation associated with dementia (Gleason and Schneider, 1990; Tariot et al., 1994). Doses as low as 50 mg twice a day have been used and, with gradual increments, the usual side effects of oversedation and ataxia have not been a major problem even in the most debilitated of nursing home residents (Tariot et al., 1994).

Electroconvulsant Therapy

While electroconvulsive therapy (ECT) is not a drug, it is often considered, together with psychotropics, among ''somatic'' or ''biological'' treatments for mental disorders. It has an important role in the treatment of geriatric depression and, in recent years, the issue of ECT in patients with underlying dementia has also been raised (Bradley et al., 1994). Many nursing home residents can benefit from this form of treatment, but little systematic research has focused on ECT as it might relate to the long-term-care environment.

The Nursing Home Environment: Implications for Treatment with Psychotherapeutic Drugs

Regardless of the particular drug used or the condition treated, several general principles should be considered having to do with the characteristics of this very old and frail group of people, and the attributes (general and individual) of the institutional setting where they live.

1. *Diagnosis.* Whenever possible, the prescribing of psychotropic medication should be postponed until a reasonable diagnostic inquiry has been undertaken. A paranoid or agitated demented resident might suffer from a urinary tract infection, and a suddenly depressed or anxious person might be reacting to the death of a roommate or the upcoming departure for a long vacation of a family member. Treatment with psychotropic medication is not curative but symptomatic; therefore, etiologic or precipitating factors must be identified and addressed first.

There are exceptions when medication will be prescribed without delay: *emergencies* (e.g., aggression in a very strong demented or psychotic resident) and *severe subjective distress,* where symptomatic relief is desirable, making further evaluation possible (e.g., rapid acting benzodiazepine for panic anxiety).

2. *Nonpharmacological interventions.* Not only regulatory pressures but common clinical sense dictates that interventions other than prescribing medication should be considered when appropriate. They include changes in the resident's environment, psychotherapy, staff education, assistance in developing workable behavioral protocols, and so forth. When successful, such interventions can obviate or at least diminish the need for pharmacotherapy, decreasing side effects and cost. It is important, however, to keep in mind that the success of nonpharmacological treatment depends to a great extent on such factors as the quality of the staff, the staff-to-resident ratio, the philosophy of care, and general conditions in each institution.

3. *Target symptoms.* It is important to identify one or several target symptoms and to have a clear indication of how to appreciate drug response over time. Ideally, objective instruments like rating scales should be used; in most cases, however, resources are limited and global evaluations by physicians, nursing staff, and families are used instead. Sleep logs, serial measurements of weight, counting the number of ''prn's'' and ''behavioral'' observations entered in the chart over a certain period of time can all help objectify efficacy.

Staff education is crucial if significant but partial improvement is to be recognized and reported. For instance, a frequently assaultive demented resident who, after treatment with ''antiagitation'' medication, has only rare outbursts, might be perceived as not improved if staff does not participate in some form of quantification of his behavior before and during treatment. It is not easy to integrate sometimes conflicting behavioral reports from staff who are differently exposed to the same resident: morning vs. evening or night shift, weekend vs. weekday, well-established staff vs. agency-hired or ''floating'' nurses who are less familiar with the resident. Describing and measuring specific goals for pharmacological treatment can, to some extent, alleviate such inconsistencies.

4. *Duration of trial and dose.* These are very important factors and subject to specific pressures and opportunities in a nursing home. In general, medicating depression or psychosis requires patience, since antidepressants and antipsychotics take weeks to become effective. Many times, physicians visit the home

infrequently and at fixed intervals, allowing patients to stay on their medications for long periods of time; thus the danger of changing doses and medications too frequently is lessened. At the same time, this feature of nursing home medical care can expose patients to drug trials in which the duration of treatment reflects caregiver availability rather than clinical need.

Obviously the well-known tenet of geriatric pharmacology to "start low, go slow" applies: many nursing home residents are likely to need very small doses of medication because of their increased neuroreceptor sensitivity, delayed liver metabolism, and changes in volume of distribution (Abernethy, 1992). It is important, however, to avoid dogmatic "dose caps" that might lead to undertreatment: it is not unusual for an elderly person to require full doses of antidepressants or antipsychotics to achieve clinical response or, where relevant, "therapeutic levels." For instance, older schizophrenic patients can show a deceptively benign "stability," only to become floridly psychotic when the benevolent but uninformed physician too rapidly reduces the "excessive" dose of antipsychotic prescribed prior to the patient's admission in the nursing home.

5. *Monotherapy.* In general, monotherapy is preferable regardless of age. It is even more desirable in nursing home residents who, as a group, have a higher prevalence of concurrent medical problems and hypersensitivity to the peripheral and central nervous system effects of drugs. In very difficult cases, combinations might still be necessary. Examples include antidepressant augmentation with lithium or stimulants, two or more drugs for aggression, and an antipsychotic plus an antidepressant for psychotic depression.

6. *Disability.* The mere presence of a target symptom or syndrome does not in itself warrant the use of psychotropics: especially in this medically fragile and mostly demented group of patients, a certain level of disability has to be present as well. For instance, an elderly woman was seeing a litter of puppies in the corner of her room and was reacting to this hallucination by talking to them and asking that they be fed. The hallucination was obviously ego-syntonic, consistent with her lifelong love of animals and occurring in a stable and relatively clear clinical context (multi-infarct dementia). It did not interfere with other activities and did not cause any disability. A decision was made not to medicate and the patient continued to remain stable. In deciding whether psychotropics are to be used, the clinician should try to describe the level of disability—such as distress to patient and others and possible negative consequences if the symptom is not treated—and to weigh it against expected side effects and risks associated with these medications.

7. *Beneficiaries.* For whom treatment with psychotropics is being prescribed should be clearly understood: many times staff relates better to pharmacological than nonpharmacological interventions, especially if the patient is aggressive or annoying. Family members might push for the use of psychotropics if the patient tends to show emotional distress combined with hostility toward them or if they have difficulty accepting the resident's cognitive, functional, or behavioral decline. Physicians might react to an agitated resident's refusal to allow physical

examination when approached. Residents themselves might insist on receiving sleeping medication despite the absence of objective insomnia. In most decent institutions, the much vilified "medicating the residents for staff convenience" does not occur systematically. Nevertheless, physicians working in nursing homes know that, in borderline clinical situations, the decision of whether to use psychotropics is complex; it should address primarily the well-being of the identified patient but also take into account the needs of other residents, of caretakers, and of the institution at large. This is not inconsistent with psychiatric practice outside the nursing home, where the negative impact of abnormal behavior resulting from mental illness—that is, duty to protect others—can be grounds for medicating a patient.

8. *Iatrogenic illness.* Elderly institutionalized residents represent a medically frail group suffering from many ailments and typically taking a number of nonpsychiatric medications. When prescribing psychotropics, one has to be mindful of possible unwanted interactions. The side effects of psychotropics might accentuate preexistent medical problems: benzodiazepines might increase preexistent confusion; drugs with anticholinergic activity make the already constipated individual more uncomfortable; orthostatic hypotension due to autonomic nervous system dysfunction is common in old age and can be accentuated by the alpha-blocking activity of low-potency antipsychotics like thorazine or thioridazine.

Many nonpsychotropic drugs have well-established effects on mental status: cimetidine is responsible for delirium, steroids for organic mood syndromes, some antihypertensives for depression, and so on.

Some medications influence the pharmacokinetics of psychotropics and vice versa: antacids delay oral absorptions of antipsychotics; barbiturates, phenytoin, and other antiepileptics increase hepatic metabolism, therefore decreasing blood levels of antidepressants; and theophylline, verapamil, and diltiazem decrease serum lithium levels while aspirin and other nonsteroidal anti-inflammatory drugs (NSAIDs) increase serum lithium levels.

There are numerous drug-drug interactions involving psychotropics and nonpsychotropics: meperidine can trigger a life-threatening syndrome characterized by rigidity, hyperreflexia, delirium, and hypertension in patients treated with MAOIs; thiazide diuretics increase lithium toxicity due to decreased renal clearance; digitalis toxicity might be more likely in patients treated with trazodone. The list of possible interactions and unintended consequences associated with the use of psychotropics in the institutionalized elderly is quite long and growing. Avoiding iatrogenic consequences in the face of such complexities requires up-to-date knowledge of geriatric pharmacology and medicine. It is in such circumstances that the value of expert psychogeriatric consultation becomes obvious (see Chapter 15).

9. *Ethical issues.* While residents' autonomy and family involvement are emphasized and their participation in decision making is encouraged, very often the nursing home finds itself involved in advocating for residents or exercising some

form of substitute judgment on their behalf. Many conflicting priorities are to be considered, posing difficult ethical questions, and some have direct relevance for the use of psychotropic medication.

For instance, the advent of new but expensive drugs like clozapine, risperidone, and some antidepressants raises for some homes questions about resource allocation, especially in today's climate of fiscal austerity.

Many demented residents are passive recipients of care, sometimes including psychotropics, and their capacity to make informed decisions in accepting or refusing such treatments is often impaired. In practice, standards for accepting treatment are lower than standards for refusing it, and residents are many times assumed to be competent simply because they do not resist treatment (Weinstock, 1987). These issues are discussed in detail in Chapters 16 and 17.

Risk/benefit analysis for the use of psychotropics can be difficult at times: Is control of episodic aggression worth the risk of sedation and increased confusion? Should an apparently terminal patient with neurovegetative signs of depression be tried on antidepressants and exposed to their side effects? Is ECT compatible with the concept of comfort care? Should paranoia in a patient with parkinsonism be controlled even if it means more neurological disability?

When institutions try to grapple with such complex issues, the psychogeriatric consultant can play a constructive role by participating in ethics committees or providing consultation to administrators and clinical staff.

Psychotropic Drug Use in the Nursing Home: Fact, Myth, and Regulation

Over the last decade, concern has been raised over the possible misuse of certain psychotherapeutic drugs in nursing home residents. Sedatives in general and antipsychotics in particular have been the most scrutinized. Media reporting of this topic has been generally unfavorable (Garrard et al., 1991).

Public policy regulating the use of psychotropics in nursing homes followed. Most notably, in 1987, Congress passed legislation affecting the use of neuroleptics in Medicaid- and Medicare-certified nursing homes, the so-called Omnibus Budget Reconciliation Act (OBRA). According to this legislation, the Health Care Financing Administration (HCFA) was instructed to develop national guidelines, which started to be implemented in October 1990. Examples of such guidelines include the following: (1) proper documentation of symptoms and diagnosis to support need for neuroleptics: (2) prohibition of neuroleptic use ''as needed'' or for behaviors like wandering; (3) once psychotropics are prescribed, attempts should be made to decrease dose gradually and to reattempt alternative interventions (HCFA, 1991).

Both before and after OBRA 1987, studies exploring the issue of psychotropic drug use in nursing homes focused on three major questions: (1) the prevalence and appropriateness of drug prescribing; (2) clinical correlations between adverse outcomes and use of psychotropics; and (3) ways to minimize the prescribing of these drugs. Following well-publicized cases of psychotropic drug overuse and inappropriate prescribing and monitoring patterns in some institutions (Avorn et al., 1989), many of these studies have tended to make the assumptions that (1) psychotropics are being used excessively in long-term care facilities; (2) psychotropic medication is by and large bad for nursing home residents; (3) "sedatives" are used as "chemical restraints" in order to satisfy the needs of caregivers; and (4) decreasing the use of psychotropics in nursing homes is intrinsically good and therefore worth pursuing as an independent goal. A critical review of research in this area reveals that these assumptions still remain to be proven.

Prevalence

There is much variability between institutions—such as levels of care and geographic location—which is reflected in sometimes divergent reports. For instance, the overall prevalence of psychotropic drug use in nursing homes ranges from a low 11% to as high as 75%. Several large-scale surveys seem to indicate that about half of nursing home residents receive psychotropics: 60% in about 20,000 Medicaid nursing home residents in Illinois in 1984 (Buck, 1988), more than 50% of 850 residents in 12 intermediate-care facilities in Massachusetts (Avorn et al., 1989), between 42 and 51% for 5 consecutive years in a 200-bed facility studied longitudinally (Lantz et al., 1990).

Antipsychotics are estimated to be used in at least 20% of nursing home residents (Ray et al., 1993). This is considered too high, but very little research has been done to determine which residents are more likely to receive these drugs or what would be an appropriate level of use for a given population mix. It is postulated that in nursing homes, antipsychotics are used primarily for agitation associated with dementia; indeed, one study showed that among agitated elderly residents, those with dementia were more likely to be treated with antipsychotics (Billig et al., 1991).

Hypnotics and anxiolytics are prescribed in an even larger percentage, up to 50% according to one study (Hasle and Olsen, 1989). The same classes of medications are used both for anxiety and insomnia. In one of the few studies that separate anxiolytic-hypnotic drugs by reason for prescribing, 13% of 1454 nursing home residents received medication for anxiety and 33% for insomnia (Tybjerg and Gullmann, 1992). Given the propensity of drugs in this category to be addictive and to lose their efficacy with continuous use, longitudinal data would be most useful, but research in this area is lacking.

The only class of psychotropic medication that is not commonly thought to be overused is that of antidepressants: in a survey of 5752 residents of 60 Medicaid-certified institutions, 868 were found to be depressed; only 15% of them, however, received antidepressants (Heston et al., 1992). Interpreting such data is difficult: it seems that the use of antidepressants is seen in a more favorable light, since it implies recognition and treatment of depression—a reversible condition. Many times, however, antidepressants are used to treat agitation, and—

even when they are given to depressed residents—their efficacy and safety have not been systematically studied in this population.

Negative Outcomes Associated with Psychotropics in Nursing Homes

Accidental falls and subsequent bone fractures in long-term-care institutions have been associated with the use of psychotropic drugs (Viskum and Juul, 1992). On motor assessments of demented nursing home residents, performance worsened with the introduction of psychotropics and improved with their discontinuation (Burgio and Hawkins, 1991). No attempts were made to study negative outcomes for nursing home residents not treated with psychotropics despite an identified need or positive outcomes of proper treatment with psychotropics in this population.

Drug Reduction Studies

The advent of OBRA regulations has stimulated efforts to minimize drug use in nursing homes, and several large studies have focused on this trend. Rovner and his group reported a 36% reduction in neuroleptic drug prescription in 17 Baltimore area nursing homes in the 6 months following implementation of regulations, as a result of an institutional quality assurance program, setting decrease in use of these drugs as a goal. Antidepressant use increased slightly in the same period of time (Rovner et al., 1992). Two large prospective, controlled drug-reduction studies, using geriatric psychopharmacological education of providers as main intervention, demonstrated significant decreases in the use of psychotropics, which was considered to be a desirable outcome (Avorn et al., 1992; Ray et al., 1993). In one of these studies, reports of depression in residents taken off medication increased (Avorn et al., 1992). Of note, in both studies, drug use decreased also in the nursing homes used as controls, but at a lower rate. This is consistent with a naturalistic study of change in prescribing patterns in a teaching nursing home in Rochester, New York, where two surveys, 12 years apart, in the absence of any organized effort to reduce medication use, revealed a decrease in the use of all psychotropics, antipsychotics, and sedative hypnotics but an increase in the use of antidepressants (Leibovici, 1993).

Institutional and regulation-driven efforts to decrease the use of psychotherapeutic drugs in nursing homes have been met with concern by clinicians working in such settings. Drug discontinuation studies were criticized for their oversimplified hypothesis—"more medication is bad, less medication is good"—and the danger of undertreating patients in need was emphasized. Three major professional organizations, the American Association for Geriatric Psychiatry, American Geriatrics Society, and the American Psychiatric Association, issued a common position paper with the goal of contrasting dogmatic beliefs about psychotropic drugs in nursing homes with a rational framework that would allow for proper use of these medications when needed while increasing the level of knowledge on the subject and curbing abusive or ignorant prescribing patterns when identified (AAGP, AGS, APA, 1992). Ideas put forward include expanding clinical training and research in the fields of geriatric psychopharmacology and psychiatry; recognizing that regulation is being developed in the absence of sufficient scientific knowledge; and affording the same opportunities for psychiatric treatment to nursing home residents as those afforded to noninstitutionalized geriatric patients with similar problems, including state-of-the-art evaluation and interventions for highly prevalent problems like dementia, depression, or psychosis.

In conclusion, the subject of treatment with psychotropic drugs in long-term-care institutions is a complex and evolving one, touching on a number of disciplines like geriatric pharmacology and medicine, psychopathology in the elderly, public policy, and systems theory. Probably, as a result of changes in these fields (new knowledge, increased resources and attention to this area, regulation) there has been progress in the last decade, but much remains to be done. More expert consultants and more education of providers are needed in many settings. Regulation will have to be refined and geared away from wholesale drug-reduction drives. Research will have to become more focused after an initial "descriptive" phase. Directions for new research in this area should include (1) prospective, longitudinal studies of the use of psychotropic agents in correlation with such variables as resident psychopathology, institutional characteristics, staff attitudes, and level of knowledge; (2) nursing home–based clinical trials of interventions for agitation, depression, insomnia, and psychosis, including both medication and, where appropriate, nonpharmacological therapies; and (3) studies comparing psychopathology and response to treatment of institutionalized and community-dwelling geriatric patients.

References

AAGP, AGS, APA. Psychotherapeutic medications in the nursing home. *J Am Geriatr Soc* 40:946, 1992.

Abernethy DR. Psychotropic drugs and the aging process: Pharmacokinetics and pharmaco-dynamics. In: Salzman C, ed. *Clinical Geriatric Psychopharmacology.* Baltimore: Williams & Wilkins, 1992: 61–73.

Aisen PS, Johanessen DJ, Marin DB. Trazodone for behavioral disturbance in Alzheimer's disease. *Am J Geriatr Psychiatry* 1:349, 1993.

Alexopoulos GS. Treatment of depression. In: Salzman C, ed. *Clinical Geriatric Psychopharmacology.* Baltimore: Williams & Wilkins, 1992:139.

Alexopoulos GS, Young RC, Lieberman KW, Shamoian CA. Platelet MAO activity in geriatric patients with depression and dementia. *Am J Psychiatry* 144:1480, 1987.

Avorn J, Dreyer P, Connelly K, Soumerai SB. Use of psychoactive medication and the quality of care in rest homes: Findings and policy implications of a statewide study. *N Engl J Med* 320:227, 1989.

Avorn J, Soumerai SB, Everitt DE, et al. A randomized trial of a program to reduce the use of psychoactive drugs in nursing homes. *N Engl J Med* 327:168, 1992.

Ball CJ. The use of clozapine in older people. *Int J Geriatr Psychiatry* 7:689, 1992.

Billig N, Cohen-Mansfield J, Lipson S. Pharmacologic treatment of agitation in a nursing home. *J Am Geriatr Soc* 39:1002, 1991.

Bradley L, Rockwell E, Jeste DV. ECT for severe agitation in dementia patients. In: *Program of the 7th Annual Meeting and Symposium of the AAGP.* Tampa, FL, 1994.

Buck J. Psychotropic drug practice in nursing homes. *J Am Geriatr Soc* 36:409, 1988.

Burgio LD, Hawkins AM. Behavioral assessment of the effects of psychotropic medication on demented nursing home residents. *Behav Modif* 15:194, 1991.

Chandler JD, Chandler JE. The prevalence of neuropsychiatric disorders in a nursing home population. *J Geriatr Psychiatry Neurol* 1:71, 1988.

Charney DS, Menkes DB, Heninger GR. Receptor sensitivity and the mechanism of action of antidepressant treatment: Implications for the etiology and treatment of depression. *Arch Gen Psychiatry* 38:1160, 1981.

Friedman R, Tal D, Gryfe CI: Doxepin in aggressive institutionalized demented patients. In: *Program of the Annual Meeting of the Royal College of Physicians and Surgeons of Canada,* 1987.

Gerrard J, Makris L, Dunham T, et al. Evaluation of neuroleptic drug use by nursing home elderly under proposed Medicare and Medicaid regulations. *JAMA* 265:464, 1991.

Georgotas A, McCue RE, Hapworth W. Comparative efficacy and safety of MAOIs versus TCAs in treating depression in the elderly. *Biol Psychiatry* 21:1155, 1986.

Gleason RP, Schneider LS. Carbamazepine treatment of agitation in Alzheimer's outpatients refractory to neuroleptics. *J Clin Psychiatry* 51:115, 1990.

Hasle H, Olsen RB. Consumption of psychopharmaceuticals by residents at nursing homes: Significance of the environment at the nursing home. *Ugskr Laeger* 151:1313, 1989.

HCFA. Medicare and Medicaid: Requirements for long term care facilities, final regulations. *Fed Reg* 56:48865, 1991.

Heylen SLE, Gelders YG, Vanden Bussche G. Risperidone (R 64 766) in the treatment of behavioral symptoms in psychogeriatric patients: Pilot clinical investigation. In: *Program of the International Symposium of Psychogeriatrics,* Lausanne, 1988.

Herrman N, Eryavec G. Buspirone in the management of agitation and aggression associated with dementia. *Am J Geriatr Psychiatry* 1:249, 1993.

Heston LL, Gerrard J, Markis L, et al. Inadequate treatment of depression of nursing home elderly. *J Am Geriatr Soc* 40:1117, 1992.

Kane MJ, Cole K, Sarantakos S, et al. Safety and efficacy of bupropion in elderly patients: Preliminary observations. *J Clin Psychiatry* 44:134, 1983.

Lantz MS, Louis A, Lowenstein G, Kennedy GJ. A longitudinal study of psychotropic prescriptions in a teaching nursing home. *Am J Psychiatry* 147:1637, 1990.

Leibovici A, Tariot PN. Agitation associated with dementia: A systematic approach to treatment. *Psychopharmacol Bull* 24:49, 1988.

Leibovici A, Weinstein-Finnefrock V, Romano-Eagan JA, Podgorski C. Psychotropic drug prescribing patterns in a teaching nursing home: Changes after 12 years. In: *Program of the 6th Congress of IPA,* Berlin, 1993.

Loebel JP, Leibovici A. The management of other psychiatric states: Hallucinations, delusions and other disturbances. *Med Clin North Am* 78:841, 1994.

Nies A, Robinson DS, Friedman MJ. Relationship between age and tricyclic antidepressant levels. *Am J Psychiatry* 134:790, 1977.

Parmalee PA, Katz IR, Lawton MP. Depression among institutionalized aged. *J Gerontol* 22:9, 1989.

Ray WA, Taylor JA, Meador KG, et al. Reducing antipsychotic drug use in nursing homes: A controlled trial of provider education. *Arch Intern Med* 153:713, 1993.

Rovner BW, Edelman BA, Cox MP, Shmuely Y. The impact of antipsychotic drug regulations on psychotropic prescribing practices in nursing homes. *Am J Psychiatry* 149:1390, 1992.

Rovner BW, Kafonek S, Filipp L, et al. Prevalence of mental illness in a community nursing home. *Am J Psychiatry* 143:1446, 1986.

Schatzberg AF, Cole JO. Antidepressants. In: *Manual of Clinical Psychopharmacology,* 2nd ed. Washington, DC: American Psychiatric Press, 1991.

Sweet RA, Mulsant BH, Gupta B, et al. Duration of neuroleptic treatment and prevalence of tardive diskinesia in late life. In: *Program of the 7th AAGP Symposium,* Tampa, FL, 1994.

Tariot PN, Erb R, Leibovici A, et al. Carbamazepine treatment of agitation in nursing home patients with dementia: A preliminary study. *J Am Geriatr Soc* 42:1160–1166, 1994.

Tariot PN, Podgorski CA, Blazina L, Leibovici A. Mental disorders in the nursing home: Another perspective. *Am J Psychiatry* 150:1063, 1993.

Teicher MH. Biology of anxiety. *Med Clin North Am* 72:791, 1988.

Tybjerg J, Gulmann NC. Use of psychopharmaceuticals in municipal nursing homes: A nationwide study. *Ugeskr Laeger* 154:3126, 1992.

Viskum B, Juul S. Accidental falls in nursing homes: A study on the role of drugs in accidental falls in nursing homes. *Ugeskr Laeger* 154:2955, 1992.

Weinstock R. Informed consent and competence issues in the elderly. In: Rosner R, Schwartz HI, eds. *Geriatric Psychiatry and the Law* New York: Plenum Press, 1987.

4

Dementia

Michael S. Mega and Jeffrey L. Cummings

The care of the nursing home patient is largely the care of the demented patient. More than half of nursing home residents are intellectually impaired. As society ages, nursing homes will provide care for a growing number of cognitively compromised elderly. Thus, physicians providing nursing home care must be expert in the assessment and management of demented patients. This chapter provides a framework for the assessment, diagnosis, and management of dementia within the nursing home setting. Dementing disorders encountered in the extended-care population are discussed, and the morbidity and mortality data pertinent to this population are reviewed. The examination of the late-stage dementia patient is described, emphasizing the clinical features of advanced Alzheimer's disease (AD). The chapter concludes with an overview of treatment options for the behavioral challenges presented by institutionalized demented patients.

Types of Dementia among Nursing Home Residents

Dementia is a syndrome that, like fever, requires a systematic evaluation to identify its many causes (see Table 4.1). The syndrome of dementia is defined as an aquired persistent intellectual decline involving at *least* three of the following domains: language, memory, visuospatial skills, cognition (calculation, abstraction, judgment, etc.), and emotion or personality (Cummings et al., 1980). This persistent decline from previous function must not be secondary to delirium. The *Diagnostic and Statistical Manual of Mental Disorders,* 4th ed. (APA, 1994)

TABLE 4.1. Major Causes of Dementia Based on Cortical, Subcortical, or Mixed Dysfunction

Cortical dysfunction
  Alzheimer's disease
  Frontal lobe degeneration

Subcortical dysfunction
  Extrapyramidal syndromes
    Parkinson's disease
    Huntington's disease
    Progressive supranuclear palsy
    Wilson's disease
    Spinocerebellar degeneration
    Fahr's disease
  Hydrocephalus
  Dementia of depression
  Demyelinating disease
  Human immunodeficiency virus
    encephalopathy
  Vascular dementias
    Lacunar state
    Binswanger's disease

Mixed dysfunction
  Multi-infarct dementia
  Infections
    Slow virus dementias
    General paresis
  Toxic/Metabolic encephalopathies
    Systemic illnesses
    Endocrinopathies
    Deficiency states
    Drug intoxications
    Heavy metal exposure
    Industrial toxins
  Miscellaneous syndromes
    Posttraumatic
    Postanoxic
    Neoplastic
    Etc.

Source: Adapted from Cummings and Benson, 1992.

defines dementia as an impairment in short- and long-term memory plus additional decline in at least one other domain (e.g., abstraction, judgment, language, praxis, visuospatial skills, or personality) that interferes with either occupational or social functioning or interpersonal relationships. The abnormalities cannot be secondary to a delirium and should not be based on "nonorganic" causes (e.g., depression). Clinical diagnostic criteria for AD (McKhann et al., 1984) and vascular dementia (VaD) (Roman et al., 1993), the two most common causes of dementia in the elderly, have helped standardize the assessment and diagnosis of these disorders. These criteria are presented in Tables 4.2 and 4.3.

The criteria for AD and VaD listed in Tables 4.2 and 4.3 underscore the characteristic dementia profiles that these two disorders manifest. The classic profile of cognitive dysfunction in AD is typically one of progressive memory loss with a fluent aphasia, poor visuospatial skills, and loss of insight into the severity or even presence of these deficits. Motor abnormalities are absent until

TABLE 4.2. Criteria for the Diagnosis of Probable Alzheimer's Disease

1. Dementia present
2. Onset between 40 and 90 years of age
3. Deficits in two or more cognitive areas
4. Progression of deficits
5. Consciousness undisturbed
6. Absence of other reasonable diagnosis

TABLE 4.3.   Criteria for the Diagnosis of Probable Vascular Dementia

1. Dementia present
2a. Focal neurological signs
2b. Vascular lesion(s) on brain imaging
3. A relationship between 1 and 2 with either:
   Onset within 3 months of a stroke
   Abrupt cognitive deterioration
   Fluctuating stepwise progression

late in the disease course. This contrasts with the typical presentation of VaD, which often has a stepwise decline, vascular risk factors (e.g., hypertension, diabetes, cardiac disease, and so on), and focal neurological signs. Focal findings may be subtle, such as a decreased arm swing on one side only during "stressed" gait when the patient is asked to walk on the toes or heels. Other common neurological signs and symptoms are dysarthria, parkinsonism, incontinence, and gait difficulty. The characteristic profiles of AD and VaD underscore the importance of approaching dementia as a *syndrome,* with the goal of distinguishing the specific diagnosis from the wide differential of possible causes.

The nursing home population includes many types of dementia. Based upon the criteria shown in Table 4.2, Rovner et al. (1990) found that 37.9% of nursing home residents had AD, 17.8% had VaD, and 11.7% had dementia secondary to other causes. These data reveal that extended-care institutions are populated mainly by patients suffering from AD, VaD, or a mixed etiology of both. Less prevalent disorders, Parkinson's and Huntington's disease, add to the numbers of cognitively impaired residents. Dementias resulting from complex medical disorders or the effect of medications are common and contribute to the cognitive morbidity of patients with advanced medical and neurological disease. Cognitive impairment resulting from intracranial masses, reversible metabolic disturbances, and the effects of nonpharmacological toxins are rare. If cognitive dysfunction develops in a resident who was intact upon nursing home admission, then treatable causes of dementia and acute confusional states must be investigated (Cummings, 1983). Moreover, the occurrence of delirium superimposed on dementia is common, particularly among debilitated patients in advanced stages of dementia. (See Chapter 5 for a thorough discussion of delirium.)

Comorbidity in Dementia Patients in Extended Care

Institutionalized dementia patients are more severely impaired than those encountered in the outpatient setting and are generally unable to survive without some assistance. Some 50% of institutionalized patients are incontinent, 70% are disoriented, and 80% need help with dressing (Dijk et al., 1992). Dependence on nursing care is highest for dementia patients and those with severe functional disability. A useful instrument to rate the functional capabilities of demented

TABLE 4.4. Global Deterioration Scale (GDS)

Stage	Functional Capability
1	No deficits
2	Subjective complaints only of memory deficit
3	Earliest evidence of memory deficit only with intensive interview
4	Clear-cut deficit on careful interview
5	Inability to survive without some assistance
6	Requires assistance with activities of daily living
7	Verbal and psychomotor skills are lost

Source: Adapted from Reisberg et al., 1982.

patients is the Global Deterioration Scale (GDS) of Reisberg et al. (1982). Most extended-care patients are in stages 5, 6, or 7 of the GDS (see Table 4.4).

Medical illness may occur along with dementia; careful monitoring is necessary to uncover such conditions. Diseases common in the elderly will have an equal prevalence in the demented population (Bernardini et al., 1993), although patients with dementia report fewer minor clinical illnesses than nondemented patients, probably from an inability to register complaints due to cognitive impairment. Visual or hearing difficulties, anemia, and dysuria that go unreported will often worsen cognitive dysfunction.

Patients with advanced dementia require continuous medical surveillance. Skin care is particularly important for the bedridden; early treatment of decubitus ulcers will reduce the morbidity related to infections and the costs of acute hospitalization. Ambulatory patients who wander may fall and are at risk for hip fractures or subdural hematomas. General care includes awareness of oral and dental disorders that may cause pain, be a source of infection, and contribute to poor nutritional intake. Close monitoring of demented patients will uncover these reversible causes of dysfunction and optimize functional capabilities.

Mortality in Dementia Patients in Extended Care

Dementia is an independent risk factor for mortality in the nursing home patient. Over an 8-year period, 606 dementia patients admitted to a psychogeriatric nursing home had a 2-year survival rate of 60 and 30% for women and men respectively, versus 85 and 80% for nondemented controls (Dijk et al., 1992). Although comorbid conditions such as heart failure, hypertension, and other chronic diseases had an adverse effect on survival, dementia had an additive effect on mortality in nursing home patients. The risk of dying from pneumonia was the same for patients with or without dementia. The 2-year survival rate for demented outpatients is 75%, compared with 50% for nursing home patients and 40% for the demented in psychiatric hospitals (Dijk et al., 1991). Such data reflect the more advanced disease of extended-care residents compared to outpatients. A recent review concluded that (1) dementia patients have an increased mortality rate as compared with the general population; (2) demented females have a better survival than their male counterparts, possibly reflecting the trend in the general population; and (3) there is no consistent difference between the survival of patients with VaD as opposed to AD (Dijk et al., 1991). The major causes of death in both AD and VaD patients (Molsa et al., 1986; Burns et al., 1990) are bronchopneumonia (50 to 70%) and cardiovascular disease (5 to 10%).

Predictors of shorter survival in patients with dementia include the degree of cognitive impairment (Heyman et al., 1987; Hier et al., 1989), especially for VaD; younger age at onset; male sex (Barclay et al. 1985); and, in AD patients, a history of hypertension (Hier et al., 1989). The stronger correlation between cognitive impairment and mortality in VaD than in AD reflects the more severe systemic vascular disease in VaD patients. In AD, the rate of cognitive decline rather than the initial impairment may be a better predictor of mortality (Hier et al., 1989).

Examination of the Dementia Patient

Initial evaluations reveal distinct clinical profiles for patients with different types of dementia (Cummings and Benson, 1992), whereas late-stage dementias of varied etiologies resemble one another as cognitive and physical impairments become severe. The essential elements of the mental status exam include assessments of attention, language, memory, and visuospatial function; if time permits, the assessment of frontal system function, praxis, and cognition (e.g., abstraction, judgment, and calculation) would provide a more comprehensive mental status evaluation.

The best test of attention is digit span; $7 +/- 2$ digits forward and $5 +/- 1$ digit backward is normal. Language evaluation should include an assessment of fluency, comprehension, naming, and repetition. Fluency is best appreciated during conversation with the patient by listening for the frequency of nonspecific words such as "it" or "thing," which may betray an "empty speech" or word-finding difficulty. Comprehension is assessed by asking the patient to follow either three-step commands or, if necessary, to answer even simple yes/no questions. Naming should assess both high- and low-frequency items, and repetition is best evaluated with the phrase "no ifs, ands, or buts."

Memory testing should distinguish between an amnestic disorder (i.e., the inability to *learn* new information) and a retrieval deficit (i.e., difficulty *accessing* newly learned material). Distinguishing between these two memory disorders is possible at the bedside by using an 8- or 10-word list and asking the patient to recite the list back after each of four presentations. The number of correctly recited items for each presentation is recorded and provides a learning curve for the task. After a 10-minute delay occupied with other mental-status tasks, the patient is asked to recall as many of the presented items as possible. Any item not produced during free recall should then be cued with a category clue. For example, if one of the words not recalled was "dog," then the examiner would ask the patient: "One of the words you missed was an animal, does that help?"

If the category clue does not help the patient retrieve the item, then the examiner should next give a multiple choice clue: "Was the animal a cat, dog, or bird?" If category or multiple-choice clues result in a significant improvement in the number of items produced by the patient over the number spontaneously recalled, then the patient is considered to have a retrieval deficit disorder, not an amnesia. New information is learned, but there is difficulty in retrieving it; thus cues help the patient. In memory testing, it is important to distinguish between amnesia and a retrieval deficit, because in AD as opposed to most other dementing disorders, amnesia is prominent (Cummings and Benson, 1992).

Visuospatial skills are easily assessed with the copying of simple two- and three-dimensional figures. Frontal-system function can be assessed throughout the entire clinical interview by noting any evidence of perseveration, disinhibition, or easy distractibility. Praxis is the ability to accurately execute a complex motor pattern on command and is best assessed by asking the patient to "pretend" to comb his or her hair, or use a toothbrush, and so on. Calculations with one- and two-digit equations and simple word problems, as well as abstractions using similarities and proverb interpretation, test the patient's ability to manipulate knowledge (i.e., cognition).

Cognitive assessment of patients with severe dementia and very limited intellectual ability is a daunting task. Standardized instruments are useful for the initial assessment and monitoring of cognitive change in nursing home patients. The Mini-Mental State Exam (MMSE) of Folstein et al. (1975) is a widely used tool that has norms adjusted for age and education (Crum et al., 1993). Unfortunately, a "floor effect" is found when applying the MMSE to the severely impaired. Patients may survive for several years beyond the time they can no longer produce a single scoreable response on the MMSE. Most demented patients in the nursing home setting will be in GDS stages 5 to 7, and many patients remain in the severely demented stage (7) for years. An instrument capable of stratifying the examination of these patients with advanced dementia is the Functional Assessment Staging (FAST) inventory (Reisberg et al., 1986; Sclan and Reisberg, 1992). The FAST (Table 4.5) provides 11 substages encompassed within GDS stages 6 and 7, enabling the clinician to assess disease progression in severely impaired AD patients. Patients with non-AD dementias can also be assessed with this instrument. The FAST provides clinical expectations for stage-specific behaviors and guides clinical responses to emerging disabilities. If, for example, a patient manifests a symptom such as urinary incontinence inconsistent with his or her other abilities, the clinician should investigate secondary causes for the incontinence and not consider it a new manifestation of the dementing illness. Using standardized instruments such as the FAST will assist in distinguishing usual from unusual findings in the examination of the severely demented. A comparison of the GDS, MMSE, and FAST scores with the stages of dementia is shown in Table 4.6.

The mental status exam of the advanced dementia patient, GDS stages 6 to 7 or MMSE score of 5 to 0, reveals a significant deficit in attention. The patient is unable to direct or maintain attention on tasks; digit span may be as short as 2 forward. Verbal output will consist primarily of echolalia (echoing the examiner's

TABLE 4.5.   Functional Assessment Staging (FAST)

Stage	Functional Capability
1	No deficits
2	Subjective complaints only of memory deficit
3	Earliest evidence of memory deficit only with intensive interview
4	Clear-cut deficit on careful interview
5	Inability to survive without some assistance
6a	Inability to dress properly without assistance or cueing
6b	Inability to bathe properly
6c	Inability to handle the mechanics of toileting
6d	Urinary incontinence
6e	Fecal incontinence
7a	Speech limited to six words or less during an intense interview
7b	Speech limited to a single word during an intense interview
7c	Inability to walk without personal assistance
7d	Inability to sit without support
7e	Loss of ability to smile
7f	Loss of ability to hold up head independently

Source: Adapted from Reisberg, 1986.

words), or the patient may repeat his or her own words (palilalia). Ths may alternate with screaming, repeating a simple three- or four-word phrase repetitively, or verbalizing only a single intelligible word and little else. Mutism may ensue. Comprehension will also be poor, as well as naming, writing, and reading comprehension. Reading aloud may be disproportionately spared; patients can often read single words presented in large block letters even in advanced stages of AD. The memory of the severely demented patient may, at best, be limited to distinguishing familiar from unfamiliar faces, touch, or sounds. Visuospatial functioning will likewise be grossly impaired. In the ambulatory patient who is prone to wander, getting lost is a major concern. Progressive motor disability will impair dressing and may make independent eating and swallowing impossible. Frontal systems dysfunction is prominent in the severely demented patient, manifested by repetitive perseverative behavior and being drawn to any object in the immediate environment (stimulus-bound behavior).

TABLE 4.6.   Comparison of Standardized Assessments of Dementia

	Stage of Dementia				
	Incipient–Mild		Moderate	Moderate–Severe	Severe
Years from	0–7	7–9	9–10.5	10.5–13	13–19
MMSE	29–25	25–19	19–14	14–0	N/A
GDS	3	4	5	6	7
FAST	3	4	5	6a–e	7a–f

Source: Adapted from Reisberg et al., 1986.

Elemental Neurological Signs and Symptoms

Cranial nerve examination of the patient with advanced dementia may reveal a supranuclear gaze palsy resulting in the loss of volitional gaze with a fixed stare overcome only by oculocephalic reflexes (demonstrated by showing reflex eye movements with head turning). Bulbar dysfunction occurs, requiring assistance with feeding and making aspiration pneumonia frequent. Some 50% of patients are unable to feed themselves within 8 years after onset of AD (Volicer et al., 1989). A 2-year prospective study of 71 institutionalized AD patients who initially fed themselves documented the emergence of four groups (Volicer et al., 1989): those who continued to feed themselves (23.9%); those who required assistance but had no difficulty swallowing (18.3%); patients who refused food but could swallow (23.4%); and those who choked on liquids or solids (32.4%). Although the progression of dementia and weight loss was greater for the patients who did not feed themselves, mortality was not significantly different among groups in spite of the use of a feeding tube in only one patient.

With disease progression, ambulation is lost and eventually the patient cannot stand or sit without assistance. The bedbound demented patient may lie in a flexed, rigid posture, losing even the ability to support his or her head. Release signs emerge. Grasp reflexes of both the hands and feet, as well as the sucking

TABLE 4.7. Percentage of Advanced Alzheimer's Disease Patients Manifesting Neurological Signs[a]

Neurological Signs	FAST Stage 6a–c	FAST Stage 6d–e	FAST Stage 7a–b	FAST Stage 7c–f
Release signs				
Paratonia	77.3	75	100	100
Tactile sucking	13.6	33.3	100	91.7
Hand grasp	9.1	41.7	100	100
Foot grasp	4.5	33.3	80	83.3
Snout	18.2	58.3	60	75
Extrapyramidal signs				
Rigidity	18.2	50	60	91.7
Decreased arm swing	90.9	75	80	NA
Slowed gait	90.9	83.3	90	NA
Small stepped gait	68.2	83.3	80	NA
Hypomimia	12.5	57.1	57.1	57.1
Flexion attitude	45.5	50	90	NA
Pyramidal signs				
Plantar response	23.8	58.3	90	81.8
Jaw jerk	0	25	50	41.7
Foot clonus	0	8.3	0	33.3

Source: Adapted from Franssen et al., 1993.

[a]All signs (except snout) showed a significant ($p < .05$) increase in both prevalence and mean activity (based on a 7-point scale) with the degree of functional decline as defined by FAST.

reflex, rooting reflex, and paratonia or gegenhalten can be elicited. The number of primitive reflexes is an observed indicator of the severity of dementia (Jenkyn et al., 1985; Franssen et al., 1991; Benesch et al., 1993). Extrapyramidal signs occur in the advanced stages of AD, specifically rigidity and bradykinesia as well as stooped posture. However, other extrapyramidal manifestations such as tremor, cogwheel rigidity, shuffling gait, or sialorrhea are uncommon. Pyramidal signs found in the late-stage patient include extensor plantar responses as well as hyperactive muscle stretch reflexes. Myoclonus occurs in a substantial number of late-stage AD patients, more often when onset of the dementia was before age 65; seizures occur in 10 to 25% of cases (Romanelli et al., 1990).

The relationships between FAST stage and various neurological signs are shown in Table 4.7 (Franssen et al., 1993).

Awareness of when such signs may be encountered in the course of AD is important. The premature appearance of an extensor plantar response in an AD patient who is not in the end stage of the disease must be evaluated as a stage-inappropriate signs of pyramidal dysfunction. The patient may have fallen and sustained a contusion or subdural hematoma, a stroke may have occurred, or cervical spondylosis may be compromising spinal cord function.

Neuropsychiatric Disturbances

Behavioral abnormalities present the most demanding management challenges in dementia. Teri et al. (1988) investigated the relationship between the level of cognitive dysfunction and the type of behavioral abnormalities in 127 AD patients. Four problems were found to increase significantly with greater cognitive impairment: incontinence, poor hygiene, agitation, and wandering. Other neuropsychiatric symptoms were independent of the level of cognitive dysfunction. Table 4.8 lists the neuropsychiatric manifestations of AD.

Personality changes occur in all AD patients and often predate cognitive dysfunction (Petry et al., 1989). Disengagement and apathy are the most common; however, disinhibition and lability may also occur (Rubin et al., 1987; Petry et al., 1988). Agitation is more common in advanced patients than in patients who are early in their course. Agitation is a management challenge and may manifest as motor restlessness or as oppositional aggressiveness. The source of agitation is often delusions produced from progressive cognitive deterioration. Delusions affect 30 to 50% of patients who are mainly in the middle phase of the illness (Cummings et al., 1987; Wragg and Jeste, 1989). Delusional patients exhibit a more accelerated cognitive decline than those without delusions (Drevets and Rubin, 1989). Hallucinations affect 5–20% of AD patients with visual being more common than auditory hallucinations; the latter often accompany delusions, while the visual type may indicate a co-occurring delirium (Cummings et al., 1987). Mood changes range from elation in 5 to 20% of AD patients (Cummings and Victoroff, 1990) to symptoms of depression in 20 to 40% (Cummings et al., 1987; Mendez et al., 1990). Expressions of tearfulness, worthlessness, and other

TABLE 4.8. Neuropsychiatric Symptoms Encountered in Alzheimer's Disease

Personality changes	Anxiety
Disengagement	Psychomotor Disturbance
Disinhibition	Agitation or combativeness
Delusions	Wandering
Persecutory	Pacing
Theft	Purposeless activity
Infidelity	Miscellaneous
Capgras syndrome	Sexual activity changes
Hallucinations	Decreased interest
Auditory	Increased interest
Visual	Appetite changes
Mood changes	Sleep disturbances
Depression	Kluver-Bucy syndrome
Euphoria	
Lability	
Catastrophic reactions	

Source: Adapted from Cummings, 1992.

depressive features in the AD patient, unlike cognitively intact patients with major depressive disorders, are usually easily redirected by the caregiver (Merriam et al., 1988). Anxiety concerning upcoming events and psychomotor agitation, wandering, or pacing pose some of the most difficult management problems. Neuroleptics may exacerbate psychomotor agitation by inducing akathisia. Occasionally, late-stage AD patients manifest symptoms of the Kluver-Bucy syndrome (Lilly et al., 1983), including sensory agnosia, hyperoral behavior with dietary changes, altered sexuality, and a persistent urge to explore stimulus items in their environment (hypermetamorphosis).

As deterioration proceeds, behavioral abnormalities such as delusions, hallucinations, and agitation may increase. With continued cognitive decline, behavioral symptoms may decrease or remit completely. Medication aimed at improving delusions or hallucinations may worsen the tenuous cognitive status of the demented patient. Recommendations for management of the behavioral disturbances of the dementia patient are presented at the end of this chapter.

Laboratory Findings

Routine laboratory assessment of patients with advanced dementia is unwarranted unless delirium is suspected. Imaging studies may reveal atrophy, which is severe in the advanced stage of most dementias (Figure 4.1). Repeated imaging studies are unnecessary unless an acute process is suspected. In AD, functional studies, such as positron emission tomography (PET) or single photon emission computed tomography (SPECT), typically show abnormalities most marked in the parietal and posterior temporal lobes bilaterally (Figure 4.2) (Haxby et al., 1986; Johnson

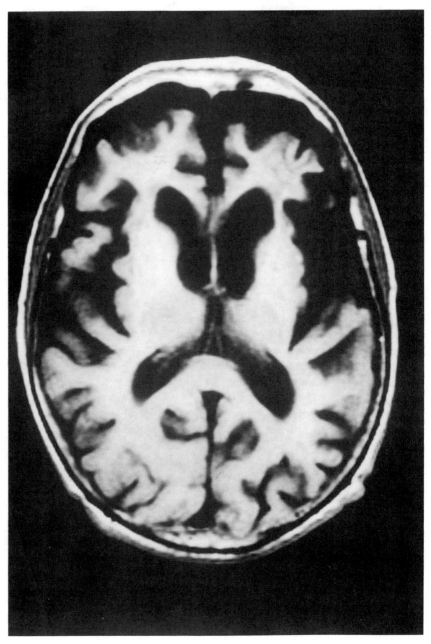

FIGURE 4.1. Magnetic resonance imaging scan of a patient with advanced Alzheimer's disease showing severe cortical atrophy.

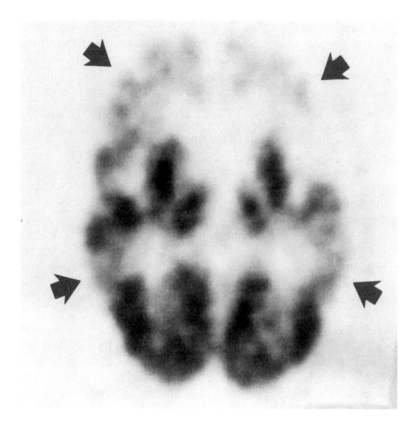

FIGURE 4.2. Positron emission tomography scan of a patient with advanced Alzheimer's disease demonstrating markedly reduced cortical metabolism in posterior temporal and frontal cortex (*arrows*).

et al., 1987). The electroencephalogram often shows frontally predominant or generalized slowing. If new neurological signs such as an extensor plantar response or hemiparesis are noted, then computed tomography (CT) of the head or magnetic resonance imaging (MRI) may be necessary to determine whether a new focal lesion has appeared.

Routine laboratory studies are most crucial when acute changes in mental function or behavior are evident. Under these circumstances, the evaluation of reversible causes of delirium must be thorough. (See Chapter 5 for a complete discussion of this topic.) Increased confusion or obtundation inappropriate for a patient's stage of dementia may be secondary to infection; thus blood and urine cultures should be obtained even in the absence of a fever or elevated white blood cell count. Dehydration is often a major cause of decompensation in the institutionalized elderly. Electrolytes should be obtained if dehydration is suspected. Patients in the advanced stages of dementia are particularly sensitive to the adverse sedative effects of medications; thus pharmacological regimes should be reviewed and drugs discontinued as appropriate. All management changes and interventions must be negotiated with the patient's family, since they often do not desire life-prolonging measures (see Chapters 16 and 17).

Treatment

There is no current treatment that reverses the course of primary degenerative dementias. Several agents are being investigated for possible utility in the treatment of the cognitive decline of AD. One currently available drug, tacrine (an acetylcholine esterase inhibitor), has been shown to provide limited cognitive benefit for a select group of patients with AD (Davis et al., 1992; Farlow et al., 1992). Treatment of VaD is directed toward controlling risk factors such as hypertension, diabetes, and vascular occlusion. Behavioral therapies may also be useful in the maintenance of skills of daily living or the learning of a new environment, especially when physical practice and multisensory feedback is employed in the training period (McEvoy and Patterson, 1986).

The clinician's major contribution will be to provide treatment options for the behavioral disturbances that often occur in the demented patient. Delusions and agitation are among the most troubling behavioral abnormalities in patients with AD. Treatment of these symptoms with low-dose neuroleptics is often useful. In addition to neuroleptics, which have dose-limiting extrapyramidal side effects, some patients may respond to treatment with trazodone, propranolol, buspirone, or thiothixene. Physostigmine has shown promise in the treatment of delusional symptoms (Cummings et al., 1993). Table 4.9 lists other typical disturbances encountered and the commonly used pharmacological agents helpful in their management. Dosages should be as low as possible in institutionalized elderly dementia patients. Drugs with anticholinergic effects may interfere with memory and cognition, thereby increasing the intellectual impairment; they should therefore be avoided. Nondemented nursing home patients with high serum anticholinergic levels have greater impairment in their capacity for self-care than those with low levels (Rovner et al., 1988). Agitation in demented patients may be increased rather than decreased by psychotropic medication; with increased dosages, an increase in agitated behavior may result.

Physical restraint becomes necessary when agitation is particularly severe or when wandering is associated with a high risk for injury. A soft ''posy'' restraint, applied in bed at night or in a sturdy geriatric chair during the day, is always preferable to individual limb restraints. Under such conditions, skin care is very important, particularly in the immobile, incontinent patient. The overreliance on physical restraints often results in excess disabilities such as nosocomical infections and even death (Sloane et al., 1991). The reader is referred to Chapters 2

TABLE 4.9. Medications Used for Symptomatic Treatment in Dementia

Symptom	Agent	Daily Dose in Milligrams (range in milligrams)
Psychosis	Haloperidol	1 (0.5–3) PO
	Thioridazine	75 (10–75)
Agitation	Neuroleptics	
	Haloperidol	1 (0.5–3)
	Thioridazine	25 (10–75)
	Molindone	75 (30–150)
	Nonneuroleptics	
	Propranolol	120 (80–240)
	Trazodone	100 (100–400)
	Buspirone	15 (15–30)
	Carbamazepine	1,000 (800–1200)
	Lithium	900 (300–900)
	Valproate	1,000 (750–1500)
	Lorazepam	1 (0.5–6)
Depression	Nortriptyline	50 (50–100)
	Desipramine	50 (50–150)
	Trazodone	100 (100–400)
	Fluoxetine	20 (5–40)
Anxiety	Oxazepam	30 (20–60)
	Lorazepam	1 (0.5–6)
	Propranolol	120 (80–240)
Insomnia	Temazepam	15 (15–30)
	Lorazepam	1 (0.2–4)
	Nortriptyline	25 (20–75)
	Trazodone	100 (100–400)
	Thioridazine	25 (10–75)
Sexual aggression (males)	Medroxyprogesterone	300 mg/week, (intramuscular)

Source: Adapted from Cummings and Benson, 1992.

and 3 for a more thorough discussion of the treatment of dementia and associated behavioral problems.

Many long-term-care facilities have developed special care units for dementia patients that attempt to limit the amount of medication given to patients while also providing safe environments. The quality of these "special" units varies widely (Ohta and Ohta, 1988), with the worst providing little more than an excuse to separate the cognitively impaired from the rest of the residents at the lowest cost. However, some units employ features such as textured, sound-absorbent, pastel-colored walls with safe outdoor wandering areas planted with nontoxic plants. Double rooms have the names, photographs, and brief biographies of the occupants on the door, and staff-to-patient ratios are high. Reduced-stimulation units (Cleary et al., 1988) eliminate television and radio, control staff and visitor access, and allow patients to wander and eat where they wish. Staff and family are educated in techniques of communicating with patients, such as speaking slowly and softly, making eye contact, touching, and allowing patients to make choices within appropriate options. Units such as these may offer a viable option for long-term care with a minimum of sedation or restraint. With an increased ability to ambulate and a less structured eating schedule, patients in these units may have a higher risk of hip fractures and dehydration, with subsequent urinary tract infections (Coleman et al., 1990). Thus close monitoring is necessary in these units to reduce acute illness.

Dementia is a common cause of death. Alzheimer's disease alone is estimated to be the fourth leading cause of mortality in the United States (Katzman, 1976). Many families do not plan the approach to end-stage care of a demented relative. A recent large survey of the families and professionals caring for demented patients (Luchins and Hanrahan, 1993) revealed that only 42% of family members had discussed end-stage planning with their demented relative. Some 70% preferred to withhold tube feeding and focus on comfort and pain control for the terminal phase of their relative's illness; 61.4% of physicians belonging to the Gerontological Society of America who responded to a questionnaire agreed with this minimum-care approach. A plan for the treatment of the patient with end-stage dementia should be discussed with the family and patient, if possible, before the terminal stage is reached and the patient is no longer able to express his or her own desires. (See Chapter 15, 16, and 17 for a review of the family's role in the care of the demented resident.)

References

APA. *Diagnostic and Statistical Manual of Mental Disorders,* 4th ed. Washington, DC: American Psychiatric Press, 1994.

Barclay LL, Zemcov A, Blass JP, Sansone J. Survival in Alzheimer's disease and vascular dementias. *Neurology* 35:834, 1985.

Benesch CG, McDaniel KD, Cox C, Hamill RW. End-stage Alzheimer's disease: Glasgow coma scale and the neurologic examination. *Arch Neurol* 50:1309, 1993.

Bernardini B, Meinecke C, Zaccarini C, et al. Adverse clinical events in dependent long-term nursing home residents. *J Am Geriatr Soc* 41:105, 1993.

Burns A, Jacoby R, Luthert P, Levy R. Cause of death in Alzheimer's disease. *Age Aging* 19:341, 1990.

Cleary AT, Clamon C, Price M, Shullaw G. A reduced stimulation unit: Effects on patients with Alzheimer's disease and related disorders. *Gerontologist* 28:511, 1988.

Coleman EA, Barbaccia JC, Croughan-Minihane MS. Hospitalization rates in nursing home residents with dementia. *J Am Geriatr Soc* 38:108, 1990.

Crum RM, Anthony JC, Bassett SS, Folstein MF: Population-based norms for the mini-mental state examination by age and educational level. *JAMA* 269:2386, 1993.

Cummings JL. Treatable dementias. In: Mayeux R, Rosen WG, eds: *The Dementias.* New York: Raven Press, 1983:165.

Cummings JL, Benson DF, LoVerme S. Reversible dementia. *JAMA* 243:2434, 1980.

Cummings JL, Benson DF. *Dementia: A Clinical Approach,* 2nd ed. Boston: Butterworth-Heinemann, 1992.

Cummings JL, Gorman DG, Shapira J. Physostigmine ameliorates the delusions of Alzheimer's disease. *Biol Psychiatry* 33:536, 1993.

Cummings JL, Miller B, Hill MA, Neshkes R. Neuropsychiatric aspects of multi-infarct dementia and dementia of the Alzheimer type. *Arch Neurol* 44:389, 1987.

Cummings JL, Victoroff JI. Noncognitive neuropsychiatric syndromes in Alzheimer's disease. *Neuropsychiatry Neuropsychol Behav Neurol* 3:140, 1990.

Davis KL, Thal LJ, Gamzu ER, et al. A double-blind, placebo-controlled multicenter study of tacrine for Alzheimer's disease. *N Engl J Med* 327:1253, 1992.

Dijk PTM van, Dippel DWJ, Habbema JDF. Survival of patients with dementia. *J Am Geriatr Soc* 39:603, 1991.

Dijk PTM van, Sande HJ van de, Dippel DWJ, Habbema JDF: The nature of excess mortality in nursing home patients with dementia. *J Gerontol* 47:M28, 1992.

Drevets WC, Rubin EH. Psychotic symptoms and the longitudinal course of senile dementia of the Alzheimer type. *Biol Psychiatry* 25:39, 1989.

Farlow M, Gracon SI, Hershey CA, et al. A controlled trial of tacrine in Alzheimer's disease. The Tacrine Study Group. *JAMA* 268:2523, 1992.

Folstein MF, Folstein SE, McHugh PR. "Mini-mental state": A practical method for grading the mental state of patients for the clinician. *J Psychiatry Res* 12:189, 1975.

Franssen EH, Kluger A, Torossian CL, Reisberg B. The neurologic syndrome of severe Alzheimer's disease: Relationship to functional decline. *Arch Neurol* 50:1029, 1993.

Franssen EH, Reisberg B, Kluger A, et al. Cognition-independent neurologic symptoms in normal aging and probable Alzheimer's disease. *Arch Neurol* 48:148, 1991.

Haxby JV, Grady CL, Duara R, et al. Neocortical metabolic abnormalities precede non-memory cognitive defects in early Alzheimer's-type dementia. *Arch Neurol* 43:882, 1986.

Heyman A, Wilkinson WE, Hurwitz BJ, et al. Early-onset Alzheimer's disease: Clinical predictors of institutionalization and death. *Neurology* 37:980, 1987.

Hier DB, Warach JD, Gorelick PB, Thomas J. Predictors of survival in clinically diagnosed Alzheimer's disease and multi-infarct dementia. *Arch Neurol* 46:1213, 1989.

Jenkyn LR, Reeves AG, Warren T, et al. Neurologic signs in senescence. *Arch Neurol* 42:1154, 1985.

Johnson KA, Mueller ST, Walshe TM, et al. Cerebral perfusion imaging in Alzheimer's disease. *Arch Neurol* 44:165, 1987.

Katzman R. The prevalence and malignancy of Alzheimer's disease. *Arch Neurol* 33:217, 1976.

Lilly R, Cummings JL, Benson DF, Frankel M. The human Kluver-Bucy syndrome. *Neurology* 33:1141, 1983.

Luchins DJ, Hanrahan P. What is appropriate health care for end-stage dementia? *J Am Geriatr Soc* 41:25, 1993.

McEvoy CL, Patterson RL. Behavioral treatment of deficit skills in dementia patients. *Gerontologist* 26:475, 1986.

McKhann G, Drachman D, Folstein M, et al. Clinical diagnosis of Alzheimer's disease: Report of the NINCDS-ADRDA Work Group, Department of Health and Human Services Task Force on Alzheimer's Disease. *Neurol* 34:939, 1984.

Mendez MF, Martin RJ, Smyth KA, Whitehouse PJ. Psychiatric symptoms associated with Alzheimer's disease. *J Neuropsychiatry Clin Neurosci* 2:28, 1990.

Merriam AE, Aronson MK, Gaston P, et al. The psychiatric symptoms of Alzheimer's disease. *J Am Geriatr Soc* 36:7, 1988.

Molsa PK, Marttila RJ, Rinne UK. Survival and cause of death in Alzheimer's disease and multi-infarct dementia. *Acta Neurol Scand* 74:103, 1986.

Ohta RJ, Ohta BM. Special units for Alzheimer's disease patients: A critical look. *Gerontologist* 28:803, 1988.

Petry S, Cummings JL, Hill MA, Shapira J. Personality alterations in dementia of the Alzheimer type. *Arch Neurol* 45:1187, 1988.

Petry S, Cummings JL, Hill MA, Shapira J. Personality alterations in dementia of the Alzheimer type: A three-year follow-up study. *J Geriatr Psychiatry Neurol* 2: 203, 1989.

Reisberg B, Ferris SH, DeLeon MJ, Crook T. The global deterioration scale for assessment of primary degenerative dementia. *Am J Psychiatry* 139:1136, 1982.

Reisberg B. Dementia: A systematic approach to identifying reversible causes. *Geriatrics* 41(4):30, 1986.

Roman GC, Tatemichi TK, Erkinjuntti T, et al. Vascular dementia: Diagnostic criteria for research studies report of the NINDS-AIREN international workshop. *Neurology* 43:250, 1993.

Romanelli MF, Morris JC, Ashkin K, Coben LA. Advanced Alzheimer's disease is a risk factor for late-onset seizures. *Arch Neurol* 47:847, 1990.

Rovner BW, David A, Lucas-Blaustein MJ, et al. Self-care capacity and anticholinergic drug levels in nursing home patients. *Am J Psychiatry* 145:107, 1988.

Rovner BW, German PS, Broadhead J, et al. The prevalence and management of dementia and other psychiatric disorders in nursing homes. *Int Psychogeriatr* 2:13, 1990.

Rubin EH, Morris JC, Storandt M, Berg L. Behavioral changes in patients with mild senile dementia of the Alzheimer's type. *Psychiatry Res* 21:55, 1987.

Sclan SG, Reisberg B. Functional assessment staging (FAST) in Alzheimer's disease: Reliability, validity, and ordinality. *Int Psychogeriatr* 4:(suppl 1):55, 1992.

Sloane PD, Mathew LJ, Scarborough M, et al. Physical and pharmacologic restraint of nursing home patients with dementia. *JAMA* 265:1278, 1991.

Teri L, Larson EB, Reifler BV. Behavioral disturbance in dementia of the Alzheimer's type. *J Am Geriatr Soc* 36:1, 1988.

Volicer L, Seltzer B, Rheaume Y, et al. Eating difficulties in patients with probable dementia of the Alzheimer's type. *J Geriatr Psychiatry Neurol* 2:189, 1989.

Wragg RE, Jeste DV. Overview of depresion and psychosis in Alzheimer's disease. *Am J Psychiatry* 146:577, 1989.

5

Delirium

Sandra A. Jacobson and Andrew F. Leuchter

Considering the characteristics of the patient population at greatest risk for developing delirium as well as the serious morbidity, mortality, and health care costs associated with this syndrome, it is not surprising that delirium is becoming a major concern in the nursing home. Delirium occurs more frequently in the elderly, particularly in patients with dementia, multiple medical problems, undernutrition, visual deficits and hearing problems, and in those receiving multiple medications. Varying incidence rates of delirium have been reported; even in one of the best long-term-care facilities, Katz and colleagues found that 6 to 12% of those with cognitive impairment were retrospectively diagnosed as delirious (Katz, et al., 1991).

When this syndrome is unrecognized, there is a significant risk of injuries such as fractures and subdural hematoma. In addition, the mortality rates associated with delirium in acute care settings are alarmingly high, far exceeding those of dementia or depression (Francis et al., 1990; Rabins and Folstein, 1982; Trzepacz et al., 1985).

Even in patients with moderately severe dementia, delirium is a treatable condition. As such, it offers some degree of hope to these patients, since appropriate treatment can at times have dramatic effects in improving functional status. For all of these reasons, timely and accurate diagnosis of delirium is critical.

Diagnosis

The syndrome of delirium is currently diagnosed on clinical grounds, using criteria of the *Diagnostic and Statistical Manual of Mental Disorders,* 4th ed. (DSM-IV) (APA, 1994). These criteria are reproduced in Table 5.1.

TABLE 5.1.   DSM-IV Diagnostic Criteria for Delirium
Due to a General Medical Condition

A. Disturbance of consciousness (i.e., reduced clarity of awareness of the environment) with reduced ability to focus, sustain, or shift attention.

B. A change in cognition (such as memory deficit, disorientation, language disturbance) or the development of a perceptual disturbance that is not better accounted for by a preexisting, established, or evolving dementia.

C. The disturbance develops over a short period of time (usually hours to days) and tends to fluctuate during the course of the day.

D. There is evidence from the history, physical examination, or laboratory findings that the disturbance is caused by the direct physiological consequences of a general medical condition.

Under the DSM-IV classification scheme, delirium is coded if the patient manifests a disturbance of consciousness with attentional impairment in conjunction with cognitive or perceptual disturbance which are not better accounted for by dementia. Although not specifically mentioned, disturbances in psychomotor activity are also frequently noted. In the elderly patient, decreased psychomotor behavior (Lipowski's "hypoactive" variant) is a much more commonly observed symptom than is increased psychomotor behavior (Lipowski, 1990).

The clinical features in delirium develop acutely (hours to days) and fluctuate over the course of a day. The acuity with which symptoms develop may in part reflect etiology; delirium may develop immediately after an insult such as head injury or more slowly in the course of metabolic derangement (Lipowski, 1990). Fluctuation, also known as *waxing and waning,* may take the form of *lucid intervals* (transient clearing) or *sundowning* (transient worsening, often observed with nightfall). Although the latter term is used by some practitioners to refer only to mental status fluctuation in dementia, it may in some cases represent repeated episodes of delirium in patients with marginally compensated cerebral function.

Within the DSM-IV framework, delirium may be coded by presumed etiology (general medical condition, substance intoxication, substance withdrawal, or multiple etiologies). All sets of criteria share the defining features set forth under A, B, and C of Table 5.1; they differ only in the etiological criteria set forth under D.

It is because of the acute onset and fluctuating course of delirium that it is important to have staff trained to recognize this disorder. Reliance on a physician who might be making weekly or monthly rounds is a dangerous practice, since many cases of delirium might go unrecognized. Useful tools for training staff in delirium diagnosis include the Confusion Assessment Method (Inouye et al., 1990) and the Delirium Rating Scale (Trzepacz et al., 1988). If educated as to the prodromal symptoms—which include new onset restlessness, anxiety, irritability, insomnia, and nightmares—clinically sophisticated staff might also be able to detect impending delirium.

The *Manual of the International Statistical Classification of Diseases,* 9th ed. (ICD-9) (WHO, 1977) offers a description of *transient organic psychotic condi-*

TABLE 5.2.   Draft ICD-10 Criteria for Delirium, Other Than Alcoholic

Symptoms, mild or severe, must be present *in each one* of the following areas:

  1. Impairment of consciousness and attention (on a continuum from clouding to coma; reduced ability to direct, focus, sustain, and shift attention)

  2. Global disturbance of cognition (perceptual distortions, illusions, and hallucinations—most often visual; impairment of abstract thinking and comprehension, with or without transient delusions but typically with some degree of incoherence; impairment of immediate recall and of recent memory but with relatively intact remote memory; disorientation for time as well as, in more severe cases, for place and person)

  3. Psychomotor disturbances (hypo- or hyperactivity and unpredictable shifts from one to the other; increased reaction time; increased or decreased flow of speech; enhanced startle reaction)

  4. Disturbance of the sleep-wake cycle (insomnia or, in severe cases, total sleep loss or reversal of the sleep-wake cycle; daytime drowsiness; nocturnal worsening of symptoms; disturbing dreams or nightmares which may continue as hallucinations after wakening)

  5. Emotional disturbances (e.g., depression, anxiety or fear, irritability, euphoria, apathy or wondering perplexity)

The onset must be rapid, the course diurnally fluctuating, and the total duration of the condition under six months.

tions that corresponds to the DSM description of delirium. In the further delineation of acute versus subacute confusional states, however, *delirium* is listed as a subtype, at the same taxonomic level as conditions such as *infective psychosis* and *organic reaction,* such that the terminology is somewhat confusing. The draft of ICD-10 in circulation sets forth criteria for *delirium, other than alcoholic,* reproduced in Table 5.2. Under these criteria, symptoms must be present in each of five domains, including consciousness/attention, global cognition, psychomotor behavior, sleep-wake cycle, and emotion. In addition, the condition must have an acute onset and fluctuating course and have a total duration of less than six months. As noted by Lindesay and others, under the latter criterion, delirium cannot be coded unless a patient has recovered or died (Lindesay et al., 1990).

In addition to the cognitive, behavioral, and emotional symptoms noted above, neurological abnormalities are often found to accompany the development of delirium. These include ataxia, tremor, myoclonus, asterixis, choreiform movements, symmetrical reflex changes, symmetrical tone changes, dysarthria, dysphasia, and dyspraxia (Lindesay et al., 1990; Lipowski, 1983).

Differential Diagnosis

Recognition of delirium in the nursing home population is greatly confounded by the prevalence of dementia, depression, debilitating medical illness, and preexisting functional disability among institutionalized patients. Of the differential diagnoses for delirium, the most important and difficult to distinguish is that of dementia. The two disorders frequently coexist, and some confusion of the two has arisen because of misattribution of symptoms of unrecognized delirium to the dementia syndrome.

Clinical features that may be useful in distinguishing delirium from dementia include the following (Lipowski, 1990; Roth, 1991):

1. Certain symptoms, such as impairment in attention and level of consciousness, are more characteristic of delirium (except perhaps in the later stages of dementia).

2. Delirium may involve impairment of both recent and long-term memory; dementia may involve impairment of recent memory more than long-term.

3. Delirium may come on acutely, dementia more insidiously. In a patient with known dementia, sudden worsening suggests that delirium is now superimposed.

4. Level of consciousness fluctuates in delirium but not in dementia.

5. Delirium may involve more prominent hallucinations than dementia.

6. Patients with delirium may appear more fearful and perplexed and patients with dementia more apathetic.

7. Delirious patients improve over time if appropriately evaluated and treated.

Etiology

Common etiologies of delirium in the nursing home setting are listed in Table 5.3. It is important to note, in reviewing this list, that most cases of delirium are multifactorial in origin (Francis et al., 1990). In patients whose cerebral function is already compromised by dementing illness, however, even minor problems such as urinary tract infections can precipitate delirium.

Although nonsteroidal anti-inflammatory drugs have been implicated in delirium (Francis et al., 1990), clearly the worst offenders in the nursing home are anticholinergic medications. Not only are anticholinergic effects found among antipsychotic medications such as thioridazine (Mellaril) and chlorpromazine (Thorazine), which were historically used in the treatment of delirium, but these effects also confound the use of certain other medications used to treat conditions such as chronic congestive heart failure. Tune and colleagues measured anticholin-

TABLE 5.3. Common Etiologies of Delirium in the Nursing Home

Medications
Anticholinergics
Sedative-hypnotics
Infection
Urinary tract
Pneumonia
Fluid/Electrolyte Imbalance
Dehydration
Third-spacing of fluid (congestive heart failure)
Metabolic Derangement
Hyper- or hypoglycemia
Hypoxia
Nutritional (including vitamin) deficiency

ergic effects of the 25 medications most commonly prescribed to the elderly and found that 9 of those medications produced levels associated with significant impairment in recent memory and attention, even in normal elderly control subjects (Tune et al., 1992). Those nine medications included ranitidine, codeine, dipyridamole, warfarin, isosorbide, theophylline, nifedipine, digoxin, and prednisolone (Tune et al., 1992).

Still another potential problem in the population of elderly patients is that the syndrome of delirium may present as dysphoria, which is sometimes mistaken for primary depression. If these patients are treated with tricyclic antidepressants, delirium may worsen significantly because of anticholinergic side effects.

Certain etiologies of delirium, although not the most common, must be considered early in the course of evaluation because of their seriousness. Wise and Brandt have suggested a mnemonic for etiologies of delirium which may be life-threatening if not diagnosed emergently (Wise and Brandt, 1992):

W	Wernicke's encephalopathy/alcohol withdrawal
H	Hypoxemia
H	Hypertensive encephalopathy
H	Hypoglycema
H	Hypoperfusion
I	Intracranial (bleed or infection)
M	Meningitis/encephalitis
P	"Poisons" or medications

Neuroleptic malignant syndrome should probably be added to this list. In the elderly, this can be caused by administration of dopamine blockers (antipsychotics) or withdrawal of dopamine agonists used in the treatment of Parkinson's disease. Although delirium is said to be found in about 50% of cases of neuroleptic malignant syndrome (Levinson and Simpson, 1986), in our experience, it is present almost invariably.

Evaluation

Whether evaluation and treatment of delirium are performed in the nursing home or in an acute care facility depends on the condition of the patient, proximity to emergency care facilities, availability of laboratory services, and the medical sophistication of the nursing home physician and staff. The patient who appears prostrate, has unstable vital signs, or has had a sudden, unexplained change in status is best managed in an acute care facility under most circumstances. On the basis of a small literature on psychological and situational factors contributing to delirium (Kennedy, 1959; Kuroda et al., 1990) as well as cost considerations, some practitioners argue that most other patients are best managed in the nursing home.

Wherever a case is managed, the following basic workup usually is indicated for every patient in whom delirium has been diagnosed:

Mental status exam: Designed to assess level of consciousness, perceptual disturbance, psychomotor activity, and severity of cognitive impairment. For quantitative assessment of cognitive status, the standardized Folstein Mini-Mental State Exam (MMSE) (Folstein et al., 1975) is recommended for brevity and ease of use but may not be helpful in patients with significant preexisting dementia. A score of less than 24 on the MMSE indicates global cognitive impairment. In the presence of dementia, delirium will produce a further worsening on this scale.

Physical exam: Includes survey of serial vital signs, neurological screening, cardiac and pulmonary exams.

    Lab exam: Hematology—complete blood count with differential, platelet count, sedimentation rate.

    Chemistry—albumin, blood urea nitrogen, calcium, CPK, creatinine, electrolytes, glucose, and liver function tests.

    Drug Analysis—as available, for all prescribed medications.

    Urinalysis

    Electrocardiogram

    Chest x-ray

If there is any doubt as to the presence of delirium, an electroencephalogram (EEG) may be useful in confirming the clinical diagnosis (Jacobson et al., 1993; Leuchter and Jacobson, 1991). Conventional (paper) EEG findings in hypoactive delirium include slowing of the posterior dominant rhythm and increased generalized slow-wave activity. Quantitative EEG (QEEG) findings in hypoactive delirium include decreased power in the alpha band and increased power in the theta and delta bands. The EEG and QEEG are especially helpful in cases of new-onset agitation in the context of dementia where a prior EEG study is available for comparison.

In addition to these nonspecific EEG findings, other EEG patterns may be found that may suggest particular etiologies of delirium. These include continuous epileptiform discharges in complex partial status epilepticus, localized delta activity in focal lesions, and triphasic waves in metabolic derangement.

Further workup of a patient with delirium depends on clinical suspicion and initial lab findings. It may include a blood gas analysis, toxic screen, magnetic resonance imaging (MRI) or computed tomography (CT), lumbar puncture, thyroid function tests, and/or thiamine and folate levels.

The basic evaluation algorithm described above may be difficult to carry out in the nursing home facility. It often is true that a brief hospitalization suffices for workup and initial treatment, with follow-up management in the nursing home itself.

Treatment

Whether treatment commences in the acute care setting or in the nursing home, the same principles apply. An understanding of the distinction between curative and palliative treatment in the context of delirium is essential. Curative treatment is directed toward the underlying disease, whereas palliative treatment is largely nonspecific and directed toward control of symptoms such as agitation. Curative treatments are as numerous as etiologies, and are not discussed further here. It is worth emphasizing, however, that since certain etiologies of delirium represent medical emergencies, it is of critical importance that appropriate and timely diagnosis take precedence over mere quieting of the agitated, delirious patient.

Treatment first involves the discontinuation or taper of all nonessential medications. The patient is moved near the nursing station and placed on close observation. Vital signs are taken frequently and fluid intake/output is monitored carefully, since these patients are usually unable to perform any self-monitoring of even the most basic bodily functions. Measures are taken to ensure adequate oxygenation, hydration, and sleep. Basic laboratory values are rechecked frequently.

The environment of the delirious patient is structured to maximize consistency and familiarity. Frequent reorientation to person, place, and time are provided by staff. Familiar personal effects are placed near the bedside. Room lighting that is neither too bright nor too dim is provided. If at all possible, the patient is placed in a room with windows so that usual diurnal cues are restored. Eyeglasses and hearing aids are returned to the patient if they have been removed.

Psychosocial support is also an important element of treatment. Family members are encouraged to stay with the patient. Some facilities even allow family members to stay overnight by providing a cot or bed in the patient's own room. The transient nature of delirium and its medical implications are discussed fully with the family.

It often is true that appropriate and timely interventions such as those described above obviate the need for psychopharmacological intervention to treat agitation in the context of delirium. In some cases, however, pharmacological treatment does become necessary. Two classes of medications are used: high-potency antipsychotics, and short-acting benzodiazepines that are not metabolized by the liver. Antipsychotics alone may be used for most etiologies of delirium. Benzodiazepines are used for alcohol/sedative withdrawal delirium, neuroleptic malignant syndrome, hepatic encephalopathy (for the latter condition at very low doses), for patients who worsen with antipsychotics, and in combination with antipsychotics in special cases of intractable agitation.

If benzodiazepines are used as sole agents in the nonspecific treatment of agitation in delirium, it should be remembered that these medications suppress respiration, invalidate cognitive status testing, and themselves cause delirium. Although the dose of benzodiazepine must be individualized, a typical regimen is lorazepam (Ativan) 0.5mg PO/IM/IV, with the dose repeated or doubled after 1 to 2 hours if symptoms are not controlled. For patients in alcohol or sedative withdrawal delirium, standing doses of benzodiazepines on a slowly tapering schedule are given rather than one-time or as-needed doses.

Among antipsychotics, high-potency agents are preferred to low-potency agents for the treatment of agitation in delirium because they have less anticholinergic and hypotensive effects and less effect on respiration (Fish, 1991). Two medications commonly used are haloperidol (Haldol) and droperidol (Inapsine), both of the butyrophenone class. Anecdotally, droperidol has been reported to be more sedating and to carry a greater risk of lowering blood pressure than haloperidol, but controlled studies have not been published to corroborate these reports. The two agents are believed to be equally efficacious, with droperidol being approximately twice as potent as haloperidol. With haloperidol, extrapyramidal side effects are minimal when used parenterally, but intravenous use has been associated with torsades de pointes tachycardia (Metzger and Friedman, 1993). Haloperidol is approved by the Food and Drug Administration for PO and IM use but not for IV use, although it has been used intravenously in many acute care settings. Droperidol is available only for parenteral use.

In elderly patients, the following dosing regimen is recommended for haloperidol: 0.5 mg PO/IM for mild agitation, 1.0 mg PO/IM for moderate agitation, and 2.0 mg PO/IM for severe agitation. The dose may be repeated (or doubled) every 30 minutes until the patient is sedated or calm. Most patients respond to three or fewer doses. If agitation continues, transfer to an acute care facility should be considered. When agitation has subsided, the medication is tapered over 3 to 5 days; if this taper is done more precipitously, delirium may recur. The reader is referred to Chapter 3 for a more complete discussion of psychopharmacological issues.

Resolution of Delirium

Delirium in the elderly may be very slow to resolve. Koponen and colleagues found a range of 3 to 81 days to resolution among their cohort, with a mean of 20 days (Koponen et al., 1989). During this phase, it is not always clear that the patient is, in fact, improving, since intraepisode waxing and waning may continue, such that behavioral and cognitive indices fail. It is in this context that the quantitative EEG (QEEG) finds its greatest utility in delirium (Jacobson et al., 1993). The QEEG in particular is sensitive to subtle changes in slow-wave activity between studies and can provide either reassurance that the patient is improving or warning that the disease process may not be responding to current treatment.

Another extremely important part of the recovery process is to ensure as far as possible that the patient and/or family understand that the episode of delirium was transient, that this is a treatable illness which might recur if the patient becomes medically unstable again, and that it does not mean that the patient is ''going crazy.'' The patient must have ample opportunity to vent concerns about recollections or specific behaviors that might have occurred during the episode.

Prevention of Delirium

Several preventive measures can be recommended to physicians practicing in the nursing home. These include the following: avoiding polypharmacy, becoming familiar with specialized medication prescribing practices for elderly patients, avoiding ''high-risk'' medications such as those with anticholinergic effects, watching carefully for prodromal signs and symptoms, and training staff in the assessment of patients for delirium (Lipowski, 1990).

Summary

Unrecognized delirium in the nursing home may place the elderly patient at significant risk. In addition to maintaining a high index of suspicion regarding the possible presence of delirium, it is important to ensure that on-site staff are trained to recognize this syndrome. For this purpose, a standardized instrument such as the Confusion Assessment Method may be helpful. Delirium is a treatable condition, and appropriate treatment may have dramatic effects in improving functional status, even in patients with moderately severe dementia.

Acknowledgments

This work was supported in part by NIMH research grant 1RO1 MH 40705 (Dr. Leuchter), training grant MH 17140 (Dr. Jacobson), the UCLA Alzheimer's Disease Center (NIA grant PHS 1P30AG10123), and the Department of Veterans Affairs. The views expressed in this manuscript reflect those of the authors and do not necessarily reflect those of the Department of Veterans Affairs. The authors wish to thank Stephen L. Read, MD, who provided helpful comments on an earlier draft of this manuscript.

References

APA: *Diagnostic and Statistical Manual of Mental Disorders,* 4th ed. Washington, DC: American Psychiatric Association, 1994.

Fish DN. Treatment of delirium in the critically ill patient. *Clin Pharm* 10:456, 1991.

Folstein MF, Folstein SE, McHugh PR. "Mini-mental state": A practical method for grading the cognitive status of patients for the clinician. *J Psychiatry Res* 12: 189, 1975.

Francis J, Martin D, Kapoor WN. A prospective study of delirium in hospitalized elderly. *JAMA* 263:1097, 1990.

Inouye SK, van Dyck CH, Alessi CA, et al. Clarifying confusion: The confusion assessment method. *Ann Intern Med* 113:941, 1990.

Jacobson SA, Leuchter AF, Walter DO. Conventional and quantitative EEG in the diagnosis of delirium among the elderly. *J Neurol Neurosurg Psychiatry* 56:153, 1993.

Jacobson SA, Leuchter AF, Walter DO, Weiner H. Serial quantitative EEG among elderly subjects with delirium. *Biol Psychiatry* 34:135, 1993.

Katz IR, Parmelee P, Brubaker K. Toxic and metabolic encephalopathies in long-term care patients. *Intern Psychogeriatr* 3:337, 1991.

Kennedy A. Psychological factors in confusional states in the elderly. *Gerontol Clin* 1:71, 1959.

Koponen H, Stenback U, Mattila E, et al. Delirium among elderly persons admitted to a psychiatric hospital: Clinical course during the acute stage and one-year follow-up. *Acta Psychiatr Scand* 79:579, 1989.

Kuroda S, Ishizu H, Ujike H, et al. Senile delirium with special reference to situational factors and recurrent delirium. *Acta Med Okayama* 44:267, 1990.

Leuchter AF, Jacobson SA. Quantitative measurement of brain electrical activity among subjects with delirium. *Int Psychogeriatr* 3:231, 1991.

Levinson DF, Simpson GM. Neuroleptic-induced extrapyramidal symptoms with fever. *Arch Gen Psychiatry* 43:839, 1986.

Lindesay J, Macdonald A, Starke I. *Delirium in the Elderly.* New York: Oxford University Press, 1990.

Lipowski ZJ. Transient cognitive disorders (delirium, acute confusional states) in the elderly. *Am J Psychiatry* 140:1426, 1983.

Lipowski ZJ. *Delirium: Acute Confusional States.* New York: Oxford University Press, 1990.

Metzger ED, Friedman RS. Torsades de pointes and intravenous haloperidol. In: *1993 New Research Abstracts of the Annual Meeting of the American Psychiatric Association,* Washington, DC: American Psychiatric Assoc., 1993:66.

Rabins PV, Folstein MF. Delirium and dementia: Diagnostic criteria and fatality rates. *Br J Psychiatry* 140:149, 1982.

Roth M. Clinical perspectives. *Int Psychogeriatr* 3:309, 1991.

Trzepacz PT, Baker WB, Greenhouse J. A symptom rating scale for delirium. *Psychiatry Res* 23:89, 1988.

Trzepacz PT, Teague GB, Lipowski ZJ. Delirium and other organic mental disorders in a general hospital. *Gen Hosp Psychiatry* 7:101, 1985.

Tune L, Carr S, Hoag E, Cooper T. Anticholinergic effects of drugs commonly prescribed for the elderly: Potential means for assessing risk of delirium. *Am J Psychiatry* 149:1393, 1992.

Wise MG, Brandt GT. Delirium. In: Yudofsky SC, Hales RE, eds. *Textbook of Neuropsychiatry.* Washington, DC: American Psychiatric Press, 1992.

WHO. *Manual of the International Statistical Classification of Diseases, Injuries, and Causes of Death,* 9th rev. Geneva: World Health Organization, 1977.

6

Mood Disorders

Soo Borson and Page Moss Fletcher

Mood disorders are psychiatric syndromes defined by prominent changes in emotional tone. To recognize disordered mood states, and to separate them from normal and expected responses to life events, one must identify sustained changes in social behavior, interest, attitudes, energy, thinking, judgment, and patterns of eating and sleeping that accompany the change in mood. The identification of mood disorders is a clinical task based on familiarity with standards of diagnosis and skilled observation and interaction with patients. Nurses' aides in long-term-care settings can be trained in the observational skills needed to report concerns about possible mood disorder in patients, but a full diagnostic assessment requires specialized interviewing skills and knowledge of the patient's history and medical status. Uncomplicated mood disorders can be evaluated by psychiatrists, general physicians, psychologists, and nurses experienced in differential diagnosis of psychiatric disorders in the elderly; more complex presentations are in the domain of the geriatric psychiatrist. In this chapter, we review the clinical features, diagnosis, prevalence, etiology, and management of manic and depressed elderly patients encountered in long-term care.

Manic and Manic-like States

Epidemiology

The relative plethora of information on depression in the nursing home contrasts with a minimal literature on mania or bipolar disorder. In this section, we briefly summarize the presentation and treatment of mania in the elderly, based on studies of elderly psychiatric inpatients and outpatients. Recent reviews (Rubin, 1988; Young, 1992; Young and Klerman, 1992; Mirchandani and Young, 1993) emphasize that manic states in the elderly are a heterogenous group of syndromes with an extensive differential diagnosis that includes not only bipolar disorder but also secondary (''symptomatic'') mood disorders, delusional disorders, paranoid schizophrenia, schizoaffective disorder, delirium, and dementia. These diagnostic distinctions are important, as they often determine the focus of treatment.

The frequency of mania in nursing home patients is unknown. Weissman et al. (1991) cited a 1-year incidence of 9.7% of bipolar affective episodes (mania or depression) among residents of nursing homes included in the Epidemiological Catchment Area Study. Current rates could be lower consequent to the enactment of the Omnibus Budget Reconciliation Act (OBRA) in 1987, mandating pre-screening of patients for mental illness requiring active treatment and permitting the exclusion of chronically mentally ill persons from nonpsychiatric facilities.

Clinical Features

Clinical diagnostic criteria for mania are presented in Table 6.1. When the elderly patient presents with affective signs and symptoms of a pressured, driven, or accelerated nature, the possibility of mania, hypomania, bipolar disorder, and other diagnoses as noted above must be considered. A prudent first step lies in careful assessment of the patient for an organic mood disorder or ''secondary mania.'' Krauthammer and Klerman (1978) defined this as a manic episode involving an elated and/or irritable mood and classic manic symptoms causally linked to a medical or pharmacological condition. Importantly, elderly patients are more likely than younger adults to have mania as a symptom of another disorder rather than of primary bipolar disorder. Secondary manic episodes are likely to begin later in life than primary bipolar disorder, and family history is less often positive for affective disorders (Krauthammer and Klerman, 1978; Rubin, 1988). Many cerebral organic pathologies have been implicated as causes of secondary mania in the elderly. Among the most important are cerebral infarction (stroke, particularly right-sided), infection (e.g., viral encephalitis, neurosyphilis), tumors, and substance abuse, including alcohol (Cummings, 1986; Starkstein and Robinson, 1989). Medications may also cause a manic syndrome, including agents such as L-dopa, corticosteroids, anticholinergics, psychostimulants, and antidepressants (Cummings, 1991; Merchandani and Young, 1993). Occasionally, a manic episode occurs as a complication of an acute nonneurological disease such as myocardial infarction.

Secondary and primary manic episodes cannot be reliably distinguished on the basis of symptoms, as manic syndromes due to medical disorders or drugs frequently meet all diagnostic criteria defining a primary manic episode except etiology (i.e., the patient has no history of primary bipolar affective disorder; Rubin, 1988). A history of prior episodes beginning in early or middle adulthood usually identifies elderly patients with primary bipolar disorder, and thorough medical assessment (including medications) usually reveals potential causes in secondary manic states.

TABLE 6.1. Diagnostic Criteria for Mania and Related States

Manic episode

  A. A distinct period of abnormally and persistently elevated, expansive, or irritable mood, lasting at least 1 week (or if any duration of hospitalization is necessary)

  B. During the period of mood disturbance, at least three of the following symptoms have persisted (four if the mood is only irritable) and have been present to a significant degree:

    1. Inflated self-esteem or grandiosity
    2. Decreased need for sleep
    3. More talkative than usual or pressure to keep talking
    4. Flight of ideas or subjective experience that thoughts are racing
    5. Distractiblity (i.e., attention is easily drawn to unimportant or irrelevant external stimuli)
    6. Increase in goal-directed activity (either socially, at work or school, or sexually) or psychomotor agitation
    7. Excessive involvement in pleasurable activities that have a high potential for painful consequences (e.g., unrestrained buying sprees, sexual indiscretions, or foolish business investments)

  C. The mood disturbance is sufficiently severe to cause marked impairment in daily functioning or in usual social activities or relationships with others, or to necessitate hospitalization to prevent harm to self or others, or there are psychotic features

  D. Not due to the direct physiologic effects of a substance (e.g., drugs of abuse, medication) or a general medical condition

Hypomanic episode

  A, B, and D, similar to manic episode

  C. The mood disturbance causes definite, uncharacteristic changes in functioning, observable by others but not severe enough to cause marked impairment in daily routine or requiring hospitalization; psychotic features are not present

Mixed manic-depressive episode

  Meets criteria for both manic episode (above) and major depressive episode (Table 6.2) for at least 1 week, with symptoms present at least nearly every day

Secondary manic episode

  Similar to manic episode except that evidence of a specific causal factor is present: substance abuse, medication or other treatment effect, or a medical condition known to be a potential direct cause (e.g., stroke, hyperthyroidism)

Adapted from the *Diagnostic and Statistical Manual,* 4th ed. (APA, 1994).

The clinical picture of mania may be muted in elderly patients. For example, Post in 1965 noted that flight of ideas is often replaced in elderly manics by ''senile anecdotal and circumstantial garrulity'' (shallow overtalkativeness). Slater and Roth (1977) observed that euphoria in elderly manics often is not ''infectious''; speech and thought are ''threadbare and repetitious,'' lacking the typical ''sparkle and versatility'' of younger patients; and that while overall severity of illness may be ''relatively mild . . . hostility and resentment'' are often marked.

Several special clinical presentations of mania in the elderly patient are note-worthy. *Confusion* may be marked, giving rise to the clinically useful concept of ''manic delirium'' or ''delirious mania.'' These terms highlight the potential for manic states to impair intellectual function in elderly patients and the difficulty of distinguishing between psychiatric and neurological causes of cognitive dysfunction in actively manic patients. In addition, *mixed bipolar episodes* are apparently more frequently encountered in elderly than in young patients with bipolar disorder. These episodes are characterized by features of both mania and depression together, admixed, or alternating in rapid succession. *Mania with psychotic features* may be difficult to distinguish clinically from other psychotic states of the elderly. *Chronic hypomanic states* occasionally occur in elderly patients but have not been well characterized. A history of long-standing primary bipolar disorder is the usual backdrop for these presentations, and narcissistic, self-centered, and demanding personality features are common.

Clinicians who treat the elderly will encounter both patients with late-onset mania and those with recurrent primary bipolar disorder beginning earlier in life. In late-onset mania, comorbid neurological disorders are much more common than in elderly patients with early-onset and multiple prior episodes of mania (Tohen et al., 1994). However, mania can cause a dementia syndrome (Charron et al., 1991). In three demented manic patients, successful lithium therapy led to complete clearing of cognitive dysfunction and abandonment of the dementia diagnosis. In both secondary and primary manic episodes, lithium is the treatment of choice when not contraindicated by other medical illness, primarily some renal and cardiac diseases. In addition, antipsychotic or benzodiazepine anxiolytic drugs may be needed in the short-term treatment of acute mania in the elderly for control of associated psychotic symptoms and sleep disorder. Other mood-stabilizing agents, such as carbamazepine and valproic acid, may be utilized in lieu of lithium when necessary or after an adequate trial of lithium has proven unsuccessful. Mirchandani and Young (1993) discuss management of mania in the elderly in depth, with attention to alternative treatments as well. Most acutely manic patients require inpatient psychiatric treatment for stabilization; a few can be managed successfully in the nursing home setting.

> *Example.* A 72-year-old man with a long history of primary bipolar disorder and binge drinking while manic was observed to be leaving his nursing home at frequent intervals to visit a local tavern. When psychiatric consultation was requested, his behavior had deteriorated to the point of chronic confusion, hyperactivity, hostility, and crawling about the floor barking like a dog, and he was sleeping less than 3 hours per day. His lithium level was 0.5 mEq/L. Antipsychotic treatment was initiated with haloperidol 2 mg bid and his lithium dose was increased to achieve a level of 1.0 mEq/L. He was confined to the nursing home with the aid of constant staff supervision. Over the course of a week, his manic episode was brought under control and no signs or symptoms of alcohol withdrawal were observed. Within 3 weeks, antipsychotic treatment was successfully discontinued and his lithium level was maintained at 0.8 mEq/L without recurrence of mania or alcohol abuse for the next several years.

Depression

Depressions are the most common remediable psychiatric disorders in elderly residents of long-term-care facilities. All depressive subtypes commonly recognized in younger and medically healthy persons are represented in this population, including major depressions with and without agitation or psychosis, chronic depressions of several kinds, and intermittent depressions of lesser severity. In addition, complex, partial, or masked expressions of depressive disorder are frequent in the frail, disabled, and often cognitively impaired population cared for in nursing homes. Diagnostic criteria for all of the depressive subtypes currently recognized in the United States are shown in Table 6.2.

TABLE 6.2. Diagnostic Criteria for Depressions

Major depressive episode

    A. At least five of the following symptoms have been present nearly every day, for most of the day, during the same 2-week period and represent a change from previous functioning; at least one of the symptoms is either (1) depressed mood or (2) loss of interest or pleasure.

        1. Depressed mood, as indicated by either subjective report or observations made by others.
        2. Markedly diminished interest or pleasure in all or almost all activities.
        3. Significant weight loss or gain when not dieting (e.g., more than 5% of body weight in a month) or decrease or increase in appetite.
        4. Insomnia or hypersomnia.
        5. Psychomotor agitation or retardation.
        6. Fatigue or loss of energy.
        7. Feelings of worthlessness or excessive or inappropriate guilt (which may be delusional; not merely self-reproach or guilt about being sick).
        8. Diminished ability to think or concentrate, or indecisiveness.
        9. Recurrent thoughts of death (not just fear of dying), recurrent suicidal ideation without a specific plan, or a suicide attempt, or a specific plan for committing suicide.

    B. The symptoms cause clinically significant distress or impairment in daily activities, social life, or other important areas of functioning.

    C. The symptoms are not due to the direct effects of a substance (e.g., drugs of abuse, medication) or a general medical condition.

    Major depressions are further classified by *severity* (mild, moderate, severe), *duration* (acute/subacute or chronic—2 years or more), *clinical features* [psychosis (hallucinations or delusions), catatonia (immobility, muteness, agitation, odd posturing, copying others' speech or movements), melancholia (severe loss of ability to feel pleasure, marked guilt, severe weight loss, and other features), typical vs. atypical pattern (striking improvement in mood when something good happens, weight gain, sleeping too much)], and *course* (fully recovered, without recovery, seasonal pattern, single vs. repeated episodes).

Dysthymic disorder

    A. Depressed or irritable mood, most of the day, more than half the time, for at least 2 years, associated with significant distress or impairment in important areas of functioning.

    B. Mood disturbance is accompanied by at least two other symptoms, including disturbed appetite or sleep, fatigue or low energy, low self-esteem, concentration problems, or hopelessness.

    C. Major depression is not present, and disturbance is not due to a major depression in partial remission.

    D. No history or mania or hypomania, and psychosis is not present.

    E. Symptoms are not due to the direct physiological effects of a substance or a general medical condition (e.g., hypothyroidism or cancer chemotherapy).

(continued)

TABLE 6.2.   Diagnostic Criteria for Depressions (*continued*)

Depression not otherwise specified

DSM-IV recognizes several depressive patterns under this category; subsyndromal depressions common in nursing home patients are classified here.

A. *Minor depressive disorder:* Episodes of 2 weeks or more of depressive symptoms, but with fewer than the five items required for Major depressive disorder.

B. *Recurrent brief depressive disorder:* Meets all criteria for major depression except duration. Episodes last from 2 days to 2 weeks and occur intermittently, but at least monthly for a year.

C. *Other depressions:* The clinician cannot determine whether depression is primary or secondary (due to direct effects of a substance or medical illness).

Adapted from the *Diagnostic and Statistical Manual,* 4th ed. (APA, 1994).

Mood disorders in nursing home patients are the outcome of multiple interacting causal factors, depicted in Figure 6.1. These include individual psychological and neurobiological vulnerabilities, ill health and disability, specific losses and stresses, and qualities of the physical and social environment that set the stage for development of depression or contribute to its chronicity. Depressions are a major cause of personal suffering among nursing home patients, impair participation in activity and social life, and impose particular burdens on families and staff caring for patients.

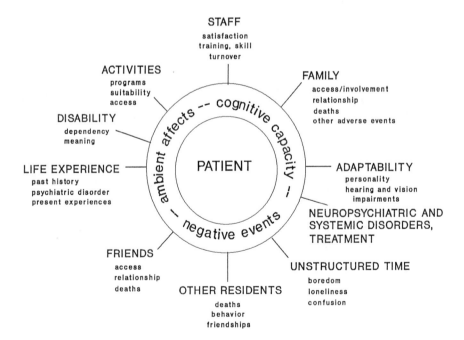

FIGURE 6.1. The causal matrix of depression in long-term care.

Epidemiology

Results of numerous studies of the prevalence of depressive disorders in nursing homes published since the late 1970s have been summarized in several recent reports and reviews (Ames, 1991; Abrams et al., 1992; German et al., 1992; Katz and Parmelee, 1992; Koenig and Blazer, 1992). The prevalence of major depressions varies across studies from 5 to 43%, while that of less severe and pervasive (subsyndromal or "minor") depressions appears much higher, at 16% to over 60%. When diagnosis is based on criteria from the *Diagnostic and Statistical Manual,* 3rd ed., the prevalence of major depressive syndromes approximates 15 to 20%, of minor depressions 25 to 40%, and of significant unhappiness and emotional suffering nearly 50% (Katz et al., 1989; Foster et al., 1991; Katz and Parmelee, 1994).

The relationship between these depressive subtypes has not been fully elucidated. Many chronically depressed elderly with apparently mild mood symptoms have serious functional impairments due to depression, indicating that mood change may not be the most prominent feature of depression. Loss of interest and the ability to experience pleasure (anhedonia) may be a more reliable indicator in some older persons and is reflected in emotional withdrawal, decreased activity, or irritability. Many mild depressions are the residue of untreated or partially treated major depressions, and major depressions often emerge against a background of chronic unhappiness. This continuum of depressive states in elderly patients has been confirmed by the longitudinal studies of Katz and his collaborators as well as others. A conservative estimate of new cases of depression in nursing home patients appears to be at least 12 to 14% per year (Katz et al., 1989; Foster et al., 1991; Katz and Parmelee, 1994), and about half of all new cases meet criteria for major depression. Follow-up of patients with mild, subsyndromal depression has shown that many are likely to become more severely depressed over time; others improve or remain mildly depressed for long periods. For some patients, depression is a progressive illness if not successfully treated; all forms of depression deserve detailed evaluation.

Among institutionalized patients with dementia, the prevalence of depressive disorders is less clear. This question is of more than academic importance: dementias are the chief cause of psychiatric morbidity in nursing homes (Goldfarb, 1962; Teeter et al., 1976; Rovner et al., 1986; Burns et al., 1988), and the presence of dementia may alter both depressive features and the approach to treatment. Several methodologically rigorous studies of depression prevalence in the United States excluded patients with moderate or severe cognitive impairment. Some studies that included both demented and nondemented subjects report lower overall prevalence of depression (Parmelee et al., 1989; German et al., 1992), but others do not provide convincing evidence that moderately demented patients are protected from depression (Rovner et al., 1986; Snowden, 1986; Kafonek et al., 1989).

Why does the prevalence of depression appear to vary so widely in different studies? Heterogeneity in methods of detecting depression, selection of patients and nursing homes for study, and classification of depressive syndromes probably accounts for most of this variation, and direct comparisons among studies cannot be made with certainty. However, both individual patient vulnerabilities and features of the nursing home environment may affect prevalence, but they have not been studied in depth. In the United States, most nursing homes participating in research are located in urban northeastern regions, enjoy substantial private support and corresponding enrichment of treatment programs, and serve mainly middle-class white populations. Particularly underrepresented in research are facilities serving the rural elderly, ethnic minorities, the poor, and patients removed from their home communities for care. However, reports from international sites in Singapore, South Africa, Australia, Italy, the United Kingdom, Scotland, and Japan (Abrams et al., 1992; Koenig and Blazer, 1992; Ames, 1993; Rovner and Katz, 1993) all support the finding that depressive morbidity is high in long-term-care settings.

Complications of Depression: Medical Morbidity and Mortality

Depression can contribute to deteriorating health in frail elderly persons. Its effects on food and fluid intake may result in weight loss, undernutrition, dehydration, impaired resistance to infection (Schleifer et al., 1989), and increased mortality from preexisting cardiac disease (Avery and Winokur, 1976), possibly mediated through excessive sympathetic nervous system arousal (Barnes et al., 1983).

Comorbid depression is associated with increased mortality rates in long-term care, with relative risks for depressed patients of 1.5 to 3 as compared to nondepressed patients (Katz et al., 1989; Ashby et al., 1991; Rovner et al., 1991; Parmalee et al., 1992a, b). However, when rigorous methods are used to control for the effects of medical illness, functional disability, and cognitive status, depression appears to contribute little or no independent mortality risk (Parmelee et al., 1992a, b). Further study is needed to resolve the question of whether depression plays a direct causal role in hastening death.

Clinical Features of Depression in Nursing Home Patients

Classic Major Depression and Other Dysphoric States

The work of Ames (1991), Katz et al. (1989), Katz et al. (1990), and Rovner and Katz (1993) has demonstrated that, in many nursing home patients, depressions can be classified using accepted diagnostic standards developed for young adults. Diagnostic ambiguity, while frequent, is no different in principle from that encountered in other groups of older patients with serious medical illness and functional disabilities, just "more so." However, factors related specifically to nursing homes require that psychiatrists, other mental health professionals, and nursing home staff become intimately familiar with presentations of affective pathology that are not straightforward. The institutional environment itself may impede recognition of depression by submerging residents' individual symptoms in the press of care. Nursing home patients rarely request treatment for depression, and the diagnostic process must often rely heavily on collateral information from staff whose knowledge of their patients' histories or inner life may be scanty. A detailed understanding of depression in individual patients may require more time and skill than staff can commit. Finally, untreated, long-lasting depressions often lose their affective hallmarks, leaving only a residue of functional impairment that obscures their original character.

Masked Depressions in Nursing Home Patients: Special Considerations

The concept of masked depression was eloquently elaborated in the original work of Lesse (1964). This classic of descriptive psychopathology is recommended reading for all who supervise the care of elderly persons in institutional settings. In a more recent, data-based study, Loebel et al. (1991) compared reasons for referral with subsequent psychiatric diagnosis in 197 patients residing in six Seattle nursing homes. Among the 38 (19%) patients found to be suffering from a depression or anxiety disorder, mood symptoms were identified by staff as the chief presenting problem in only 61%. Behavior problems were predominant in 34%, and "staff concern" with no specific problem stated was noted in 24%. Psychotic features were primary in 13%, somatic symptoms or signs in 11%, impaired function in 3%, and a mixed group of symptoms (including suicidal ideas or acts, cognitive impairment, and nursing home adjustment failure) in 13%. These data emphasize that "masking" of depressive syndromes in the nursing home setting is common and takes many forms.

Extreme social withdrawal, accompanied by voluntary efforts to reduce human contact and sensory stimulation, descriptively termed "cocooning" by Baker and Miller (1991), is strongly associated with depressive disorder and its improvement with antidepressant treatment.

Anxiety, agitation, uncooperativeness, and aggressive or abusive behavior can mask depression. Anxiety in its many forms (including panic disorder, other anxiety diagnoses, and psychological and somatic symptoms of anxiety) is strongly associated with depression in elderly nursing home patients. Three-quarters of anxious patients are depressed, and the majority of patients with major depression are anxious (Parmelee et al., 1993). (For a further discussion of anxiety symptoms in nursing home residents, see Chapter 7.) Depressed affect and clinical depression, and several of their correlates—such as sleep disturbance, pain, recent life-threatening experience, and poor quality of relationships—are predictors of a variety of agitated behaviors or uncooperativeness (Cohen-Mansfield et al., 1990; Rovner et al., 1992; Cohen-Mansfield et al., 1992). In patients with advanced dementia, agitated behaviors such as screaming, verbal and physical aggression, and dysphoric motor overactivity can represent the behavioral expression of a depressive syndrome that cannot be verbally articulated. Regardless of cognitive status, anxious or agitated patients should be carefully examined for clinical features of a depressive syndrome. Even when the clinical picture is not typical, antidepressant pharmacotherapy (Friedman et al., 1992; Schneider and Sobel, 1992) may improve behavioral symptoms. Important and useful psychodynamic and psychotherapeutic perspectives are provided in the edited volume of Brink (1987).

Pain has recently been identified as an important mask for depression among nursing home residents. Chronic pain, a common problem in geriatric care settings, is undetected by physicians in at least two-thirds of affected patients who can describe it clearly. With cognitively impaired patients who may express their pain only through behavioral symptoms, failure rates are even higher (Sengstaken and King, 1993). The presence of chronic pain should be treated as a potential marker for depression. Parmelee et al. (1991) reported that, after controlling for medical causes, patients with major depression have both more intense pain and a greater number of pain complaints than do those with subsyndromal or no depression. This finding has been replicated using caregiver reports by Cohen-Mansfield and Marx (1993). In this study, special attention was given to assessing demented patients, whose self-reported pain complaints are often discounted and ignored (Parmelee et al., 1993).

Other somatic symptoms and signs may obscure the presence of depression in patients with significant medical illnesses. Depression amplifies symptoms of chronic medical disorders (Katon, 1984; Borson et al., 1986; Wells et al., 1989). In medically ill elderly, effective treatment of depression can reduce physical symptoms and disability usually attributed to the underlying medical disorder (Borson et al., 1992). Depression in chronically ill patients is frequently assumed to be a normal reaction to illness, a bias that leads to underrecognition of treatable depression in the chronically ill generally (Zung et al., 1984). A more appropriate view is that chronic illness is a risk factor for comorbid depression (Borson et al., 1986; Kukull et al., 1986; Koenig and Blazer, 1992), and dysphoria accompanying disabling medical illness should prompt thorough psychiatric diagnostic evaluation.

Eating disorders may be the primary presenting symptom of depression and, when severe, may resemble anorexia nervosa (Price et al., 1985; Hsu and Zimmer, 1988; Miller et al., 1991). Weight loss is common in elderly persons residing in long-term care (Silver et al., 1988); significant undernutrition has been reported in 30 to 60% (Asplund et al., 1981; Ridman and Feller, 1989; Kersteller et al., 1992) and carries the potential for serious impairment of resistance to disease and even death in this population. Depression and food intake interact in a complex fashion. Undereating can cause mild depression, and depression can cause reduced food intake by a variety of mechanisms. Some depressed patients stop eating as a form of passive suicide, and others refuse to eat as a way of influencing caregivers (''hunger strike''). Perhaps most commonly, depressed people eat less due to direct effects of depression on appetite: these patients may require special attention at meals and provision of favorite foods in addition to antidepressant treatment.

Alcohol abuse (McCullough, 1991) and *overuse of sedatives* may reflect an underlying depression. The widespread prescription of sedatives in nursing homes has raised questions as to the proper indications for their use and prompted experimental efforts to reduce overuse. Two important studies have examined the effects on patients of facilitywide reductions in sedative prescribing. Avorn et al. (1992) found that depressive symptoms increased, but Salzman et al. (1992) found that cognitive function improved. These results suggest that many depressed patients are treated for only the associated anxiety and accept oversedation, at the expense of their cognitive capacity, to reduce their suffering.

> *Example.* A 73-year-old woman, demented after an episode of herpes encephalitis, presented with dysphoria, agitation, confusion, crying spells, and addiction to alprazolam. A gradual drug taper resulted in marked improvement of cognitive function and emergence of profound and disabling agitated depression.

Cognitive impairment (depressive "pseudodementia") was first described in withdrawn nursing home patients assumed to be demented but found, upon clinical examination, to be suffering from depression (Kiloh, 1961). The severe cognitive impairments seen years ago in nondemented depressed patients have fortunately become rare, owing to improvements in nursing home care and the availability of antidepressant pharmacotherapy, but cognitive complaints remain common in depressed patients. Poon (1992), in a recent review of evidence for the existence of a dementia syndrome due to primary depression, emphasizes that, when psychological testing is a part of a clinical diagnostic evaluation, cognitive deficits due to depression can usually be distinguished from those due to primary dementing disorders. The use of simple bedside cognitive screening tests (such as the Mini-Mental State Exam) may be sufficient. Depressive cognitive dysfunction preferentially affects attention, motivation, and energy to engage in activities requiring mental effort; access to and use of stored information is impaired as a result. New learning can be impeded by distractibility in patients with anxious depressions, due to marked forgetfulness, short attention span, and spells of apparent confusion, about which they may complain bitterly, convinced that "their minds are gone." Patients with severe depressive retardation may appear quite dull and apathetic, have great difficulty recalling information they knew just a short time before the development of their affective illness, or be unable to participate effectively in diagnostic interviews. These cognitive deficits, due to the psychobiology of depression itself, typically develop in tandem with the onset or worsening of the mood disorder and are reversible with effective treatment. In contrast, patients with cognitive defects due to dementing illness can usually pay attention, try their best to perform (often becoming frustrated with the effort), and minimize their mental difficulties. Their cognitive problems develop and persist regardless of the presence of mood disorder, often appearing after a known brain insult or displaying a pattern characteristic of a specific dementia diagnosis. (See Chapter 4 for a discussion of clinical features and diagnosis of dementia.)

In actual geriatric practice, varying degrees of dementia and depression often coexist, and most research data support the view of experienced geropsychiatrists that patients who present with prominent signs of both dementia and depression probably have both disorders. In patients with a primary dementia, the development of a depression amplifies the impact of brain dysfunction on day-to-day life, and antidepressant drugs or other treatments can improve function. In addition, a typical treatment-responsive depression may be the first presenting problem seen in patients who are developing a dementing illness.

It is not usually necessary (nor is it always possible) to determine in advance whether depression accounts for all of the cognitive deficits observed in a given patient; far more important is the clinician's recognition of the depression and appropriate therapeutic response to it. The issue will usually be clarified in time by the response of cognitive impairment to effective treatment. The standard of care in nursing homes must include provision of sufficiently competent psychiatric services to ensure that both dementia and depression are accurately diagnosed and adequately managed.

Cognitive, neurological, and behavioral disturbances in brain disease can influence the way depression manifests itself. In patients with diffuse or multifocal brain disease, damage to the integrity of the central nervous system may prevent the development of the most easily recognized features of syndromal depressions, obscuring them beneath cognitive, motor, or other behavioral deficits more readily observed by caregivers. Both verbal and nonverbal expression of affect may be impaired in patients with brain disease (Ross and Rush, 1981); as a result, observable behavioral indicators of depression assume special salience in brain-damaged patients. Fogel and Stone (1992) and Cummings (1985) have emphasized the involvement of multiple brain structures, from brainstem through frontal cortex, in generating specific features of the depressive syndrome. Cummings (1985) has provided a comprehensive review of the literature on the nature and pathophysiology, where known, of depressions and other affective disturbances associated with brain disease and dysfunction.

Neurological damage itself can be a direct cause of depressive syndromes when it affects brain pathways important in mood and psychomotor or neurovegetative function. Parkinson's disease, stroke (frontal, deep lacunar, and brainstem infarction especially), Huntington's disease, Shy-Drager syndrome, progressive supranuclear palsy, and other disorders are commonly associated with depressive disorders as a result of neural damage. In Alzheimer's disease, sustained depression usually reflects neuropathological involvement of subcortical structures; this conclusion is supported by postmortem examination of the brain (Chan-Palay and Asan, 1989). Other nondepressive disorders of affect regulation, such as lability of mood and emotional expression, occur in neurological diseases; here antidepressant pharmacotherapy may be helpful. Any sustained period of emotional distress should be viewed as potentially reflecting a treatable depression. It is important to note that a neurological cause for depression does not imply unresponsiveness to antidepressant pharmacotherapy or other somatic or psychosocial treatments.

Excess disability and motivational failure are core components of depressions in patients in long-term care and may be their chief presenting symptom. For individual patients, determining how much disability is "excessive" and how much motivation should be expected (and to what end) can be difficult in the presence of disabling medical conditions and in the setting of the under- or overstimulating environments frequently prevailing in nursing homes. Detailed assessments and sophisticated clinical skills are usually required to identify the presence of and reasons for excess disability and rehabilitation failures; the intimate familiarity with patients and the clinical psychiatric assessment needed for this task are often beyond the reach of direct-care staff. It is important that such problems not escape the attention of those at higher levels.

> *Example.* A 79-year-old married African-American woman was admitted to an inner-city nursing home after amputation of a leg because of severe burns caused when she rushed to remove a pan of flaming motor oil from the stove. Discharge home was planned once she had learned to walk with a prosthesis. When 3 months passed with little progress in rehabilitation, she was referred for psychiatric consultation to improve her motivation. She was found to be experiencing a major depressive episode, precipitated by the loss of her leg. Her motivational failure was due to desire to avoid returning home to her demented husband, who had put the oil on the stove to warm it. The discovery of this previously hidden problem led to placement of her husband in a nursing home, rapid progress in her rehabilitation, resolution of her depression without other treatment, and successful return to her life in the community.

Risk Factors for Depression in Nursing Home Patients

Medical illness and disability are primary risk factors for the development of both major and minor depressive syndromes. Rates of depression in long-term-care settings generally exceed those reported in samples of elderly persons residing in the community, including those with chronic diseases (reviewed by Koenig and Blazer, 1992) and increase with functional dependency and level of care (Gurland et al., 1983; Parmelee et al., 1989; Katz and Parmelee, 1994). A *prior history of depression, dysphoric response to change, or high level of need for personal intimacy* probably elevates risk following institutionalization, but this has not been studied. A fruitful area for future investigation is the relative power of individual vs. institutional variables in predicting onset and persistence of depressions.

Nursing home placement is a major life event rarely undertaken happily. Indeed, patients awaiting nursing home admission appear to have rates of depression comparable with those in patients actually admitted (Zemore and Eames, 1979), and anticipation of nursing home placement appears to be a risk factor for completed suicide (Loebel et al., 1991). Admission to a nursing home usually results from important prior losses and brings new ones: the decision for nursing home care is the result of loss of capacity for independent function and lack of available, adequate in-home care, and placement adds losses of personal control, privacy, and proximity to remaining family and friends (Osgood, 1992). This suggests that it is not the transition to institutional life itself that confers added risk for depression but the nature and personal significance of the disability that make placement necessary.

Life in a nursing home might, in principle, ameliorate mood disorders in frail older persons by simplifying burdensome daily chores and providing easy access to support and assistance, medical care, and opportunities for friendship, social interaction, and activities appropriate to functional ability. There is conflicting evidence about whether a supportive nursing home environment can in fact achieve this goal. Snowden and Donnelly (1986) found that severity of depressive symptoms was lower in long-term residents than recently admitted patients. Parmelee et al. (1992b) found, in a facility providing clinical care for depression, that about half of patients with major depression at the time of admission were improved a year later, but most continued to experience some degree of depressive symptomatology; in this study, long-stay residents fared no better than newly admitted patients. Among patients admitted with milder depressions, half were improved a year later, but the other half were unchanged or worse (Parmelee et al., 1992b). Ames et al. (1991) reported low recovery rates (<30%) after 1 year, despite the availability of psychiatric consultation and management. This suggests that psychiatric treatment alone is not sufficient to improve the outlook for depression in the nursing home setting and that nursing homes have not currently realized their potential as therapeutic environments.

What *environmental factors* might make a difference? For depression, no studies have been designed to relate the prevalence or clinical picture of depression in residents to institutional factors, although both clinical and theoretical considerations suggest that they are important. For suicide, Osgood (1992) has identified several institutional factors associated with risk in long-term care, including larger facility size, less privacy for residents, higher staff turnover, lower charges for care (possibly reflecting fewer available services and a less enriched environment), and religious affiliation. Because suicide is most commonly associated with depression, particularly among the elderly (Conwell et al., 1994; Conwell and Caine, 1991), it is likely that environmental factors figure prominently in suicide through their effects both on psychosocial risks for development of depression (Brant and Osgood, 1990) and on its recognition and treatment.

We propose that an institutional factor important in initiating or maintaining depression in residents of some long-term care facilities is *contagion of dysphoria and dysfunction* among patients and staff. Especially important are residents' relationships with nurses' aides, which are among the most intimate and sustaining that patients in long-term care have. Some 80 to 100% of personal care is provided by relatively untrained and unskilled workers who come from sociocultural, linguistic, and economic backgrounds often far different from those of their patients; patient contact with a nurse averages only 12 minutes per day (Institute of Medicine, 1986). The high aide turnover rates common in many facilities, estimated at 45 to 70% per year (Waxman et al., 1984) or even 70 to 100% (Libow and Starer, 1989) add recurring emotional losses to those experienced by patients as a result of nursing home placement, poor health, and attrition of family and friends.

Not unexpectedly, research has shown a correlation between residents' emotional well-being and satisfaction with care and the level of job satisfaction among nurses' aides. Aides' length of employment, wages, level of benefits, and perceptions of the fairness and competence of the charge nurse all correlate with patient satisfaction (Kruzich et al., 1992). Even when job assignments are stable, aides' many responsibilities often limit the more time-consuming emotional aspects of personal care (Bowers and Becker, 1992). It is interesting that vulnerability to the disruptive effects of high staff turnover is highest among the most functionally impaired residents, who are also most vulnerable to depression.

Sources of poor morale and job dissatisfaction among aides are several. As a group, aides are often multiply burdened by adversity at home and at work in ways that create a cycle of distress and indignity in their own lives (Tellis-Nayak and Tellis-Nayak, 1989). On the job, high workload, inadequate skills—especially in the care of cognitively impaired patients with disruptive behavior—and the physical and emotional demands built into the care of disabled elderly persons contribute to feelings of pressure, burden, and burnout and set the stage for a cycle of abuse that reverberates throughout staff and patients. These factors have been explored in depth in the ground-breaking studies of Troner (1994), using anthropologic fieldwork methods.

Abusive behavior of aides toward residents is disturbingly prevalent in nursing homes and probably contributes to depression as well as general misery among residents. In an important series of studies, nursing assistants disclosed high rates of abusive behavior toward patients—40% acknowledged at least one act of psychological abuse in the previous year and 10% at least one act of physical abuse (Pillemer and Moore, 1989, 1990; Pillemer and Bachman, 1991). Missing from these studies is the fact that abuse is rarely habitual: most abusive acts appear in a flash of anger reflecting aides' exhaustion and repeated mistreatment by patients whose social restraint has been lost due to mental impairments (Foner, 1994). Episodes of purposeful taunting and humiliation of residents by angry aides also occur and are likely to cluster around patients whose reputation for insulting, threatening, and otherwise ugly and aggressive behavior has spread throughout the facility and affected many caregivers. Regular scapegoating of the most vulnerable residents by aides may signify a response to habitual mistreatment by their superiors, inadequate or insensitive supervisory practices, or frank psychopathology.

Several models of intervention to reduce patient abuse have been developed. Pillemer and Hudson (1993) have described a brief curriculum for abuse prevention, based on increasing staff awareness of the dynamics of abuse, ability to recognize abuse-prone situations, and capacity for conflict avoidance and resolution. A study conducted in 10 very diverse nursing homes in the greater Philadelphia area confirmed high base rates of self-reported abusive behavior by staff. In the month preceding training, yelling in anger at a resident was reported by 51% and insulting or swearing at a resident by 23%. Threats of physical harm and actual physical abuse (including excessive restraint; pushing, shoving, grabbing, or slapping; throwing something at a resident; kicking; and hitting with the fist) were also reported, but at substantially lower rates. Following abuse prevention training, positive effects were noted on aides' attitudes toward patients and caregiving, levels of conflict experienced, resident aggression toward aides, and number of abuse events. Although patient satisfaction with care and mood were not examined in this study, reduction in abusive interactions with caregivers can be expected to improve both—at least in relation to day-to-day care. Institutional changes to reduce workload and explicit skills training have been shown to reduce aide burnout (Chappell and Novak, 1992), a major causal factor in patient abuse. Other forms of aide training focused on interactional dynamics have been known, for nearly 20 years, to improve aides' job satisfaction (Goldman and Woog, 1975; Moses, 1982).

Patient welfare on a day-to-day basis is clearly dependent on the well-being of aides. Therefore, the function and fate of these primary caregivers may be fundamental to the psychogenesis of despondency, disengagement, and clinical depression in residents; to the failure of staff to recognize and intervene in them; and to the failure of psychiatric care of patients to solve the epidemiological problem. Much more attention should be given to developing mechanisms for improving aides' satisfaction and safety from emotional and physical abuse by patients who are no longer in control of their own behavior. Among these mechanisms may be such diverse activities as unionization of aides with the anticipated result of improved working conditions, wages, and benefits (Foner 1994), interpersonal training, open recognition by nurses and administrators of the effects on aides of the personally stressful nature of the work, and institutional efforts to provide regular, constructive ways of discharging accumulated job tensions before they are played out in abusive behavior toward patients. Conversely, habitual abuse of aides by a patient should be made an explicit and valid reason for psychiatric consultation and management and not merely couched in vague terms such as "agitation." Recognition of the needs of both aides and patients for a humane, supportive, and safe environment is an important step toward its realization.

Detection of Depression and Utilization of Mental Health Services

Heston et al. (1992) examined medical records of nearly 6000 nursing home patients admitted to 60 Minnesota nursing homes during the 1970s and 1980s and reported that primary physicians had made a diagnosis of depression or affective psychosis in about 15% of these, a rate of about half that reported from epidemiological surveys for all depressions combined. Of the *depressed* patients, only *10%* were receiving an antidepressant drug and over half received no psychotropic medication. Recognition of depression by nurses and awareness of treatment options are likely to be critical to improvements in patient care; however, Rovner et al. (1992) found that nurses' ratings of patients' depressive symptoms were neither sensitive to nor specific for clinically diagnosed depression. Rovner et al. (1991), studying a cohort of patients admitted in the late 1980s, reported prior recognition of depression in only 14% of patients diagnosed as depressed by psychiatrists and active treatment in only one-quarter of patients so diagnosed. Even when primary care internists identify depressive symptoms in their elderly patients and formulate appropriate treatment plans, they often do not implement them (Barsa et al., 1986). In contrast to these discouraging findings, Conn and Goldman (1992) reported that 10 to 12% of 544 patients in a Toronto long-term geriatric center with an active psychiatric consultation-liaison service were receiving an antidepressant, for indications that appeared generally appropriate. However, for most community nursing homes, which lack intensive psychiatric support services and staff training in recognition of depressive states, it is a safe assumption that much depression still goes undetected and untreated.

In the first large-scale systematic study of mental health service utilization by nursing home patients, Burns et al. (1993) reported that only 6% of all patients with a mood disorder diagnosis received any mental health treatment, and only 3.5% had contact with a speciality-trained mental health provider. Geographic factors and age influenced mental health treatment. Patients residing in the north-eastern part of the country and younger geriatric patients were most likely to be treated by specialists. Unfortunately, the oldest patients—who are most likely to be severely functionally impaired, who present complex clinical problems, and who are in greatest need of evaluation and management by geropsychiatrists—appear least likely to get it.

What will remedy this state of affairs? Effective methods for identifying depressed persons are a priority for health services research and application. Provisions of OBRA recognizing that mental health diagnosis and treatment are integral to high-quality nursing home care are a significant step. However, the utility of the mandated Minimum Data Set (MDS) and Resident Assessment Profiles (RAPs) as screens for depressive disorders has not been established and at best can be only as good as the skills of the staff who complete them.

Inclusion of psychiatric nurse clinicians as members of the nursing home staff can have an important impact, and nurse gerontologists are a valuable and underutilized resource in assessment and treatment (Kolcaba and Miller, 1989). Santmyer and Roca (1991) reported that a psychiatric nurse consultant can evaluate and manage about 50% of nursing home patients with psychiatric problems, requiring the help of a geropsychiatrist for the remainder. Several alternative models for providing comprehensive psychiatric service to nursing home patients have been described but not yet tested for their contribution to quality of care. Libow and Starer (1989) have emphasized that the best nursing homes nationwide are characterized by the ready availability of expert geropsychiatric consultation; meeting this manpower needs within current mandates for cost containment is a significant challenge.

Caring for Depressed Patients in Long-Term Care

Clinical Assessment and Treatment Planning

Depressed patients usually look sad, worried, or withdrawn when observed unobtrusively. Many try hard to conceal their distress. Some respond to staff interest by seeming brighter, only to withdraw again when left alone. Many patients make frequent calls for help or complain loudly about lack of assistance. Staff often respond by insisting that these patients can do more for themselves than they do. Patients may pick at their food, refuse to go to meals, or disparage the quality of food served. They may wake frequently at night, ask for sleeping pills, seem too tired to function during the day, or complain loudly about physical symptoms for which medical treatment has already been optimized. When asked about what interests them, they may be unable to think of anything.

Diagnostic criteria for the various subtypes of depression are provided in Table 6.2. It is important to note that many medical illnesses and disabilities can give rise to some of the symptoms of depression but not all of its features. Most nondepressed patients adapt to their physical limitations by developing new sources of stimulation, enjoyment, and meaning in their lives.

The elements of comprehensive diagnostic assessment are shown in Table 6.3. A clinical judgment must be made as to the *possible contribution of medical factors* to the depressive syndrome. Early undiagnosed pneumonia, poorly controlled congestive heart failure or excessive diuresis, overtreatment of hypertension, inappropriate polypharmacy (either medical or psychotropic drugs), inability to eat because of swallowing problems, specific neurological disorders, respiratory insufficiency requiring adjustment of medications, electrolyte imbalance, or sensory deficits such as hearing and visual loss can all contribute to some of the signs and symptoms of depression. These should be considered and appropriately treated. In general, drug regimens should be simplified whenever this is consistent with good medical practice.

Psychosocial, environmental, and psychological factors with the potential to affect mood should be assessed with the help of nursing and aide staff, family when available, social worker, and activities therapist. Practical interventions can be developed from this information; they include help in resolving conflictual relations between patient and roommate or aide, prescription of an activity program, or planning a regular program of visitation by family members or volunteers. Environmental modifications may be pertinent, especially for patients with sensory, motor, or cognitive deficits and those who have become severely withdrawn from others. Staff and visitors should be educated about ways to improve communication with hearing- or vision-impaired patients (e.g., audibly identifying all visitors to a blind patient's room; speaking to the ''good ear'' of a hearing-impaired patient). Frequent, brief, but personal contacts are helpful with confused or fearful patients, and providing adequate light can partly compensate for some visual impairments. Predictable assignment of compatible aides furnishes great comfort to depressed patients.

Medical treatments for depression are required when depression is severe enough to interfere with day-to-day activities, causes intense personal suffering, or is beyond the reach of psychological and psychosocial interventions. This is almost always the case when mood disturbance takes the form of a major depression, is associated with sustained changes in physical function (sleep, appetite, energy, psychomotor agitation or retardation), or is accompanied by anxiety, fearfulness, or psychotic features. Milder chronic depressions frequently require medical therapy as well. Many such illnesses cause protracted but relatively invisible suffering and represent the residue of untreated prior major depressive episodes. Medical treatments for depression include prescription of antidepressant drugs and electroconvulsive therapy.

TABLE 6.3. Psychiatric Evaluation and Treatment Planning for the Depressed Patient

Identify patient with possible mood disorder

Consolidate history and observations made by staff: symptoms, behavior changes, duration, effects
    on others

Examine patient
    Define depressive symptoms and signs
    Assess cognitive and behavioral problems
    Determine medical, neurological, and functional status
    Inquire about prior psychiatric history
    Identify specific relationship problems
    Evaluate attitudes towards care, awareness of problem, emotional understanding

Review medical record
    Diagnoses present and omitted
    Psychiatric, psychosocial history
    Recent physical examination
    Physicians' orders and medication sheets
    Nursing notes: sleep, eating, mood, behavior
    Social work, physical and activity therapy notes
    Minimum Data Set/Preadmission Screening and Annual Review evaluations

Synthesize and record data
    Are further tests needed?
    Assign best-estimate psychiatric diagnosis
    Formulate reasonable pathogenetic hypotheses
    Identify risks relevant to treatment planning: medical, pharmacological factors; suicide

Develop and record treatment plan
    Is hospitalization needed?
    Psychosocial, environmental, and sensory approaches
    Antidepressant drug therapy
    Electroconvulsive therapy

Specify how results will be evaluated
    Responsibility for treatment components—who?
    Monitors for treatment response and adverse effects—what, how often?
    Plan for follow-up

Antidepressant Pharmacotherapy

Katz et al. (1990) reported the superiority of active treatment with nortriptyline over placebo in nursing home patients with major depression. With a conventional dosing paradigm, about half of patients who tolerated the drug experienced useful benefit, while placebo response was negligible. However, 11 of the 32 patients receiving active drug treatment and 1 of 14 receiving placebo experienced adverse events necessitating discontinuation. Additional clinical trials are needed to define the full spectrum of drug-responsive depressions in nursing home patients, develop strategies for reducing side effects, and assess the efficacy of newer antidepressants that may be better tolerated by some frail elderly (such as paroxetine and other selective serotonin reuptake inhibitors, or venlafaxine).

All classes of antidepressant drugs have been used safely in clinical treatment of individual patients, including tricyclics, newer serotonergic agents, monoamine oxidase inhibitors, and psychostimulants such as methylphenidate or dextroamphetamine. The choice of drug should be made on the basis of risks and side effect profiles and the patient's prior response to a particular agent (if any). Some antidepressant drugs may be hazardous for patients with specific medical vulnerabilities. Examples include tricyclic antidepressants, which are inadvisable for patients with cardiac conduction defects, and monoamine oxidase inhibitors, which are contraindicated in patients taking meperidine for pain. The compatibility of specific antidepressants with medically essential drugs must be considered before initiating treatment. Once a drug is chosen, treatment is initiated with the lowest appropriate dose. A conservative program of incremental dosing, based on contingencies of response and anticipated or observed side effects, can be scheduled in advance. Specific nursing staff should be assigned to supervise and monitor treatment. Concrete guidelines for monitoring should be spelled out and must include side-effect detection strategies (e.g., serial blood pressures and electrocardiograms in patients at risk, constipation, and behavioral and cognitive assessments). Details of the overall treatment plan and requisite monitors should be spelled out clearly in the patient's chart. When psychiatrists provide only intermittent consultation, telephone monitoring via nursing staff is necessary and usually sufficient, provided the next visit is scheduled no longer than 1 month away. (See Chapter 16 for the role of the consulting psychiatrist.)

The reader is referred to recent comprehensive reviews (McCue, 1992; Salzman et al., 1993) for detailed discussion of principles and the still relatively scant literature relevant to antidepressant treatment of frail older persons. (See Chapter 3 for a discussion of antidepressant medication use.)

Electroconvulsive Therapy

Electroconvulsive therapy (ECT) is indicated and underutilized for treatment of severe depression in nursing home patients for whom antidepressant pharmacotherapy is unsafe or ineffective. Nursing home staff may be unaware of the indications for, or the safety and efficacy of, ECT, and thus be unable to support reluctant patients or family members in considering a recommendation for its use.

> *Example.* A 93-year-old man had progressively withdrawn from personal contact and lost 20 pounds in the year prior to his first evaluation by a psychiatrist. He was found to have a delusional depression with profound psychomotor retardation but no severe medical illnesses. Cognitive testing revealed mild dementia consistent with a diagnosis of Alzheimer's disease. Sequential treatment by his primary physician with fluoxetine and nortriptyline in maximal tolerated doses had failed. He and his family were unwilling to consider hospitalization for ECT, and nursing staff showed little enthusiasm. Methylphenidate was prescribed with significant benefit for 2 months, at which time his depression relapsed. The patient died of pneumonia 1 month later.

Psychosocial Treatments

Few psychological or psychosocial treatments for depression have been tested rigorously in nursing home populations. However, several group treatment approaches have shown promise in controlled trials in patients with self-reported depressive symptoms. Of six controlled studies using cognitive-behavioral therapy, reminiscence, problem-solving training, or current topics discussion groups, five found significant improvements in mood and one (which included depressed, demented patients) reported improvements in cognitive function (Hussian and Scott, 1981; Goldwasser et al., 1987; Rattenbury and Stones, 1989; Youssef, 1990; Zerhusen et al., 1991; Abraham et al., 1992). None of these studies included a clinical diagnostic interview for depressive disorders, and it is possible that the interventions were most effective for patients suffering from low morale rather than a depressive illness. Future research should include psychiatric diagnostic assessment of patients selected for treatment. Therapeutic trials employing combined or sequential biomedical and psychosocial interventions as well as caregiver training are badly needed.

Multidisciplinary mental health teams working under psychiatric supervision can provide a full spectrum of individual and group therapies for patients who can benefit from these approaches, as well as staff training and support. Frequently, psychologically trained social work and nursing staff employed by the long-term care facility, working in conjunction with biomedical treatment, can help to bring isolated, withdrawn patients back into the social milieu. Individual professional psychotherapy for depressed nursing home patients is most often prohibited by time and cost constraints, and, apart from case reports, has not been established as an effective treatment in this setting. Nevertheless, skill in assessing the psychodynamics of depression and rapid formulation of individualized psychotherapeutic interventions can sometimes have dramatic effects. (See Chapters 13 and 14 for a more complete treatment of psychotherapeutic techniques.)

> *Example.* An 89-year-old wheelchair-bound widow, a former stage entertainer, had been mildly but persistently depressed since admission to a nursing home 2 years earlier. She was lonely, isolative, and reluctant to participate in social activities. Clinical evaluation identified no significant anxiety, other behavioral symptoms, or neurovegetative signs of depression, but inquiry into psychological factors disclosed that she was intensely ashamed of her aged appearance, of her dependence on others for help with personal care, and especially of exposure in front of male aides. She hated the fact that she could no longer rely on her stage presence to excite others' interest in her. Open discussion of these issues with a psychiatrist provided her great and immediate relief. Measures employed to reinforce these gains included regular visits to the beauty shop for makeup, assigning only female aides for bathing and toileting, and involving her as a leader in designing special group activities based on her theatrical career. Staff reported with surprise the sustained amelioration of her chronic depression.

Programmatic Changes in Nursing Home Care

Depressions in their protean forms are usually the product of multiple causal factors that include individual psychodynamics and psychobiology, systemic and neuropsychiatric illness, functional disability (including sensory impairments), concurrent drug treatments, and social and institutional factors affecting the giving and receiving of daily care (Figure 6.1). Viewed from the perspective of the nursing home as a health care institution, the high depressive morbidity found there demands focused programmatic change to improve its detection, accurate differential diagnosis, and treatment. Individual nursing homes, like individual patients, may need different approaches based upon resident profiles, staffing patterns, existing services, and commitment to improvement in the quality of care. Several such approaches have been alluded to in the preceding sections, such as systematic attention to the needs of aides. Others may include periodic facilitywide professional review of the use of psychotropic medications, changes in administrative structure, annual staff retreats, creation of a new staff position for a geriatric psychiatrist, mandatory continuing education of physicians and nurses in the art and science of recognizing and treating depression, and regular interactive staff meetings to review the nursing home mission.

Conclusions

Mood disorders are prevalent in elderly nursing home patients and can usually be effectively diagnosed using conventional psychiatric methods. Evaluation of mania and depression in patients with severe dementias, mixed behavioral syndromes or atypical presentations, or multiple major medical comorbidities is more difficult and is a task for specialty-trained geropsychiatrists and continuing geropsychiatric research. Medical, neurobiological, psychological, social, environmental, and administrative dimensions form a causal matrix for depression in the nursing home setting, interacting to create affective illness in ways that are unique for each patient. Effective interventions may be derived from consideration of each of these causal domains, and combinations of several approaches are generally the most effective. While psychiatrists must participate actively and often take the lead in developing effective institutional programs and providing treatment for patients, no single clinical discipline can be entrusted with the full responsibility for this fundamentally collaborative task. Substantial improvements are needed in recognition of the spectrum of depressive morbidity, timely and well-targeted treatment and follow-up, and application of programmatic innovations that can reduce the burden of depressive morbidity noted worldwide in the setting of long-term care.

References

Abraham IL, Neundorfer MM, Currie LJ. Effects of group interventions on cognition and depression in nursing home residents. *Nurs Res* 41:196, 1992.

Abrams RC, Teresi JA, Butin DN. Depression in nursing home residents. *Clin Geriatr Med* 8:309, 1992.

Ames D. Depression in elderly residents of local-authority residential homes: Its nature and efficacy of intervention. *Br J Psychiatry* 156:667, 1990.

Ames D. Epidemiological studies of depression among the elderly in residential and nursing homes. *Int J Geriatr Psychiatry* 6:347, 1991.

Ames, D. Depressive disorders among elderly people in long-term institutional care. *Aust N Z J Psychiatry* 27:379, 1993.

Ashby D, Ames D, West CR, et al. Psychiatric morbidity as a predictor of mortality for residents of local authority homes for the elderly. *Int J Geriatr Psychiatry* 6:567, 1991.

Asplund K, Normark M, Pettersson V. Nutritional assessment of psychogeriatric patients. *Age Ageing* 10:87, 1981.

Avery D, Winokur G. Mortality in depressed patients treated with electroconvulsive therapy and antidepressants. *Arch Gen Psychiatry* 33:1029, 1976.

Avorn J, Soumerai SB, Everitt DE, et al. A randomized trial of a program to reduce the use of psychoactive drugs in nursing homes. *N Engl J Med* 327:1683, 1992.

Baker FM, Miller CL. "Cocooning": A clinical sign of depression in geriatric patients. *Hosp Comm Psychiatry* 42:845, 1991.

Barnes RF, Veith RC, Borson S, et al. High levels of plasma catecholamines in dexamethasone-resistant depressed patients. *Am J Psychiatry* 140:1623, 1983.

Barsa J, Toner J, Gurland B, Lantigua R. Ability of internists to recognize and manage depression in the elderly. *Int J Geriatr Psychiatry* 1:57, 1986.

Borson S, Barnes RA, Kukull WA, et al. Symptomatic depression in elderly medical outpatients. *J Am Geriatr Soc* 34:341, 1986.

Borson S, McDonald GJ, Gayle T, et al. Improvement in mood, physical symptoms, and function with nortriptyline for depression in patients with chronic obstructive pulmonary disease. *Psychosomatics* 33:190, 1992.

Bowers B, Becker M. Nurses' aides in nursing homes: The relationship between organization and quality. *Gerontologist* 32:360, 1992.

Brant BA, Osgood N. The suicidal patient in long-term care institutions. *J Gerontol Nurs* 16:15, 1990.

Brink TL. *The Elderly Uncooperative Patient.* New York: Haworth Press, 1987.

Burns BJ, Larson ID, Goldstrom WE, et al. Mental disorder among nursing home patients: Preliminary findings from the national nursing home pretest. *Int J Geriatr Psychiatry* 3:27, 1988.

Burns BJ, Wagner HR, Taube JE, et al. Mental health service use by the elderly in nursing homes. *Am J Public Health* 83:331, 1993.

Chan-Palay V, Asan E. Alterations in catecholamine neurons of the locus ceruleus in senile dementia of the Alzheimer type and in Parkinson's disease with and without depression. *J Comp Neurol* 287:373, 1989.

Chappell NL, Novak M. The role of support in alleviating stress among nursing assistants. *Gerontologist* 32:351, 1992.

Charron M, Fortin L, Paquette I. De novo mania among elderly people. *Acta Psychiatr Scand* 84:503, 1991.

Cohen-Mansfield J, Marx MS. Pain and depression in the nursing home: Corroborating results. *J Gerontol* 48:P96, 1993.

Cohen-Mansfield J, Marx MS, Werner P. Agitation in elderly persons: An integrative report of findings in a nursing home. *Int Psychogeriatr* 4(suppl 2):221, 1992.

Cohen-Mansfield J, Werner P, Marx MS. Screaming in nursing home residents. *J Am Geriatr Soc* 38:785, 1990.

Conn DK, Goldman Z. Pattern of use of antidepressants in long-term care facilities for the elderly. *J Geriatr Psychiatry Neurol* 5:228, 1992.

Conwell Y. Suicide in the elderly. In: Schneider LS, Reynolds CF III, Lebowitz BD, et al., eds. *Diagnosis and Treatment of Depression in Late Life.* Washington DC: American Psychiatric Press, 1994.

Cummings JL. Organic psychoses: Delusional disorder and secondary mania. *Psychiatr Clin North Am* 9:293, 1986.

Cummings JL. Behavioral complications of drug treatment of Parkinson's disease. *J Am Geriatr Soc* 39:708, 1991.

Cummings JL. Disturbances of mood and affect. *Clinical Neuropsychiatry*. Needham Heights, MA: Allyn and Bacon, 1985:183.

Fogel B, Stone A. Practical pathophysiology in neuropsychiatry: A clinical approach to depression and impulsive behavior in neurological patients. In: Yudofsky SC, Hales RE, eds. *Textbook of Neuropsychiatry,* 2nd ed. Washington DC: American Psychiatric Press, 1992:329.

Foner N. Nursing home aides: Saints or monsters? *Gerontologist* 34:245, 1994.

Foster JR, Cataldo JK, Boksay IJE. Incidence of depression in a medical long-term care facility: Findings from a restricted sample of new admissions. *Int J Geriatr Psychiatry* 3:13, 1991.

Foster JR, Cataldo JK. Prediction of first episode of clinical depression in patients newly admitted to a medical long-term care facility: Findings from a prospective study. *Int J Geriatr Psychiatry* 8:297, 1993.

Friedman R, Gryfe CI, Tal DT, Freedman M. The noisy elderly patient: Prevalence, assessment, and response to the antidepressant doxepin. *J Geriatr Psychiatry Neurol* 5:187, 1992.

German PS, Rovner BW, Burton LC, et al. The role of mental morbidity in the nursing home experience. *Gerontologist* 32:152, 1992.

Goldfarb AI. Prevalence of psychiatric disorders in metropolitan old age and nursing homes. *J Am Geriatr Soc* 10:77, 1962.

Goldman EB, Woog P. Mental health in nursing homes training project. *Gerontologist* 15:119, 1975.

Goldwasser AN, Auerbach SM, Harkins SW. Cognitive, affective, and behavioral effects of reminiscence group therapy on demented elderly. *Int J Aging Hum Dev* 25:209, 1987.

Heston LL, Garrard J, Makris L, et al. Inadequate treatment of depressed nursing home elderly. *J Am Geriatr Soc* 40:1117, 1992.

Hsu LKG, Zimmer B. Eating disorders in old age. *Int J Eating Disord* 7:133, 1988.

Hussian RA, Scott LP. Social reinforcement of activity and problem-solving training in the treatment of depressed institutionalized elderly patients. *Cog Ther Res* 5:57, 1981.

Institute of Medicine. *Improving the Quality of Care in Nursing Homes.* Washington DC: National Academy Press, 1986.

Johnson JC. Delirium in the elderly. *Emerg Med Clin North Am* 8:255, 1990.

Kafonek S, Ettinger WH, Roca R, et al. Instruments for screening for depression and dementia in a long-term care facility. *J Am Geriatr Soc* 37:29, 1989.

Katon W. Depression: Relationship to somatization and chronic medical illness. *J Clin Psychiatry* 45:4, 1984.

Katz IR, Lesher E, Kleban M, et al. Clinical features of depression in the nursing home. *Int Psychogeriatr* 1:5, 1989.

Katz IR, Parmelee PA. Depression in elderly patients in residential care settings. In: Schneider LS, Reynolds CF III, Lebowitz BD, Freidhoff AJ, eds. *Diagnosis and Treatment of Depression in Late Life.* Washington DC: American Psychiatric Press, 1994:437.

Katz IR, Simpson GM, Curlik SM, et al. Pharmacologic treatment of major depression for elderly patients in residential care settings. *J Clin Psychiatry* 51:41, 1990.

Kerstetter JE, Holthausen BA, Fitz PA. Malnutrition in the institutionalized older adult. *J Am Dietetic Assoc* 92:1109, 1992.

Kiloh LG. Pseudodementia. *Acta Psychiatr Scand* 37:336, 1961.

Koenig HG, Blazer DG. Epidemiology of geriatric affective disorders. *Clin Geriatr Med* 8:235, 1992.

Kolcaba K, Miller CA. Behavior problems: Geropharmacology treatment: Extend nursing responsibility. *J Gerontol Nurs* 15:29, 1989.

Krauthammer C, Klerman GL. Secondary mania: Manic syndromes associated with antecedent physical illness or drugs. *Arch Gen Psychiatry* 35:1333, 1978.

Kruzich JM, Clinton JF, Kelber ST. Personal and environmental influences on nursing home satisfaction. *Gerontologist* 32:342, 1992.

Kukull WA, Koepsell TD, Inui TS, et al. Depression and physical illness among general medical clinic patients. *J Affect Disord* 10:153, 1986.

Lesse S. *Masked Depression.* New York: Jason Aronson, 1964.

Libow L, Starer P. Care of the nursing home patient. *N Engl J Med* 231:93, 1989.

Loebel JP, Borson S, Hyde T, et al. Relationships between requests for psychiatric consultations and psychiatric diagnoses in long-term care facilities. *Am J Psychiatry* 148:898, 1992.

Loebel JP, Loebel JS, Dager SR, et al. Anticipation of nursing home placement may be a precipitant of suicide among the elderly. *J Am Geriatr Soc* 39:407, 1991.

McCue RE. Using tricyclic antidepressants in the elderly. *Clin Geriatr Med* 8:323, 1992.

McCullough PK. Geriatric depressions: Atypical presentations, hidden meanings. *Geriatrics* 46:72, 1991.

Miller DK, Morley JE, Rubenstein LZ, Pietruszka FM. Abnormal eating attitudes and body image in older undernourished individuals. *J Am Geriatr Soc* 39:462, 1991.

Mirchandani IC, Young RC. Management of mania in the elderly: An update. *Ann Clin Psychiatry* 5:67, 1993.

Moses J. New role for hands-on caregivers: Part-time mental health technicians. *J Am Health Care Assoc* 8:19, 1982.

Osgood N. Environmental factors in suicide in long-term care facilities. *Suicide Life-Threat Behav* 22:98, 1992.

Parmelee PA, Katz IR, Lawton MP. Depression among institutionalized aged: Assessment and prevalence estimation. *J Gerontol* 44:M22, 1989.

Parmelee PA, Katz IR, Lawton MP. The relation of pain to depression among institutionalized aged. *J Gerontol* 46:P15, 1991.

Parmelee PA, Katz IR, Lawton MP. Depression and mortality among institutionalized aged. *J Gerontol* 47:P3, 1992a.

Parmelee PA, Katz IR, Lawton MP. Incidence of depression in long-term care settings. *J Gerontol* 47:M189, 1992b.

Parmelee PA, Katz IR, Lawton MP. Anxiety and its association with depression among institutionalized elderly. *Am J Geriatr Psychiatry* 1:46, 1993.

Parmelee PA, Smith B, Katz IR. Pain complaints and cognitive status among elderly institution residents. *J Am Geriatr Soc* 41:517, 1993.

Pillemer K, Bachman R. Helping and hurting: Predictors of maltreatment of patients in nursing homes. *Res Aging* 13:74, 1991.

Pillemer K, Hudson B. A model abuse prevention program for nursing assistants. *Gerontologist* 33:128, 1993.

Pillemer K, Moore DW. Abuse of patients in nursing homes: Findings from a survey of staff. *Gerontologist* 29:314, 1989.

Pillemer K, Moore DW. Highlights from a study of abuse of patients in nursing homes. *J Elder Abuse Neglect* 2:5, 1990.

Poon LW. Toward an understanding of cognitive functioning in geriatric depression. *Int Psychogeriatr* 4(Suppl 2):241, 1992.

Post F. *The Clinical Psychiatry of Late Life.* Oxford: Pergamon Press, 1965.

Price WA, Gianini AJ, Collella J. Anorexia nervosa in the elderly. *J Am Geriatr Soc* 37:184, 1985.

Rattenbury C, Stones MJ. A controlled evaluation of reminiscence and current topics discussion groups in a nursing home context. *Gerontologist* 29:768, 1989.

Ridman D, Feller AG. Protein-calorie undernutrition in the nursing home. *J Am Geriatr Soc* 37:173, 1989.

Robinson RG, Starkstein SE. Current research in affective disorders following stroke. *J Neuropsychiatry Clin Neurosci* 2:1, 1990.

Ross ED, Rush AJ. Diagnosis and neuroanatomical correlates of depression in brain-damaged patients. *Arch Gen Psychiatry* 38:1344, 1981.

Rovner BW, Kafonek S, Filipp L, et al. Prevalence of mental illness in a community nursing home. *Am J Psychiatry* 143:1446, 1986.

Rovner BW, German PS, Brant LJ, et al. Depression and mortality in nursing homes. *JAMA* 265:993, 1991.

Rovner BW, Katz IR. Psychiatric disorders in the nursing home: A selective review of studies related to clinical care. *Int J Geriatr Psychiatry* 8:75, 1993.

Rovner BW, Steele CD, German P, et al. Psychiatric diagnosis and uncooperative behavior in nursing homes. *J Geriatr Psychiatry Neurol* 5:102, 1992.

Rubin EH. Aging and mania. *Psychiatr Dev* 4:329, 1988.

Salzman C, Fisher J, Nobel K, et al. Cognitive improvement following benzodiazepine discontinuation in elderly nursing home residents. *Int J Geriatr Psychiatry* 7:89, 1992.

Salzman C, Schneider L, Lebowitz B. Antidepressant treatment of very old patients. *Am J Geriatr Psychiatry* 1:21, 1993.

Santmyer KS, Roca RP. Geropsychiatry in long-term care: A nurse-centered approach. *J Am Geriatr Soc* 39:156, 1991.

Schleifer SJ, Keller SE, Bond RN, et al. Major depressive disorder and immunity. *Arch Gen Psychiatry* 46:81, 1989.

Schneider LS, Sobin PB. Non-neuroleptic treatment of behavioral symptoms and agitation in Alzheimer's disease and other dementia. *Psychopharm Bull* 28:71, 1992.

Sengstaken EA, King SA. The problem of pain and its detection among geriatric nursing home residents. *J Am Geriatr Soc* 41:541, 1993.

Shulman K, Post F. Bipolar affective disorder in old age. *Psychiatry* 136:26, 1980.

Silver AJ, Morley JE, Strome S, et al. Nutritional status in an academic nursing home. *J Am Geriatr Soc* 36:487, 1988.

Slater E, Roth M. *Clinical Psychiatry,* 3rd ed. London: Bailliere, Tindall, and Cassell, 1977.

Snowden J, Donnelly N. A study of depression in nursing homes. *J Psychiatric Res* 20:327, 1986.

Snowden J. Dementia, depression, and life satisfaction in nursing homes. *Int J Geriatr Psychiatry* 1:85, 1986.

Starkstein SE, Robinson RG. Affective disorders and cerebral vascular disease. *Br J Psychiatry* 154:170, 1989.

Stone K. Mania in the elderly. *Br J Psychiatry* 155:220, 1989.

Strahan G, Burns BJ. *Mental Health in Nursing Homes: United States 1985. Data from the National Health Survey.* Vitaland Health Statistics, Series 13, no. 105, DHHS Publication no. (PHS) 91-1766, 1988.

Teeter RB, Garetz FK, Miller WR, Heiland WF. Psychiatric disturbances of aged patients in skilled nursing care. *Am J Psychiatry* 133:1430, 1976.

Tellis-Nayak V, Tellis-Nayak M. Quality of care and the burden of two cultures: When the world of the nurse's aide enters the world of the nursing home. *Gerontologist* 29:307, 1989.

Tohen M, Shulman KI, Satlin A. First-episode mania in late life. *Am J Psychiatry* 151:130, 1994.

Waxman HM, Garner EA, Berkenstock G. Job turnover and job satisfaction among nursing home aides. *Gerontologist* 24:503, 1984.

Weissman MM, Bruce ML, Leaf PJ, et al. Affective disorders. In: Robins LN, Regier DA, eds. *Psychiatric Disorders in America: The Epidemiological Catchment Area Study.* New York: Free Press, 1991:53.

Wells KB, Stewart AL, Hays RD, et al. The functioning and well-being of depressed patients. *JAMA* 262:914, 1989.

Young RC, Klerman GL. Mania in late life: Focus on age at onset. *Am J Psychiatry* 149:867, 1992.

Young RC. Geriatric mania. *Clin Geriatr Med* 8:387, 1992.

Youssef FA. The impact of group reminiscence counseling on a depressed elderly population. *Nurse Pract* 15:34, 1990.

Zemore R, Eames N. Psychic and somatic symptoms of depression among young adults, institutionalized adults, and noninstitutionalized aged. *J Gerontol* 34:716, 1979.

Zerhusen JD, Boyle K, Wilson W. Out of the darkness: Group cognitive therapy for depressed elderly. *J Psychosoc Nurs* 29:16, 1991.

Zung WWK, George DR, Woodruff WW. Symptom perception by nonpsychiatric physicians in evaluating for depression. *J Clin Psychiatry* 45:26, 1984.

7

Anxiety Disorders

Timothy Howell

In ways analogous to depression, anxiety may be protean in its manifestations, ranging from mild, fleeting apprehension to immobilizing panic. Our very familiarity with this "all-too-human" emotion can sometimes interfere with our understanding of how it may be affecting our nursing home (NH) patients, and this may hinder accurate assessment and treatment. Through misplaced empathy, for example, we may try to place ourselves in the shoes of our patients in the effort to ascertain how they are experiencing an anxiety-provoking situation, but then we forget to "age ourselves" in the process. For example, the prospect of arthroplasty may seem much less anxiety-provoking to a young or middle-aged health professional than to an octogenarian.

To avoid missing the diagnosis of an anxiety disorder, or unwittingly trivializing it as "expectable under the circumstances," one must become objectively familiar with the landscape of anxiety. In this chapter we review ways to approach the assessment and treatment of elderly nursing home patients with anxiety disorders—ways that can help in dealing with the diagnostic and prognostic ambiguities endemic to psychiatric problems with this patient population.

Prevalence

There are essentially no published studies on the prevalence of anxiety disorders in NH populations that have made use of random patient samples, systematic examination by psychiatrists, and well-established diagnostic criteria. Two such rigorous studies (Rovner et al., 1986; Tariot et al., 1993) of randomly selected NH residents found 91 to 94% of them to be suffering from dementia, depression, other organic mental disorders, affective disorders, or psychoses, but not anxiety disorders. It is unclear, however, whether such disorders were screened for. The Epidemiological Catchment Area (ECA) study conducted by the National Institute of Mental Health (NIMH) included a survey of nursing homes in the Baltimore area. This revealed an 11.6% prevalence of phobias among NH residents with a stay of less than a year, while the figure was 2.1% for those whose length of stay was a year or more. This study employed the Diagnostic Interview Schedule, which generated diagnoses according to standardized (DSM-III) criteria (German et al., 1986).

Another study looking at the prevalence of anxiety and depression in a large (N=791) sample of elderly (61+ years old) residents in nursing homes and congregate housing found a prevalence for generalized anxiety or panic disorder to be 3.5%, with another 13.2% reporting anxiety symptoms not sufficient to warrant a specific diagnosis. This study employed a checklist of symptoms derived from the Schizophrenia and Affective Disorders Schedule (SADS), with diagnostic criteria established by modifying those according to the DSM-III-R. Significantly, however, certain somatic symptoms of anxiety (e.g., trembling, dry mouth) were omitted on the grounds that these were likely to be reflective of concurrent medical problems. As a consequence, organic anxiety disorders may have been missed and other anxiety disorders underestimated. Anxiety was found to be strongly associated with the presence of depression, poor physical health, functional disability, and cognitive impairment but not age or length of stay (Parmelee et al., 1993).

A recent study (Junginger et al., 1993), in which trained doctoral candidates in psychology administered the Structured Clinical Interview (SCID) for DSM-III-R to 100 residents selected at random in a suburban NH, found 20% of the sample to have anxiety disorders: 6% met DSM-III-R criteria for generalized anxiety disorder (GAD), 5% each for panic disorder and obsessive-compulsive disorder (OCD), 4% for agoraphobia without panic, and 1% for simple phobia. The generalizability of these findings is probably limited, however. For example, no mention is made of patients with dementia or organic anxiety syndrome in this study; such omissions make the results less likely to be representative of the usual NH population.

Some data are available on the prevalence of anxiety symptoms in community-dwelling elderly. The NIMH ECA study (Regier et al., 1988) found the 1-month prevalence of all anxiety disorders in those above 65 years of age to be 5.5% (vs. 7.3% for adults of all ages), with phobic disorder making up 4.8%; obsessive-compulsive disorder, 0.8%; and panic disorder, 0.1%. By gender, the rates for all anxiety disorders were 3.6% for men and 6.8% for women, with phobias at 2.9% and OCD at 0.7% for men and phobias at 6.1%, panic disorder at 0.2%, and OCD at 0.9% for women.

Even these data, however, must be interpreted cautiously, given the possibility of underreporting by older subjects in the study or cohort effects reflective of different circumstances associated with different generations. There are other dilemmas confronting the establishment of accurate prevalence rates for anxiety disorders in the elderly, whether in the community or NH setting. Accurate diagnosis of anxiety in the elderly may be confounded by significant overlap between symptoms of anxiety disorder and anxiety symptoms associated with concurrent medical problems and/or treatments for those problems. Anxiety can also be a prominent component of other psychiatric disorders, including dementia, depression, psychosis, adjustment disorder, personality disorder, substance abuse, chronic pain syndromes, and chronic insomnia.

Clinical Presentation

The phenomenology of anxiety can conveniently be divided into four categories of signs and symptoms: psychological features, psychomotor signs, autonomic signs, and vigilance (see Table 7.1). These include a multitude of ways in which patients may present with anxiety and account for why, in the elderly, the diagnosis may be missed or delayed. Like the mythical Proteus, anxiety syndromes in the elderly, particularly those prone to somatization, may present with confusing sets of complaints that may wax and wane or even change over a short period of time.

It is possible that the current cohort of elderly in the United States is less comfortable with talking about feelings and hence more likely to focus on somatic symptoms of anxiety. Such a phenomenon could lead to more medical evaluations before the anxiety disorder is recognized.

TABLE 7.1.   Symptoms and Signs of Anxiety

A. Psychological features	Dysphoric apprehension or expectation
B. Psychomotor signs	Tremulousness, twitching, feeling shaky
	Muscle tension, aches, soreness
	Restlessness
	Easily fatigued
C. Autonomic signs	Shortness of breath, ''smothering''
	Palpitations, increased heart rate
	Sweating, cold/clammy feeling
	Dry mouth
	Dizziness, light-headedness
	Nausea, vomiting, GI distress
	Flushing, hot flashes, chills
	Frequent urination
	Dysphagia, ''lump in throat''
D. Vigilance	Feeling keyed up, on edge
	Exaggerated startle response
	Poor concentration, ''mind goes blank''
	Insomnia
	Irritability

Types of Anxiety

Situational Anxiety

In older NH patients, this type of anxiety is likely to be similar to that experienced by younger adults with the exception that, for the elderly, it is more likely to occur in unfamiliar situations. Examples of such situations might include sudden nonroutine events (e.g., a false fire alarm) or a need to undertake a task that the individual has not had any need to perform or practice for some time (e.g., to balance a financial account or to spell a word backwards as part of a mental status exam).

Adjustment Disorder with Anxiety

This condition occurs in response to a known stressor. It can occur in response to a crisis: e.g., NH placement, illness in family, death of a roommate, financial setback, and so on. It may also occur with less severe stressors, such as relocation from one wing of a NH to another or even from one room to another. A new medical problem, even if it is not severe or disabling, may precipitate an anxious mood. It is in this context that one must be sensitive to how the stressor is experienced by the NH resident, in terms of his or her own values and perspectives rather than one's own, so as to avoid responses and interventions based on misplaced empathy. Another diagnostic pitfall to beware of in assessing elderly patients in the NH is premature closure. It may well be that some of an elderly patient's anxiety may be the result of a new or recent stressor, but something else could also be contributing to or exacerbating his or her anxious mood, such as a concurrent anxiogenic medical problem (see below) and/or psychiatric disorder with associated anxiety. With younger patients, the simplest hypothesis that accounts for the most of a patient's symptoms is usually the most elegant and correct solution to the differential diagnosis. But with the elderly, in psychiatric as well as medical situations, there is, more often than not, more than one thing going on at the same time. Furthermore, when a problem such as anxiety turns out to be multifactorial, the different factors often have a tendency to interact with one another.

Phobic Anxiety

Phobic anxiety involves a persistent fear of a specific object or situation that is of sufficient intensity to cause significant subjective distress or avoidant behavior and which interferes with the individual's normal routine or social activities. The subjective distress may be experienced in the anxiety provoked by confrontation with the object or situation (i.e., specific phobia) or with a social or performance situation involving unfamiliar people, scrutiny by others, or potential embarrassment (i.e., social phobia). Agoraphobia is characterized by a fear of going into places from which escape could be difficult or embarrassing or where there would not be help if feelings of panic set in. In the NH setting, this disorder could become manifest in a resident who was fearful of leaving the facility or even her room.

As with younger patients, specific or social phobias may be of long standing. But with new-onset phobias, careful assessment is required. It may turn out that such fear in a certain situation is not so unrealistic after all. For example, a NH resident may have become apprehensive regarding certain social events due to the onset of incontinence or cognitive impairment. Out of embarrassment, perhaps, such a resident may not volunteer this information; hence the development of the phobia may be the first indicator of the underlying problem.

Obsessive-Compulsive Disorders

The defining feature of these disorders is the presence of obsessions or compulsions. The former can be characterized as persistently recurring ideas, images, or impulses that intrude into the consciousness of the patient. These seem to make no sense and often are morally or physically repugnant (not only to others but to the patient as well). Such obsessions are ego-dystonic in the sense that they are experienced as invasive and not voluntarily originating from the individual's own mental process. Furthermore, they are often resistant to conscious suppression by the patient and thus a source of considerable, sometimes extraordinary, anxiety and distress. The most common obsessions (in descending order of frequency) involve contamination, pathological doubt, somatic concerns, need for symmetry, aggression, and sexual images or impulses (Rasmussen and Eisen, 1992). One patient in the author's experience asked repeatedly for the police to be called, because, as she explained with much consternation, she was having repeated thoughts and impulses to stab someone and wanted to be sure that no one was hurt. The same patient also suffered from a compulsion to mop the floors of the facility and would wander about in search of a mop.

Compulsions are actions that are analogous to obsessions and are often the behavioral response to obsessions. They include repetitive behaviors that superficially may seem purposeful, performed according to specific rules or in a stereotypic manner. A prototypic example is the OCD patient who washes his or her hands in a rigid fashion according to a strict schedule up to scores of times each day. But, in fact, such activities are not ends in themselves; rather, they are means to bring about or prevent something else (e.g., repeated hand-washing to avoid morbid contamination). Thus a NH patient may anxiously labor at some meaningless activity (e.g., wander about systematically touching all the doorknobs) to ward off a calamity, such as to prevent all the other residents from dying. As with obsessions, affected individuals initially recognize the compulsions to be irrational, but they feel unable to resist performing them, however much they try. The most common compulsions are checking on certain things, washing, needing to ask or confess something, arranging objects precisely, and hoarding (Rasmussen and Eisen, 1992).

One phenomenon to be aware of in working with elderly NH residents with this disorder is that long-standing OCD symptoms may become ego-syntonic. That is, to the extent that their obsessions or compulsions have been present to some degree for years, such patients may have become used to them and may even have incorporated them into their sense of identity. Hence, they may no longer be viewed by these patients as irrational. A diagnostic dilemma arises in that the obsessions or compulsions may therefore have come to resemble psychotic symptoms, such as thought insertions or delusional behavior. Hence one must assess the individual's earlier history to clarify this possibility. Collateral sources of information, particularly those who have known the patient for at least as long as the symptoms have been present, can be helpful in this regard. Another not uncommon variant of this condition that may be seen in this population is the occurrence of transient OCD symptoms in the context of major affective disorders, with or without psychotic features.

Late-onset OCD appears to be very rare, but patients may present for treatment of long-standing OCD for the first time in late life due to age-related changes or age-associated medical/psychiatric problems. Jenike (1989) reported that only 1% of 100 consecutive patients at the Massachusetts General Hospital OCD Clinic dated the onset of their illness after age 50, while 4% were 60 years old or older when they initially presented to the clinic as part of a later cohort.

Panic Disorders

Panic disorders are marked by recurrent attacks of acute anxiety that generally arise in an unpredictable fashion. Such attacks usually manifest themselves by an intense feeling of terror, fear, or doom, which initially occurs suddenly and spontaneously. The most common somatic symptoms of a panic attack are dyspnea, palpitations, light-headedness, chest pain/pressure, smothering/choking sensations, paresthesia, hot/cold flashes, perspiration, and nausea or other gastrointestinal distress. In addition, a panicked individual may feel imminently out of control—"going crazy" or about to die. Panic attacks may lead to the formation of phobias, with patients seeking to avoid the situations in which they have experienced panic attacks. Thus a NH resident, having initially experienced one or two panic attacks in the dining room, may link the attacks with being in that location and subsequently avoid eating there (or endure meals there with much dread of a recurrence).

Initially, late-onset panic attacks are likely to be mistaken for a possible myocardial infarction, transient ischemic attack (TIA), or other acute problem. The usual scenario involves several panic attacks, with negative workup (physical exam, laboratory tests) before the psychiatric nature of problems is recognized. Elderly patients and their families are often reluctant to accept this diagnosis and thus may require careful counseling. Furthermore, significant anticipatory anxiety may persist after amelioration of the panic attacks and require considerable reassurance or even supportive psychotherapy.

Posttraumatic Stress Disorder

The essential nature of posttraumatic stress disorder (PTSD) is the development of a cluster of characteristic symptoms after an extreme, psychologically painful experience that engendered feelings of intense fear, horror, or helplessness (e.g., events involving actual or threatened death, serious injury, or destruction of property, as in war, accidents, crimes, or natural disasters). Typical symptoms include persistent, intrusive thoughts, memories, dreams, or even flashbacks, through which the traumatic event is relived. These may occur spontaneously or may be triggered by everyday events that in some way remind the individual, through association or similarity, of the initial trauma. When unusually intense, the reexperience of the traumatic event may involve dissociative states.

One consequence of these distressing, unwanted recollections is that an individual with PTSD tends to avoid thoughts or situations that evoke them. He or she may thereby become withdrawn from significant activities. Other diagnostic sequelae include feelings of estrangement, constriction of affect, or undue pessimism. Associated signs of autonomic hyperarousal include insomnia, irritability, hypervigilance, exaggerated startling, and difficulty concentrating. Posttraumatic stress disorder may sometimes be delayed in onset, when it develops (by convention) more than 6 months after the traumatic event. The delay may sometimes be measured in years or even decades. Late-onset PTSD may be triggered by a late-life stressor, such as retirement, widowhood, or a medical problem (Kaup et al., 1994). Nursing home placement might precipitate PTSD in a concentration camp survivor, for example (Herrmann and Ergavec, 1994). Another example in this author's experience was that of an elderly veteran who experienced PTSD symptoms when he developed an acute arthralgia. The traumatic event behind his relapse was his experience 50 years earlier, in combat during World War II, when he injured the same knee, diving to escape the attack of a strafing fighter plane in which a close friend was killed.

Generalized Anxiety Disorder

Generalized anxiety disorder (GAD) is characterized by persistent (i.e., 6 months or longer), excessive or unrealistic apprehension that occurs on more days than not, which are affected individual finds difficult to control. The anxiety focuses on situations where such a degree of apprehension is unwarranted. For example, a NH resident may be very worried about her financial status, despite having substantial resources that are more than adequate for her needs, and about some disaster befalling a favorite granddaughter, despite the fact that the child is well and safe.

By DSM-IV criteria (APA, 1994), the diagnosis of GAD requires that the patient have at least three of the following six symptoms: restlessness, irritability, muscle tension, disturbed sleep, poor concentration, and easy fatigability. If the NH resident has another major psychiatric disorder concurrently, the pervasive anxiety must be about different, unrelated issues. Thus, to make the diagnosis of GAD in someone with a concurrent panic disorder, the anxiety would have to involve things other than having a panic attack. Likewise, the focus of the generalized anxiety would have to be other than public embarrassment in someone with a social phobia or other than contamination, for example, in someone with OCD. Other exclusion criteria include the anxiety being due to a demonstrable organic cause or occurring only in the context of an affective or psychotic disorder.

Organic Anxiety Disorders

These disorders are now referred to in DSM-IV as anxiety disorders due to a general medical condition and substance-induced anxiety disorders. These are a major concern with the elderly, whether in the community, NH, or hospital. Table 7.2 summarizes medical problems and drugs that can give rise to both psychological and somatic symptoms of anxiety.

Even where patients clearly have one of the above anxiety disorders, it is sound practice to consider routinely whether some additional acute or chronic medical conditions may not be contributing to the clinical picture of anxiety. Not infrequently, there is more than one factor involved/interacting in the presentation of anxiety with older patients, each a source of excess morbidity. Consider, for example, a patient with a history of GAD who is in the early stages of a dementia, has chronic obstructive pulmonary disease (COPD) being treated with theophylline, and has been forced to retire early with consequent financial difficulties, who now requires placement in a NH for rehabilitation following open reduction and internal fixation of a left hip fracture. Such a patient may have multiple reasons to be anxious. In addition to addressing his psychiatric and psychosocial issues, a useful step would be to minimize his theophylline dosage to the lowest effective level (or to implement a potentially less anxiogenic medication regimen); this may contribute in a small but significant way to optimizing treatment of his anxiety. Likewise, should he develop an uncharacteristic intense attack of anxiety during the night, prompting an urgent call from nursing staff, consideration should be given to the possibility of a pulmonary embolus.

Anxiety may also occur in the context of other major psychiatric disorders (Winokur, 1988; Flint 1994). These include depression, dementia, delirium, mania, schizophrenia, and substance abuse. The reader is referred to the other chapters in this book for information on the assessment and treatment of these disorders.

TABLE 7.2.   Medical Causes of Anxiety

1. Cardiovascular disorders
     Congestive heart failure
     Arrhythmias
     Myocardial infarction
     Mitral valve prolapse
     Angina
     Cardiomyopathy
     Syncope

2. Respiratory disorders
     Chronic obstructive pulmonary disease
     Pneumonia
     Hypoxia
     Pulmonary embolus
     Sleep apnea
     Asthma
     Pneumothorax
     Pulmonary edema

3. Endocrine disorders
     Hyperthyroidism/hypothyroidism
     Cushing's disease
     Hypoglycemia
     Hypocalcemia/hypercalcemia
     Pheochromocytoma
     Carcinoid syndrome
     Hypokalemia
     Insulinoma

4. Nutritional deficiency
     Vitamin B_{12}

5. Neurologic disorders
     CNS infections
     CNS masses
     Parkinson's disease
     Movement disorders
     Focal seizures
     Postconcussion syndrome
     Toxins
     Multiple sclerosis
     Vertigo

6. Drugs
     Anticholinergic toxicity
     Digitalis toxicity
     Excessive thyroid supplementation
     Antihypertensive side effects
     Stimulants
       Amphetamines
       Methylphenidate
       Cocaine
       Caffeine
       Steroids
     Sympathomimetics
       Decongestants
       Bronchodilators
     Antidepressants
       Selective serotonin reuptake
         inhibitors (SSRIs)
       Tranylcypromine
       Tricyclics

7. Other
     Neuroleptic-induced akathisia
     Withdrawal
       Alcohol
       Sedative-hypnotics
     Chronic pain syndromes

Etiologies

Psychological theories of anxiety view it as a signal of a problem that an older person can no longer manage with his or her usual coping strategies. Anxiety may originate in an intrapsychic conflict, when the affected individual experiences a conflict between the demands of conscience, some reality-imposed limitations, and/or certain impulses. Alternatively, psychosocial issues involving stage-of-life circumstances may predominate. For example, an elderly NH patient may be acutely aware of a gap between his or her present and past capabilities, the prospect of incompetence increasing with time, or the proximity and reality of illnesses and death. A combined theory postulates that anxious individuals may be neurophysiologically vulnerable to experiencing fear in unfamiliar situations, and this biological predisposition may be augmented by the experience of frightening behaviors by parents or significant others during childhood. When such individuals encounter meaningful stressors later in life, they experience an erosion of their sense of safety and, with that, the neurophysiological disturbances associated with a sense of loss of control. If they also become increasingly anxious over their experience of anxiety symptoms (both psychological and somatic), a vicious cycle may be initiated, culminating in panic attacks (Shear et al., 1993). Where these are the primary kinds of issues, supportive therapy, with a focus on coming to terms with these issues, and problem solving may be quite helpful.

Neurobiological theories of anxiety focus on neurotransmitter systems in the central nervous system, which are postulated to form the biological substrates of fear and anxiety, the body's "flight or fight" mechanisms. One such system involves the neurotransmitter norepinephrine. More than half the cerebral noradrenergic neurons are found in the locus ceruleus, a bilateral nucleus of cell bodies in the dorsolateral tegmentum of the pons. From this structure, axons ascend to the cortex, hippocampus, hypothalamus, limbic area, and forebrain. Descending neurons modulate peripheral sympathetic activity. Animal research has demonstrated evidence that this system plays a major role in the regulation of cerebral arousal. It is postulated that alterations in this system may predispose to the development of panic attacks (Margraf and Ehlers, 1990).

In addition, much work in the past decade has elaborated our understanding of benzodiazepine (BZ) receptors, located on the cell membranes of certain neurons. The BZ receptor has been found to be linked to a receptor complex composed of a gamma-aminobutyric acid (GABA) receptor and chloride ion channel. The binding of a BZ to the BZ receptor facilitates ability of the GABA receptor complex to open the chloride channel. Negatively charged chloride ions thereby enter the cell, hyperpolarizing it and reducing its reactivity to stimulation (Wolkowitz and Paul, 1985). These receptors appear to be involved in the modulation of anxiety for a number of reasons. In addition to BZs having demonstrable anxiolytic effects, BZ antagonists have been found to cause arousal states in primates similar to human anxiety. The anxiolytic efficacy of BZs corresponds to their receptor-binding affinities. Finally, a number of animal models for anxiety have been shown to involve changes in BZ receptor binding or density (Joffe and Swinson, 1990).

Treatment

The treatment of anxiety disorders in the NH begins with a careful assessment of all the biopsychosocial factors potentially contributing to them. A high tolerance of ambiguity is helpful, as there is significant potential in elderly patients for overlapping situations where different concurrent problems cause similar symptoms. Initially, it may not be clear, for example, how much of a patient's apprehensiveness, tachycardia, chest tightness, and tremulousness is due to his or her angina, painful osteoarthritis, generalized anxiety disorder, coffee drinking, or brother's recent death. But by addressing each potential source of excess morbidity, the overall anxiety can be optimally addressed. Even with subsequent improvement in the patient's symptoms, it may still be difficult to ascertain in retrospect how much of the improvement was due to which intervention.

The basic principles of such a biopsychosocial approach are outlined in Table 7.3.

Psychological interventions for anxiety can include both general support and psychotherapy. The former is implemented to mobilize resources intended to reduce identified stress. Psychotherapy of various types may be helpful (see Chapter 14). Psychodynamic psychotherapy may be clinically indicated where the individual's anxiety stems in large part from conflicts that require uncovering and working through. Supportive psychotherapy is frequently applicable and can help a patient to learn problem-solving techniques and strengthen his or her coping styles. Cognitive psychotherapy is another often helpful approach, through which individuals can learn about the ways in which they frame situations and then make incorrect (e.g., overly generalized) assumptions, thus contributing to the generation of anxious feelings. Behavioral therapy includes such techniques as progressive relaxation or systematic desensitization. The former may be particularly helpful where muscular tension is a significant part of a patient's anxiety and the latter for phobias. Desensitization therapy consists of exposing a patient gradually to a series of stimuli, of which each successive situation is closer in nature to the object of the phobia. By gradually having the duration and intensity of their exposure to the feared situation increased, the patients' anxieties, fears, or compulsions are gradually extinguished (Dar and Greist, 1992).

The use of anxiolytic medication should be reserved for those situations when nonpharmacological measures do not suffice and the patient's symptoms interfere with his or her ability to function, cause significant subjective distress, or make other illnesses worse. Benzodiazepines with short half-lives are generally the first choice. These include (with approximate half-life in elderly patients in parenthesis) oxazepam (5 to 15 hours) and lorazepam (10 to 20 hours). Both these BZs are metabolized by glucuronidation, which is not significantly affected by aging. Hence they have no active metabolites, can provide more flexible dosing, and help to avoid cumulative toxicity. They may, however, cause rebound anxiety when tapered or discontinued quickly, and they do interact with other sedating medications (e.g., alcohol, tranquilizers). Benzodiazepines with long half-lives are primarily metabolized by oxidation, which is affected by the aging process. Thus, these BZs have active metabolites that also have long-half lives. Examples of these include (with approximate half-lives of parent drug/active metabolite in elderly patients in parenthesis) diazepam (26–53/36–200 hours), chlordiazepoxide (8–28/36–200 hours), prazepam (30–200/36–200 hours), clorazepate (30–200/36–200 hours), and halazepam (14/36–120 hours). These BZs

TABLE 7.3.   Treatment of Anxiety

A. Eliminate/minimize use of anxiogenic substances
B. Modify medications that may be causative/exacerbating factors
C. Treat underlying acute/chronic medical problems
D. Treat concurrent psychiatric disorders
E. Nonpharmacological approaches:
    1. Psychosocial support—eliminate/modify stressors
    2. Psychotherapy
F. Pharmacological treatment with anxiolytic agents

are best reserved for use with compliant, stable patients, where once-a-day dosing is preferable and cumulative toxicity is less likely. Like their short-acting cousins, the long-acting BZs have additive effects when combined with other sedating medications. Unlike them, however, they are also, because of the way they are metabolized, more likely to interact with other medications. Thus, for example, concurrent use of cimetidine can result in higher BZ levels, while concurrent use of anticonvulsants can lower BZ levels. (For an excellent summary of potentially adverse drug interactions involving anxiolytic medications, see Salzman, 1992). In emergency situations that require parenteral administration of an anxiolytic, lorazepam is the most reliably absorbed BZ.

With both classes of BZs, it is important to monitor for the development of tolerance (due to the induction of hepatic enzymes) as well as signs of drug dependency. Noncompliance, with a patient using either too much or too little of the medication, is probably less likely to be problematic in the NH setting, but situations in which patients have been found to be "borrowing" pills from peers or visiting family and friends are not unheard of. There is some literature suggesting that elderly patients are not likely to abuse BZs (Pinsker and Petchel, 1984). Hence there may be somewhat less of a need with the elderly to be overly cautious in prescribing BZs and thereby risk undertreatment. Since withdrawal symptoms can occur upon discontinuation of BZs, it is best to taper them gradually.

When considering potential side effects of BZs in the elderly, one must, as a general principle, be alert to the fact that older patients may be relatively more unstable in their sensitivity to the effects of these drugs. Progression of a vascular dementia or an intercurrent medical problem causing decreased hepatic function, for example, may lead a previously effective and well-tolerated dose to become toxic. Side effects of BZs include cognitive impairment (which can mimic dementia or the progression of a dementia) and sedation. Some elderly patients, particularly those with brain damage, may be vulnerable to becoming disinhibited on even small doses of a BZ. This may result in agitation and even aggression, which may be indistinguishable from the behavioral complications of the brain disease for which the BZs were initially prescribed.

Psychomotor impairment due to BZs can be manifested by signs of slowed reaction time, diminished hand-eye coordination, and poor motoric accuracy.

Elderly NH residents may be more vulnerable to BZ-induced cerebellar toxicity, signs of which include ataxia, dysarthria, incoordination, unsteadiness, and falls. Epidemiological research has suggested that the use of long-acting BZs in long-term-care facilities is more likely to be associated with falls than the shorter-acting ones (Ray et al., 1989). Benzodiazepines should be avoided in patients with demonstrable or suspected sleep apnea, as they may exacerbate this disorder.

There are as yet no methodologically rigorous outcome studies on the use of BZs with elderly nursing home patients, and this is reflected in the lack of consensus regarding their use with this population, even among seasoned clinicians. Some, emphasizing their potential adverse side effects, advocate that BZs be reserved for limited use in acute situations. Other relate that for some chronically anxious patients, judicious dosing can provide considerable long-term relief while avoiding significant toxicity.

Buspirone is a nonbenzodiazepine anxiolytic that has the advantage of being less sedating than the BZs. It is a partial serotonin agonist, and its elimination half-life appears not to be significantly altered by the aging process or concurrent liver disease. It also is not associated with dependence, tolerance, or addiction. Unlike the BZs, buspirone requires 2 or more weeks for the onset of its effectiveness. Its primary indication is for GAD, but its lack of significant effect on respiration has led some to recommend it as the anxiolytic agent of choice in patients with chronic anxiety associated with respiratory disease or sleep apneas (Stoudemire and Moran, 1993; Goldberg, 1994). Thus far, there have been relatively few data on use with elderly.

Beta blockers represent another class of medications for consideration with elderly, anxious NH patients, but again, data on their use in this context are quite sparse. Most of the experience with beta blockers for anxiety has been younger patients with anticipatory or performance anxiety or akathisia. The anxiolytic effects of beta blockers have been attributed to their peripheral blockade of the ''adrenergic overdrive'' in anxiety states. The presence of congestive heart failure, bradycardia, bronchospastic disease, and diabetes are relative contraindications for beta blockers.

Antidepressants have been shown to be effective for the treatment of panic disorders in younger patients, but there are still no data on this use with the elderly. Double-blind, controlled studies have shown clomipramine to be helpful with OCD in younger patients. To establish maximum effectiveness, a trial at doses up to 250 mg/day for at least 10 to 12 weeks is recommended (Jenike, 1992). Elderly NH residents, however, may not be able to tolerate such high doses and thus may achieve only partial benefit from this drug. Other medications that show some promise with OCD include the selective serotonin reuptake inhibitors (e.g., fluoxetine, sertraline) and monoamine oxidase inhibitors (MAOIs).

Antihistamines have sometimes been employed as antianxiety agents, but, especially for the elderly, they can be quite troublesome insofar as they are nonspecifically sedating and associated with significant central and peripheral anticholinergic side effects, including increased confusion, blurred vision, dry mouth, urinary retention, and constipation. Even at relatively low doses, antihistamines may cause delirium in the elderly and cause or exacerbate agitation in patients with dementia.

Antipsychotics are rarely used in the treatment of anxiety, and rightly so. Because of their potential for significant side effects (especially tardive dyskinesia), they are best reserved for unusual, refractory patients with whom alternative treatments have failed and where the benefits outweigh the risks. Potential side effects are multiple and include sedation, orthostatic hypotension, anticholinergic symptoms, and extrapyramidal signs (dystonias, akathisia, parkinsonism) as well as tardive dyskinesia. (The reader is referred to Chapter 3 for a more thorough discussion of psychopharmacology.)

Summary

In the NH setting, depression, delirium, psychoses, and dementia with behavioral complications are all pressing problems. But in the genuine concern to address these issues, those raised by anxiety disorders may be overlooked or given short shrift. While the problems associated with most of the other major psychiatric disorders may be more objectively manifest, the anxiety disorders often entail considerable subjective distress. By becoming more familiar with the landscape of anxiety, more skilled at recognizing its varied clinical presentations, and treating it, we can do more to reduce its toll on our nursing home patients.

References

APA. *Diagnostic and Statistical Manual of Mental Disorders,* 4th ed. Washington DC: American Psychiatric Association, 1994.

Dar R, Greist JH. Behavior therapy for obsessive compulsive disorder. *Psychiatr Clin North Am* 15:885–894, 1992.

Flint AJ. Epidemiology and comorbidity of anxiety disorders in the elderly. *Am J Psychiatry* 151:640–649, 1994.

German PS, Shapiro S, Kramer M. Nursing home study of the eastern Baltimore Epidemiological Catchment Area Study. In: Harper MS, Lebowitz BD, eds. *Mental Illness in Nursing Homes: Agenda for Research.* Rockville MD: Department of Health and Human Services, 1986:27–40.

Goldberg RJ. The use of buspirone in geriatric patients. *J Clin Psychiatry Monogr* 12:31–35, 1994.

Herrmann N, Eryavec G. Posttraumatic stress disorder in institutionalized World War II veterans. *Am J Geriatr Psychiatry* 2:324–331, 1994.

Jenike MA. *Geriatric Psychiatry and Psychopharmacology: A Clinical Approach.* Chicago: Year Book Medical Publishers, 1989:339.

Jenike MA. Pharmacologic treatment of obsessive compulsive disorders. *Psychiatric Clin North Am* 15:895–919, 1992.

Joffe RT, Swinson RP. Drug studies and biochemical etiology of anxiety. In: Burrows GD, Roth M, Noyes Jr R, eds. *Handbook of Anxiety.* Vol 3. *The Neurobiology of Anxiety.* Amsterdam: Elsevier, 1990:407–416.

Junginger J, Phelan E, Cherr K, et al. Prevalence of psychopathology in elderly persons in nursing homes and the community. *Hosp Comm Psychiatry* 44:381–383, 1993.

Kaup BA, Ruskin PE, Nymen G. Significant life events and PTSD in elderly World War II veterans. *Am J Geriatr Psychiatry* 2:239–243, 1994.

Margraf J, Ehlers A. Biological models of panic disorder and agoraphobia: Theory and evidence. In: Burrows GD, Roth M, Noyes Jr R, eds. *Handbook of Anxiety.* Vol 3. *The Neurobiology of Anxiety.* Amsterdam: Elsevier, 1990:79–139.

Parmelee PA, Katz IR, Lawton MP. Anxiety and its association with depression among institutionalized elderly. *Am J Geriatr Psychiatry* 1:46–58, 1993.

Pinsker H, Suljaga-Petchel K. Use of benzodiazepines in primary-care geriatric patients. *J Am Geriatr Soc* 32:595–597, 1984.

Rasmussen SA, Eisen JL. The epidemiology and clinical features of obsessive compulsive disorder. *Psychiatr Clin North Am* 15:743–758, 1992.

Ray WA, Griffen MR, Downey W. Benzodiazepines of long and short term elimination half-life and the risk of hip fractures. *JAMA* 262:3303–3307, 1989.

Regier DA, Boyd JH, Burke JD, et al. One-month prevalence of mental disorders in the United States. *Arch Gen Psychiatry* 45:977–986, 1988.

Rovner BW, Kaphonek S, Filipp L, et al. Prevalence of mental illness in a community nursing home. *Am J Psychiatry* 143:1446–1449, 1986.

Salzman C. *Clinical Geriatric Psychopharmacology,* 2nd ed. Baltimore: Williams & Wilkins, 1992.

Shear MK, Cooper AM, Klerman GL, et al. A psychodynamic model of panic disorder. *Am J Psychiatry* 150:859–866, 1993.

Stoudemire A, Moran MG. Psychopharmacologic treatment of anxiety in the medically ill: Special considerations. *J Clin Psychiatry* 54(5, suppl):27–33, 1993.

Tariot PN, Podgorski CA, Blazina L, et al. Mental disorders in the nursing home: another perspective. *Am J Psychiatry* 150:1063–1069, 1993.

Winokur G. Anxiety disorders: Relationship to other psychiatric illnesses. *Psychiatr Clin North Am* 11:287–294, 1988.

Wolkowitz OM, Paul SM. Neural and molecular mechanisms in anxiety. *Psychiatr Clin North Am* 8:145–158, 1985.

8

Schizophrenia and Other Psychotic Disorders

William E. Reichman and Peter V. Rabins

Psychotic symptoms frequently complicate the care of nursing home residents. These symptoms consist of delusions, or unshared beliefs that are clearly false; hallucinations, or false sensory experiences; and thought disorders such as loosening of associations and flight of ideas. Morriss and colleagues (1990) reported that 21% of newly admitted nursing home residents, all of whom were cognitively impaired were found to have delusions. Chandler and Chandler (1988) reported a 12% prevalence of delusions in the nursing home setting; more recently. Junginger and coworkers (1993) reported a 10% prevalence of psychotic disorders in 100 nursing home residents screened for psychopathology. Delusional beliefs generally reflect persecutory (paranoid), somatic, or grandiose themes. In some conditions, such as paranoid schizophrenia, delusions can be systematized and quite detailed, while in dementia they are often relatively simple (Cummings, 1985b; Wragg and Jeste, 1989). Occasionally, delusions consist of notions that are clearly outside the realm of everyday experience, such as believing that one is receiving communications from an unidentified flying object or that one's thoughts are being controlled. Some delusions consist of unfounded yet relatively elaborate persecutory or paranoid fears regarding neighbors, the federal government, or other powerful agencies. In rare instances, the beliefs are plausible (e.g., of being physically abused) and must be investigated for accuracy. In other cases, relatively simple, fragmented beliefs, such as delusions of theft, evolve when the demented or delirious resident misplaces something. Grandiose delusions may occur in the setting of a manic episode, while, conversely, delusional beliefs related to guilt or somatic functions can complicate major depression.

Hallucinations can occur in any sensory modality but are most typically visual and auditory and, in the long-term-care setting, frequently emerge during the course of dementia (Chapter 4) or delirium (Chapter 5). They are ubiquitous in schizophrenia, and, like delusions, are also noted in severe mood disorders such as major depression or mania with psychotic features (Chapter 6). In the elderly, hallucinations occasionally develop independent of any other psychiatric condition but secondarily to the presence of significant sensory impairment, medication, or a medical disorder. Regardless of cause, psychotic symptoms are often stressful to affected residents, upsetting to visiting family members, and burdensome to attending nursing home staff. Although significant data remain scarce, clinical experience suggests that the presence of these symptoms contributes to functional decline, disruptive behavior (Rovner et al., 1986), excessive morbidity, and disruption of the nursing home residential milieu.

This chapter reviews the phenomenology of delusions and hallucinations in the long-term-care setting with attention directed to the occurrence of these symptoms in schizophrenia and delusional disorder. Psychotic symptoms arising secondarily to identifiable medical conditions are also highlighted. Treatment of psychosis with neuroleptic medications is covered in greater detail in Chapter 3, while supportive psychotherapeutic techniques for such symptomatology are reviewed in Chapter 13.

Schizophrenia

The clinical presentation of schizophrenia has not been systematically studied within the nursing home environment. There are essentially two populations of nursing home residents who meet diagnostic criteria for schizophrenia as outlined by the *Diagnostic and Statistical Manual of Mental Disorders,* 4th ed. (DSM-IV) (APA, 1994); those with early-onset schizophrenia (EOS), who have aged and require long-term care, and elderly nursing home residents with late-onset schizophrenia (LOS). Diagnostic criteria for schizophrenia are presented in Table 8.1.

There has been continuing debate over the clinical differences between EOS and LOS in the elderly. The presence of hallucinations and delusions is common to both groups. In LOS, however, Schneiderian first-rank symptoms such as thought withdrawal, thought broadcasting, and thought insertion may be less common than in EOS (Grahame 1984; Holden 1987; Harris and Jeste, 1988; Pearlson et al., 1989). Evident in both groups are prominent persecutory beliefs frequently accompanied by auditory hallucinations (Jeste et al., 1991). Negative symptoms (withdrawal, affective blunting, apathy), formal thought disorder (loosening of associations or grossly illogical thinking), and bizarre or inappropriate affect appear to be more common in younger patients with EOS than in the elderly with EOS or LOS (Pearlson et al., 1989; Jeste et al., 1991; Castle and Howard, 1992). A variety of risk factors have been associated with LOS, including a family history of schizophrenia, sensory impairment, premorbid personality

TABLE 8.1.   Diagnostic Criteria for Schizophrenia

A. Characteristic symptoms: Two (or more) of the following, each present for a significant portion of time during a 1-month period (or less if successfully treated):

    1. Delusions
    2. Hallucinations
    3. Disorganized speech (e.g., frequent derailment or incoherence)
    4. Grossly disorganized or catatonic behavior
    5. Negative symptoms, i.e., affective flattening, alogia, or avolition

Note: Only one criterion A symptom is required if delusions are bizarre or hallucinations consist of a voice keeping up a running commentary on the person's behavior or thoughts or two or more voices conversing with each other.

B. Social/occupational dysfunction: For a significant portion of the time since the onset of the disturbance, one or more major areas of functioning such as work, interpersonal relations, or self-care are markedly below the level achieved prior to the onset (or when the onset is in childhood or adolescence, failure to achieve expected level of interpersonal, academic, or occupational achievement).

C. Duration: Continuous signs of the disturbance persist for at least 6 months. This 6-month period must include at least 1 month of symptoms (or less if successfully treated) that meet criterion A (i.e., active-phase symptoms) and may include periods of prodromal or residual symptoms. During these prodromal or residual periods, the signs of the disturbance may be manifested by only negative symptoms or two or more symptoms listed in criterion A present in an attenuated form (e.g., odd beliefs, unusual perceptual experiences).

D. Schizoaffective and mood disorder exclusion: Schizoaffective disorder and mood disorder with psychotic features have been ruled out because either (1) no major depressive, manic, or mixed episodes have occurred concurrently with the active-phase symptoms or (2) if mood episodes have occurred during active-phase symptoms, their total duration has been brief relative to the duration of the active and residual periods.

E. Substance/general medical condition exclusion: The disturbance is not due to the direct physiological effects of a substance (e.g., a drug of abuse, a medication) or a general medical condition.

F. Relationship to a pervasive development disorder: If there is a history of autistic disorder or another pervasive development disorder, the additional diagnosis of schizophrenia is made only if prominent delusions or hallucinations are also present for at least a month (or less if successfully treated).

---

disorder, female sex, lower socioeconomic status, and having never married or been a parent (Pearlson and Rabins, 1988; Pearlson and Petty, 1994). In nearly all patients with schizophrenia, the presence of psychotic symptoms is associated with decline in the activities of daily living, poor social adjustment, and maladaptive interpersonal skills.

For many elderly schizophrenic patients who had been living alone, entry into the communal setting of a nursing home may be particularly stressful and lead to increased paranoid thoughts and an exacerbation of psychotic symptomatology. Some residents may have been admitted to the nursing home after many years of living in a public psychiatric hospital. Such "deinstitutionalized" patients may manifest relatively severe tardive dyskinesia secondary to extensive exposure to neuroleptic medications or may appear exceptionally withdrawn or disheveled.

The seemingly "odd" behavior of newly admitted residents with chronic schizo-phrenia may contribute to further social isolation within the long-term care setting. Mosher-Ashley and colleagues (1991) reported that nearly 75% of surveyed administrators of nursing and rest homes felt that they did not have adequate support services to adequately care for previously admitted chronic mentally ill elderly and were thus not inclined to pursue additional admissions of a similar type.

Delusional Disorder

A number of investigators have highlighted the occurrence of persistent delusional thinking of late onset in the relative absence of prominent hallucinations and thought disorder (Kay and Roth, 1961; Flint et al., 1991). While the most promi-nent beliefs are persecutory, some patients primarily voice erotomanic, jealous, or somatic delusional themes. The delusions are generally nonbizarre—i.e., the delusional belief is something that could potentially occur in a real-life situation (spouse is unfaithful, patient is being watched by a neighbor, and so on). The relationship of this disorder to LOS or occult medical conditions such as subclini-cal cerebrovascular disease remains open to further clarification.

Mood Disorders with Psychotic Features

Delusions occasionally complicate the course of a severe major depressive episode that has been evolving for at least several weeks. Delusional beliefs in this context are typically described as "mood-congruent," emphasizing their relationship to a dysphoric or sad mood. Patients will characteristically voice the delusional belief that they have committed some unpardonable sin, express unremitting guilt about an imagined act, or perhaps complain that they are dying from an undiscovered ailment. Delusions of poverty in which individuals incorrectly believe that they have no money, clothing, or insurance are also seen. Occasion-ally, there may be mood-congruent paranoid thoughts. Hallucinations in this context are uncommon, but when they are present, they most typically consist of voices admonishing the patient. Other symptoms of major depression such as anhedonia, alterations in sleep and appetite, recurrent thoughts of death, and psychomotor retardation are invariably present and dominate the clinical presentation.

During a manic episode, the patient may endorse grandiose delusions in which there is the false belief that he or she possesses extraordinary talents, has excep-tional wealth, or has been given a "special mission in life." Occasionally, such patients voice paranoid concerns as well. There is often evidence of associated pressured speech, hyperactivity, irritability, flight of ideas, and diminished need for sleep. Patients may also acknowledge that their thoughts are racing. (The reader is referred to Chapter 6 for a more thorough discussion of mood disorders in the long-term-care setting.)

Medical Causes of Psychosis

Psychotic symptoms in the elderly nursing home resident may arise from a variety of systemic medical illnesses (Cummings, 1985b; Nasrallah, 1992), sensory impairment (Pearlson and Rabins, 1988), and stroke (Robinson and Forrester, 1987) (Table 8.2). Most commonly, delusions and hallucinations in the long-term-care setting accompany dementing disorders such as Alzheimer's disease and vascular dementia (Rovner et al., 1986; Morriss et al., 1990). In this context, delusional themes largely revolve around theft, abandonment, and the belief that one must leave the facility in order to see deceased parents or children. (A more detailed discussion of psychosis complicating dementia appears in Chapter 4.) In delirium, the onset of visual or auditory hallucinations is often quite abrupt and is accompanied by deterioration and fluctuation in the patient's arousal level, attentional abilities, sleep/wake cycle, psychomotor activity, and cognitive capacity. Other signs of delirium are also frequently present. In dementia, the emergence of hallucinations is rarely as acute and fulminant as in delirium. (The reader is referred to Chapter 5 for more information about delirium.)

TABLE 8.2.   Medical Causes of Psychosis

Cerebrovascular disease
Head trauma
Neoplasms
Seizures
Alzheimer's disease
Pick's disease
Extrapyramidal disorders
CNS infections
Demyelinating disorders
Hydrocephalus
Uremia
Liver failure
Collagen vascular disorders (systemic lupus erythematosus, temporal arteritis, sarcoidosis)
Electrolyte imbalance
Hypo- and hyperthyroidism
Hypo- and hyperparathyroidism
Hypo- and hyperadrenocorticism
Thiamine deficiency
Folic acid deficiency
Vitamin B_{12} deficiency
Niacin deficiency

TABLE 8.3.   Medications That Cause Psychosis

Anticholinergics
Dopaminergics
Steroids
Stimulants
Digoxin
Cimetidine
Benzodiazepines
Anticonvulsants
Lidocaine
Procainamide

Occasionally, medications can also give rise to psychotic symptoms in the elderly without overt evidence of delirium (Cummings, 1985; Nasrallah, 1992) (Table 8.3).

The role of sensory impairment in the etiology of psychotic symptoms warrants additional consideration. Specifically, the presence of hearing impairment (particularly conduction loss) and visual deficits (e.g., occurring secondarily to cataracts or macular degeneration) facilitate the emergence of auditory and visual hallucinations respectively. Coupled with social isolation, sensory misperceptions and hallucinations may give rise to delusional thoughts (Pearlson and Rabins, 1988; Pearlson and Petty, 1994).

Evaluation of Psychosis

The assessment of delusions and hallucinations requires consistent observation of the resident's verbal and nonverbal behavior complemented by the conduct of a formal mental status examination. The resident's cognitive ability, mood state, thought content, thought process, insight, and judgment must all be thoroughly evaluated and documented. This procedure should be performed by a sufficiently trained professional upon the individual's admission to the nursing home and at regular intervals thereafter. For some residents, the presence of paranoid thoughts may initially be manifest by an increasing tendency to remain in one's room and avoid contact with others. In other affected individuals, paranoid concerns may first appear as antecedents to aggressive behavior directed toward other residents or staff. Those residents who are still able to express themselves relatively clearly may voice their concerns directly; others may appear especially guarded, hypervigilant, or anxious. Unless residents are specifically queried, many delusional beliefs will go unnoticed by nursing home personnel (Morriss et al., 1990). Thus, hallucinations and delusions should be considered in the differential diagnosis of any unusual behavior or behavior change that occurs in the nursing home.

TABLE 8.4.   Evaluation of Psychosis

Review of present and past psychotic symptoms

Review of medical history
    Mental status examination to assess
      Cognitive ability (including arousal and attention)
      Mood state
      Content of psychosis
    Physical and neurological examinations to identify
      Systemic illnesses
      Focal neurological features
      Sensory impairment
    Review of medications
    Laboratory studies, including
      Electrolytes
      Urinalysis
      Liver functions
      Renal functions
      Nutritional status
      Hematological status
    Neuroimaging studies (computed tomography or magnetic
      resonance imaging of brain) to evaluate for
      Stroke
      Tumor
      Hydrocephalus

Many residents will not spontaneously report their hallucinatory experiences. Often, nursing home staff will notice that a resident is having a discussion with himself, perhaps signifying the presence of auditory hallucinations. Other residents may appear to be seeing something that has commanded their attention but is invisible to observers. Once it has been established that psychotic symptoms are present, it is imperative that, prior to defining treatment, a differential diagnosis be generated. This typically consists of identifying whether the symptoms are primary manifestations of dementia, delirium, schizophrenia, delusional disorder, or major mood disturbance or are secondary to the toxic effects of medication, sensory impairment, or an occult medical illness. (See Table 8.4.)

Treatment Considerations

Treatment of psychotic symptoms involves psychotherapeutic supportive techniques aimed at reducing the resident's associated anxiety (Chapter 13) and, if necessary, the judicious use of neuroleptic medications (Chapter 3). This latter intervention is appropriate only if the symptoms are of sufficient intensity to consistently upset the individual, place the patient or others at risk of harm, or significantly disrupt the nursing home milieu. It is essential that nursing home staff recognize that individuals experiencing psychotic symptoms are often quite anxious, fearful, distressed, and bewildered by their experiences.

It is rarely helpful to attempt to confront or contradict a delusional belief directly. Usually this has been tried several times without effect by staff or family. A more desirable approach is for the staff to acknowledge the distress the resident is experiencing as a result of the psychotic symptoms, offer reassurance, and distract the individual's attention to another matter. Treatment of any identified underlying cause of psychosis is paramount and may consist of the optimization of hearing and visual acuity, management of a systemic illness, dose reduction or termination of offending medications, or aggressive treatment of a major mood disorder.

References

APA. *Diagnostic and Statistical Manual of Mental Disorders,* 4th ed. Washington, DC: American Psychiatric Association, 1994.

Castle DJ, Howard R. What do we know about the aetiology of late-onset schizophrenia? *Eur Psychiatry* 7:99–108, 1992.

Chandler JD, Chandler JE. The prevalence of neuropsychiatric disorders in a nursing home population. *J Geriatr Psychiatry Neurol* 1:71–76, 1988.

Cummings JL. *Clinical Neuropsychiatry.* Orlando, FL: Grune & Stratton, 1985a.

Cummings JL. Organic delusions: Phenomenology, anatomical correlations and review. *Br J Psychiatry* 146:184–197, 1985b.

Flint AJ, Rifat SL, Eastwood MR. Late-onset paranoia: Distinct from paraphrenia? *Int J Geriatr Psychiatry* 6:103–109, 1991.

Grahame PS. Schizophrenia in old age (late paraphrenia). *Br J Psychiatry* 145:493–495, 1984.

Harris MJ, Jeste DV. Late-onset schizophrenia: An overview. *Schizophr Bull* 14:39–55, 1988.

Holden NL. Late paraphrenia or the paraphrenias? A descriptive study with a 10 year follow-up. *Br J Psychiatry* 150:635–639, 1987.

Jeste DV, Manley M, Harris MJ. Psychoses; In: Sadavoy J, Lazarus L, Jarvik L, eds. *Comprehensive Review of Geriatric Psychiatry.* Washington, DC: American Psychiatric Press, 1991:353–368.

Junginger J, Phelan E, Cherry K, et al. Prevalence of psychopathology in elderly persons in nursing homes and in the community. *Hosp Commun Psychiatry* 44:381–383, 1993.

Kay DWK, Roth M. Environmental and hereditary factors in the schizophrenias of old age (''late paraphrenia'') and their bearing on the general problem of causation in schizophrenia. *J Mental Sci* 107:649–686, 1961.

Morriss RK, Rovner BW, Folstein MF, et al. Delusions in newly admitted residents of nursing homes. *Am J Psychiatry* 147:299–302, 1990.

Mosher-Ashley PM, Turner BF, O'Neill D. Attitudes of nursing and rest home administrators toward deinstitutionalized elders with psychiatric disorders. *Commun Mental Health J* 27:241–253, 1991.

Nasrallah HA. Neuropsychiatry of schizophrenia. In: Hales RE, Yudofsky SC eds. *Textbook of Neuropsychiatry.* Washington DC: American Psychiatric Press, 1992: 621–638.

Pearlson GD, Petty RG. Late-life-onset psychoses. In: Coffey CE, Cummings JL, eds. *Textbook of Geriatric Neuropsychiatry*. Washington DC: American Psychiatric Press, 1994:261–277.

Pearlson GD, Rabins PV. The late onset psychoses: Possible risk factors. *Psychiatr Clin North Am* 11:15–33, 1988.

Pearlson GD, Dreger L, Rabins PV, et al. A chart review study of late-onset and early onset schizophrenia. *Am J Psychiatry* 146:1568–1574, 1989.

Robinson RG, Forrester AW. Neuropsychiatric aspects of cerebrovascular disease. In: Hales RE, Yudofsky SC, eds. *Textbook of Neuropsychiatry*. Washington DC: American Psychiatric Press, 1987:191–208.

Rovner BW, Kafonek S, Filipp L, et al. Prevalence of mental illness in a community nursing home. *Am J Psychiatry* 143:1446–1449, 1986.

Wragg R, Jeste DV. An overview of depression and psychosis in Alzheimer's disease. *Am J Psychiatry* 146:577–587, 1989.

9

Sleep Disorders

Donald L. Bliwise

The sleep patterns of patients in nursing homes are often profoundly disturbed. In fact, sleep disturbance has been shown in several studies to be a powerful predictor of eventual institutionalization (Pollak et al., 1990; Pollak and Perlick, 1991). It creates a major burden for caregivers (Gallagher-Thompson et al., 1992)—one that may exceed cognitive loss as a stressor. The separation of the many factors that may affect observed sleep disturbance in the nursing home is complicated and requires consideration of obvious influences, such as the impact of neurodegenerative disease per se on sleep patterns, and also of less easily appreciated factors characteristic of the experience of institutionalization, including prolonged bed rest, decreased exposure to outdoor sunlight, unvarying routine, and frank boredom (see Table 9.1).

The Effects of Institutionalization on Sleep

Few studies have actually examined the effects of institutionalization per se on sleep patterns or circadian rhythms in elderly demented patients. Some literature on young adults, however, has documented the disruptive effects of prolonged bed rest on polysomnographically recorded sleep patterns. Campbell (1984) reported that when young, healthy adults were confronted with having to spend 60 consecutive hours in bed, their sleep became fragmented and they underwent shorter sleep "bouts." In an earlier study over a much longer period of time (56 days), Winget et al. (1972) noted that prolonged bed rest was associated with a decline in the robustness of the circadian body temperature cycle. Additionally, absence of exercise in young adults who were typically physically active was

Table 9.1.   Causes of Disturbed Sleep in Nursing Home Residents

Degenerative neurologic disease
Chronic pain
Medications, particularly those with stimulant properties
Nocturia
Restless legs syndrome
Anxiety and depression
Insufficient daytime light exposure
Minimal physical activity
Inadvertent noise
Greater susceptibility to external arousal
Increased sympathetic tone
Parasomnias (REM behavior disorder, nocturnal paroxysmal dystonia)

associated with greater wakefulness at night (Baekeland, 1970). The implications of these studies in healthy young adults subjected to restrictions in daytime activity for the infirm geriatric population in long-term-care environments are profound. Aerobic exercise and even simple physical activity are powerful synchronizers of the sleep-wake cycle. Without access to such stimuli, the sleep of nursing home patients is likely to fragment (Ancoli-Israel et al., 1989b). It is important to stress that access to activity as a potential synchronizing influence on the sleep/wake cycle is fundamentally a biological and only secondarily a social/psychological effect. For example, elegant animal models have been developed that show a desynchronizing influence of activity restriction in rodent species induced merely by locking a running wheel (Edgar and Dement, 1991).

Another model for the sleep disturbance observed in nursing home patients is the disturbed sleep seen in patients in the acute care hospital setting. Following surgery, for example, patients have been shown seldom to obtain more than 20 to 30 minutes of uninterrupted sleep at a time (McFadden and Giblin, 1971). In a later study in a surgical intensive care unit (ICU), Aurell and Elmqvist (1985) reported that during the first few days in such units, patients averaged less than 2 hours of sleep per night, due to frequent interruptions. Although patients in the nursing home environment might be expected to be subjected to far less frequent staff interruptions than patients in the ICU, the frequent interruptions caused by staff and other disruptive patients can lead to sleep fragmentation. Furthermore, at least two recent studies of nursing home patients suggest that the commonly accepted practice of bed checks every 2 hours may lead directly to disruptive behavior (Evans, 1987; Cohen-Mansfield, 1990a). More recently, Schnelle et al. (1993a,b) have raised the possibility that some of these awakenings, typically made to prevent pressure sores secondary to incontinence, could be eliminated or dramatically reduced, thereby increasing the potential for uninterrupted sleep in the nursing home environment.

A final potent environmental influence on the disturbed sleep of the patient in the nursing home environment is reduced illumination. High levels of illumination, typically 2500 lux, are typically required in humans to suppress melatonin and drive the sleep-wake cycle. Animals subjected to dim light over long periods of time demonstrate considerable disruption of their circadian sleep/wake cycle, and the human circadian system has been shown to be extremely sensitive to brief pulses of light, although that sensitivity appears related to phase of the temperature cycle and adequate transduction through the retina (Czeisler et al., 1989). Patients indoors in the typical nursing home environment receive low levels of light (Ancoli-Israel et al., 1991a). In our own data, the highest recorded illumination level in nursing home patients during the autumn was 1258 lux. During the winter, the highest light level detected was 554 lux (Bliwise et al., 1993). In fact, increases in agitation and reductions in observed sleep during the winter months may have been due to such alterations in illumination. Even ambulatory Alzheimer's disease patients not living in institutions, who presumably have greater access to the outdoors, are exposed, on average, to far lower levels of illumination than are nondemented elderly controls (Campbell et al., 1988). The implications of this decreased exposure to light, together with decreased physical activity, increased bed rest, and frequent interruptions by staff experienced by the typical nursing home patient, are to make sleep disturbance in this environment a highly prevalent phenomenon. It is, therefore, not surprising that, up until the recent Omnibus Budget Reconciliation Act (OBRA) guidelines were established, the prevalence of hypnotic medication use in the nursing home environment approximated 35% (Morgan, 1987).

Sleep in Normal Aging and Dementia

Polysomnographic sleep characteristics in dementias have been reviewed in detail elsewhere and are reviewed only briefly here (Bliwise, 1993, 1994). To summarize, most of these studies have demonstrated that patients with Alzheimer's disease (AD) have significantly less slow-wave sleep (SWS) than age-matched controls and also have lower sleep efficiency (i.e., the proportion of time in bed actually spent asleep). Changes in rapid-eye-movement (REM) sleep, at least as quantified as the proportion of sleep spent in REM (REM %), show only equivocal changes in AD, though other aspects of REM sleep (density of eye movements in REM, time to initial REM period at the beginning of the night, REM latency) may show reductions or diminutions, consistent with widespread cholinergic deterioration characteristic of AD. Some studies have even demonstrated that the decreases in SWS and sleep efficiency seen in AD show direct parallels with the severity of dementia as revealed by the Folstein Mini-Mental State Exam or the Mattis Dementia Rating Scale (Prinz et al., 1982b; Vitiello et al., 1990). Generally speaking, sleep architecture in other types of dementia common for the geriatric population (Parkinson's disease, vascular dementia) shows similar changes, although in the case of Parkinson's disease (PD), confounds from medication status often make it difficult to examine the disease-related changes in sleep per se. For example, one recent study examining 26 drug-free PD patients showed far fewer changes in sleep architecture than prior studies that included patients receiving medication (e.g., levodopa/carbidopa) (Ferini-Strambi et al., 1992).

Data conflict as to whether patients with vascular dementia differ in the extent of their sleep disturbance relative to patients with Alzheimer's disease, with one study showing few differences (Allen et al., 1987) and another study suggesting greater sleep fragmentation in vascular cases (Aharon-Peretz et al., 1991).

Although degenerative conditions of the central nervous system play a major role in the sleep disturbance seen in nursing home patients, it should not be assumed that other psychiatric disorders can be ignored. For example, Reynolds et al. (1988a) reported that patients with depressive pseudodementia typically have more disturbed sleep than patients with dementia and that this difference was detectable on brief bedside examination. Polysomnographic studies have also confirmed that depressed geriatric patients have more disturbed sleep than Alzheimer's patients (Reynolds et al., 1988b).

In addition to studies of polysomnographically defined sleep stages and sleep architecture, a small number of studies have attempted to examine circadian rhythms in demented patients (e.g., Touitou, 1982). These studies have shown that, in the small number of patients and physiological variables studied to date, circadian rhythms of body temperature, melatonin, cortisol, luteinizing hormone (LH), and follicle-stimulating hormone (FSH) appear intact in dementia (typically AD) cases.

With rare exception, the studies cited above have involved noninstitutionalized individuals residing at home with spouse and/or other caregiver(s). Far fewer studies of sleep and circadian rhythms have been performed in nursing home patients. An obvious issue in all research studies of sleep and rhythms in dementia is the issue of compliance. Profoundly demented patients in long-term care are not likely to accept wearing electrodes and other sensors for overnight polysomnography. Similarly, use of rectal temperature probes to record the body temperature rhythm or placement of indwelling venous catheters for studies of circadian rhythms of hormone release are not likely to be well tolerated by most nursing home patients.

Sleep Apnea in the Nursing Home

Sleep apnea is a disorder characterized by impaired respiration in sleep. Frequent episodes of apnea or hypopnea (the latter defined by reduction in tidal volumes) occur repetitively throughout the night and are often associated with hypoxemia and cardiac arrhythmias. Large negative intrathoracic pressures, generated during inspiratory efforts against a closed upper airway, may result in increased work of the left ventricle. The two cardinal symptoms of sleep apnea are (1) snoring, choking, or gasping for breath during sleep and (2) tiredness, fatigue, and excessive sleepiness during the day. For both of these sets of symptoms, reports of family members or caregivers may be as valuable as the patient's own history, this being particularly true in the nursing home setting.

Over the last 10 years there has been increased recognition that the prevalence of sleep apnea increases with age (Bliwise et al., 1992). The first evidence of such an age-related prevalence were the snoring data of Lugaresi et al. (1980), who noted that the prevalence of self-reported snoring increases with age in both men and women, although the prevalence was higher for males at every age. The best evidence of the actual prevalence of sleep apnea in geriatric populations comes from a study of Ancoli-Israel et al. (1991c). Using an ambulatory recording system, they reported that among an independently living population of individuals over the age of 65 residing in San Diego, about 1 in 4 evidenced an Apnea Index of greater than 5 events per hour of sleep. Perhaps more relevant for an institutionalized population are data suggesting that the corresponding figure for sleep apnea prevalence in a nursing home population is 43% (Ancoli-Israel et al., 1989a). Moreover, the presence of sleep apnea in this particular nursing home population was associated with mortality; residents with sleep apnea died sooner after testing (about 200 days) than residents without sleep apnea (about 1200 days). Whether sleep apnea itself was the relevant risk factor for this excess mortality or whether some other set of risk factors may have been responsible could not be evaluated in this study.

Regardless of the status of these inconclusive results, it is quite clear that disturbed respiration in sleep is a common event in nursing home patients. In our own studies, relying on careful behavioral observations of sleeping residents and not involving physiological monitoring (Carroll et al., 1989; Bliwise et al., 1990b), we were able to reliably and easily detect such events in these patients. A prior study comparing observations of sleep apnea and polysomnography in inpatients showed that false positives were rare in making such identifications, though observations missed a good deal of the apnea that occurred (Haponik et al., 1984). Among the variables investigated, observed sleep apnea was the most powerful and consistent predictor of quantity of sleep in the nursing home (Bliwise et al., 1990b). This relationship (individuals with sleep apnea sleeping more) was seen both during nocturnal and daytime hours. These results were independent of level of dementia and use of psychoactive/analgesic medication. The findings imply that much of the daytime sleepiness and excessive napping seen in nursing home patients could be due to this specific pathophysiological cause, though factors such as sleep fragmentation and disruption of circadian rhythms cannot be discounted.

The reasons why sleep apnea is associated with excessive daytime sleepiness have been debated vigorously throughout the years but probably involve some combination of two separate factors: nocturnal oxygen desaturation and sleep fragmentation. When an individual experiences minute after minute of repetitive oxygen desaturation, each event ending in an arousal, the cumulative effect of hundreds of such episodes, occurring night after night, year after year, can result in profound and disabling impairment of daytime alertness. Neither of these phenomena in themselves, however, can be totally responsible for daytime sleepiness. Individuals may be chronically hypoxemic without hypersomnolence—such as patients with chronic obstructive pulmonary disease (COPD) (Orr et al., 1990)—just as there are individuals who incur severe sleep fragmentation (chronic insomniacs) who are not at all hypersomnolent (Seidel et al., 1984).

There is some very preliminary evidence that sleep apnea, if left untreated in the geriatric population, may result in a syndrome of mental impairment (Bliwise, 1989, 1991, 1993). In fact, in the study of nursing home patients mentioned above, measures of sleep apnea were correlated with scores on the Dementia Rating Scale (Ancoli-Israel et al., 1991b). Nonetheless, the situation may actually be quite complicated, since several studies of sleep apnea in Alzheimer's disease have not demonstrated a higher rate of sleep apnea than in aged-matched controls (Smallwood et al., 1983; Bliwise et al., 1987). Other studies have suggested higher rates of sleep apnea in AD in women (Hoch et al., 1986), though the magnitude of the effect was small (Bliwise, 1993). A more likely possibility is that sleep apnea could be related to stroke or vascular dementia (Bliwise, 1993).

Given the range of morbidity and possible mortality associated with sleep apnea and its widespread occurrence in the nursing home population, the obvious question arises as to whether diagnosis and treatment of the probably vast numbers of individuals in long-term care who have the condition is necessary, advisable, or even possible. The availability of pulse oximetry opens the possibility that suspected patients could be screened easily relative to study with full overnight polysomnography (Douglas et al., 1992; Series et al., 1993). Despite the relative ease of this type of screening, considerable controversy exists as to whether sufficient information is obtained with such approaches and whether such procedures are ultimately cost-effective (Pack, 1993). Apart from these diagnostic issues, a decision to actually treat sleep apnea in an institutionalized geriatric patient must be based on quality-of-life issues and the likelihood that the patients and their families would benefit from such a decision. Controlled clinical trials for sleep apnea treatment are not yet available.

If the decision is made to treat, the most unambiguously successful treatment for sleep apnea is the use of nasal continuous positive airway pressure (CPAP), which provides a pneumatic splint to the upper airway in order to maintain patency during negative inspiratory pressure. For the institutionalized geriatric population, CPAP represents the only aggressive treatment option. Other procedures (uvulopalatopharyngoplasty or other soft tissue surgery or hyoid suspension with mandibular advancement), which may be options in younger patients, are simply not advised for the frail and infirm geriatric population. Conservative measures such as avoidance of the supine position may also be considered in mild cases, but it is effective only if the apnea is known to have a positional component. Weight loss is another option, though weight loss in the frail elderly may be a harbinger of declining physical health and may not always be a desired outcome.

Descriptive Studies of Sleep in Nursing Home Patients

There have been a number of descriptive studies of the sleep of institutionalized patients. It should be emphasized that many of these studies have relied upon alternative methods for their data collection, though at least a few studies using polysomnography have been reported (Prinz et al., 1982a; Allen et al., 1983, 1987). As with polysomnographic studies of ambulatory, independently living demented patients, these polysomnographic studies confirm absence of stages 3 and 4 sleep, highly fragmented nocturnal sleep, and a tendency for greater daytime napping. In one report (Allen et al., 1987), the quantity of daytime sleep exceeded the quantity of nighttime sleep in 3 of 30 patients. This observation is consistent with a reduction in the amplitude of the circadian sleep/wake rhythm due to changes in the endogenous "biological clock," which is seen to a less dramatic extent in normal aging (Bliwise, 1993). No polysomnographic studies have documented changes in sleep/wakefulness prior to and after institutionalization.

Studies examining sleep patterns of geriatric patients residing in nursing homes and other long-term-care facilities have used a variety of techniques. Several studies have used the self-report of presumably nondemented nursing home patients to inquire about sleep patterns. Cohen et al. (1983), for example, reported that nurses' judgments and residents' reports were often considerably different regarding the quality of sleep experienced. Ferm (1974) also reported that nurses' global judgments of patients' sleep quality were unrelated to level of dementia, a finding since disproven by the carefully performed polysomnographic work of Prinz and Vitiello and colleagues (Prinz et al., 1982a,b; Vitiello et al., 1990). The only study presenting empirical data on sleep patterns prior and subsequent to institutionalization was that of Clapin-French (1986), who reported that self-reports of daytime napping, nocturnal sleep disturbance, and earlier bedtimes were associated with institutionalization in a group of 102 relatively cognitively intact aged individuals following admission to a long-term-care environment. Most of these alterations in sleep were attributed to adaptation to the noise, lighting, and invariant routine of the facility. These self-report data are in essential agreement with the data on lighting and confined bed rest presented above.

For obvious reasons, reliance upon nursing home patients' self-reports, particularly when patients may be demented and unable to communicate clearly, may be of questionable validity. Another approach used to examine sleep patterns in nursing home patients has involved systematic behavioral observations. For example, following the early study of Webb and Swinburne (1971), who reported extensive napping among nursing home residents, a number of studies have relied upon behavioral observations to investigate sleep in such environments. In their early study of the circadian rhythms of a wise variety of physiological functions in nursing home patients, Scheving et al. (1974) reported that these patients appeared to have considerable asynchrony among peak levels of body temperature; blood pressure and urinary potassium; as well as sodium, chloride, and norepinephrine relative to younger individuals. Among the more recent studies, a number of results relevant for long-term care have emerged. In one study observing patients once an hour, Regestein and Morris (1987) reported that sleep at night and sleep during the day appeared to be positively correlated. However, in a later study using more frequent behavioral observation (four times an hour, totaling over 240 hours of observation), Bliwise et al. (1990a) reported that observed sleep during the day was inversely related to sleep at night. Thus, not only did a daytime nap portend greater likelihood of wakefulness on the subsequent night, but observed episodes of wakefulness at night predicted greater sleepiness the subsequent day. Daytime sleepiness and nocturnal awakenings represent components of a vicious cycle, the consequences of which are disrupted and fragmented alertness throughout the 24-hour day. It is of considerable interest that in nondemented elderly individuals living independently, avoidance of daytime napping together with a curtailment of excessive time in bed over a period of 1 month was effective in increasing reported total sleep time by nearly an hour (Friedman et al., 1991). With careful supervision and monitoring by nursing staff, there is no reason why such a behavioral intervention might not work well in an institutionalized population, though the curtailment of daytime sleep may take substantial ''hands-on'' efforts by staff (Bliwise et al., 1990c).

Other behavioral observations of sleep in nursing home patients have confirmed that substantial individual differences in such sleep patterns exist (Meguro et al., 1990), with some patients demonstrating substantially greater amounts of sleep around the 24-hour day relative to other patients. In another study, we showed that sleep apnea was a major predictor of amount of observed sleep in nursing home patients, followed to a lesser degree by presence of cardiovascular/pulmonary disease, higher level of dementia, and higher rather than lower functional capacity, the latter thought to reflect the disruptive influence of the higher number of staff interactions required in more incapacitated patients (Bliwise et al., 1990b). Curiously, in this study, use of psychotropic/analgesic medication was not predictive of amount of observed sleep, even though, in ambulatory geriatric populations, use of benzodiazepines with long elimination half-lives, for example, has been associated with excessive daytime somnolence (Carskadon et al., 1982).

Systematic behavioral observations of sleep/wakefulness have thus seen considerable usage in the nursing home environment. Such observations can be made reliably (Carroll et al., 1989; Bliwise et al., 1990a), and they avoid ambiguous interpretation of electroencephalographic patterns of diffuse theta and delta. Furthermore, they have received some validation with use of ambulatory activity and respiratory sensors (Cohen-Mansfield et al., 1990b). Nonetheless, other approaches to the measurement of sleep/wakefulness in nursing home patients have been made. Ancoli-Israel and colleagues have performed extensive studies of sleep patterns in nursing home patients using wrist actigraphy (Ancoli-Israel et al., 1989b; Jacobs et al., 1989). The results of these studies compliment the behavioral observation studies to the extent that, for the subset of patients studied over periods of 24-hours, not a single patient remained awake an entire hour during the day and not a single patient remained asleep an entire hour during the night (Jacobs et al., 1989).

The Problem of Sundowning

That certain patients become more confused, agitated, and delirious at night has been recognized since the time of Hippocrates (Lipowski, 1980, 1989). In the nursing home, the term "sundowning" has been used extensively to refer to the phenomenon of agitation seemingly caused by, or at least strongly associated with, darkness. Although many textbooks continue to use this term (e.g., Kane et al., 1984), definitions of what sundowning is, whom it affects, precisely when it occurs (near the actual time of sunset or at night in general), why it occurs, and, indeed, if the phenomenon exists at all are absent in the existing literature. Though some have disputed the existence of the phenomenon (Exum et al., 1993), the persistent issue of nocturnal behavioral disturbance in the long-term-care environment permeates the nursing literature (e.g., Gress et al., 1981; Gall et al., 1990; Paiva, 1990) and suggests and empiric basis for its occurrence.

A discussion regarding sundowning invariably raises the issue of delirium. "Delirium" is a psychiatric diagnosis, not a description of behavior. As such, DSM-IV (APA, 1994) defines this state as one of disturbed consciousness and changed cognition subject to and even defined by diurnal variability and refers to presumed etiology for the condition. While some convergence with sundowning is undeniable, "delirium" is more descriptive and less explanatory. In addition, even in its most precise operationalization, this term requires that symptoms be present at any time over a 24-hour period (Liptzin et al., 1991). With such a broad time referent, the diagnosis of delirium cannot be examined over brief periods of time—e.g., hours or minutes. (The reader is referred to Chapter 5 for a more detailed discussion of delirium.)

The simplest and most direct way to investigate sundowning would be to use reliable behavioral rating scales in order to systematically and repeatedly observe demented individuals. Such rating scales by necessity must be temporally precise and delimited, since, in fact, time itself becomes the independent variable of primary interest. There exist few studies that have attempted to use temporal delineation in such behavioral ratings. Evans (1987) reported that 11 of 89 nursing home patients could be classified as demonstrating sundowning; however, her data were based on two 10-minute observation windows occurring at any point between 1000 and 1200 hours and between 1600 and 1800 on two separate days. It was unclear what happened to patients during the remainder of the 2-hour window when observations were not made, the remaining hours of the 24-hour day outside the 2-hour window, and over the days when observations were not performed. Nonetheless, this study revealed a number of interesting findings, including the demonstration of an association between sundowning and recent room transfers, more severe level of dementia, incontinence, and greater number of medical diagnoses. Although limited in data collection, the Evans study represented the first attempt to evaluate the prevalence and factors associated with sundowning since the early anecdotal observations of Cameron (1941), who claimed that sundowning could be induced by bringing demented patients into a dark room during the daytime. This latter study was poorly controlled and has never been replicated.

More recently Cohen-Mansfield and colleagues, working with the construct of agitation in nursing home patients, have reported data on time-of-day effects with possible relevance for sundowning. In one study based on retrospective

2-week ratings with the Cohen-Mansfield Agitation Inventory (CMAI), the investigators examined prevalence of agitation as a function of shift (Cohen-Mansfield et al., 1988). Results indicated that all types of agitation were more common on the day shift than on the evening and night shifts. Because patients were more likely to be asleep at night, however, it is unclear whether these results might have been secondary to this. Using a somewhat different approach involving the Agitated Behavioral Mapping Instrument (ABMI), which was used to make ratings 3 minutes of every hour over 24 hours a day, Cohen-Mansfield et al. (1989) reported that 2 of 8 AD patients showed a distinctively nocturnal pattern of agitation, 2 patients showed a predominantly morning pattern, and the remainder showed no time-linked pattern. In a later study of 24 patients, Cohen-Mansfield et al. (1992) reported similar grouping of patients. Using a time-lapse videotape monitoring system, Martino-Saltzman et al. (1991) reported that "inefficient" travel behavior in nursing home patients (i.e., wandering) was most likely to occur from 1900 to 2200. A recently reported study of home-residing Alzheimer's patients whose behaviors over a 48-hour period were recorded by caregivers suggested that maladaptive, repetitive physical behaviors were most likely between 1600 and 2000 (O'Leary et al., 1993).

In our own studies employing systematic around-the-clock observations of nursing home patients (Bliwise et al., 1990a)—using specially trained research assistants observing 24 nursing home residents four times an hour, 24 hours a day, over a 10-day period—we noted that sleep was less likely in the 1500-to-1900 time block. These times included sunset over the weeks of observation, and this suggested apparent corroboration for the notion that sunset itself may be a vulnerable period for agitation. Another more mundane possibility to account for this pattern was that dinner served during that period represented a disruptive influence. The argument against this possibility was that a similar pattern was not seen during the time blocks when lunch was served. Similar vulnerability of the late afternoon hours for wakefulness in nursing home patients was noted by Jacobs et al. (1989) using a wrist actigraph and in Alzheimer's patients residing at home as reported by caregivers (O'Leary et al., 1993).

Our original studies did not assess agitation, only sleep and wakefulness. However, more recently, we have found (Bliwise et al., 1993), using a 12-hour observation window (from 1300 to 0100) and a similar frequency of behavioral observation, that while wakefulness was less likely during the period of sunset (sunset +/− 2 hours), agitation was no more likely to occur at that time than earlier in the afternoon or later at night. Thus, these results did not confirm the existence of sundowning in a group of 9 agitated patients using a reliable, temporally specific rating of patients' behavior. Using a systematic analysis of "as needed" (prn) medication intake, Exum et al. (1993) were also unable to document the existence of this phenomenon and instead attributed sundowning to shift changes, number of staff, and existing standing medication orders. (See Chapter 2 for a complete discussion of disruptive behavior.)

Despite the Exum et al. (1993) results suggesting otherwise, medication, typically neuroleptics, have been used on a prn basis in the nursing home to treat episodes of nocturnal agitation. Medications such as haloperidol (0.5 mg to 1.0 mg) or thioridazine (25 mg) are often used; however, both have unfavorable side effects. Long-term use of haloperidol has been associated with tardive dyskinesia and thioridazine usage has been associated with orthostatic hypotension. It is important to note that benzodiazepines are typically unsuccessful and, in fact, may exacerbate confusion and disorientation. Some clinicians have noted anecdotal success with beta blockers such as propranolol or pindolol, particularly if the disruptive behaviors are aggressive. Regardless of the type of medication employed, compelling evidence exists that psychotropic medication in the nursing home environment is often associated with injurious falls (Granek et al., 1987) and should be used cautiously. (The reader is referred to Chapter 3 for a thorough discussion of pharmacological agents.)

Suggestions for nonpharmacological management of sundowning have been mentioned throughout this chapter but can be reiterated here (Table 9.2). Avoidance of frequent awakenings by staff has been mentioned and should be carefully considered on a case-by-case basis. Second, avoidance of daytime napping can play a major role in promoting sleep at night. The homeostatic regulation of sleep and wakefulness appears to be preserved, even in profoundly demented nursing home patients (Bliwise et al., 1990a). Third, increased exposure to illumination, typically at levels in excess of 2500 lux, may also be of help, and a number of very recent studies are now confirming the utility of such an intervention (Castor et al., 1991; Okawa et al., 1991; Satlin et al., 1992; Campbell et al., 1993). Last, if dysfunction of the circadian timing system is shown to underlie sundowning, this would imply that regulation of this system, perhaps through administration of exogenous melatonin or growth hormone releasing hormone, may also prove of benefit. Several research groups are starting preliminary trials with such substances and results should be forthcoming.

As a final note, management of the nocturnal disruptive behavior of nursing home patients may well depend upon the flexibility of facility itself to adapt to an otherwise difficult situation. Some institutions now regularly hold early morning activities therapy (e.g., 2:00 A.M.) for their patients who may otherwise be disruptive to other residents and the typically understaffed night shift. Such creative environmental solutions may well be the most expeditious solution to this recalcitrant management problem.

TABLE 9.2.   Behavioral Interventions Useful for Demented Nursing Home
Patients Agitated at Night

Prevention of daytime napping
Exposure to outdoor sunlight
Mild physical activity
Prevention of awakenings by staff or other disruptive patients
Establishment of nocturnal activity program for those patients refractory to other treatment

References

Aharon-Peretz J, Masiah A, Pillar T, et al. Sleep-wake cycles in multi-infarct dementia and dementia of the Alzheimer type. *Neurology* 41:1616–1619, 1991.

Allen SR, Seiler WO, Stahelin HB, Spiegel R. Seventy-two-hour polygraphic and behavioral recordings of wakefulness and sleep in a hospital geriatric unit: Comparison between demented and nondemented patients. *Sleep* 10:143–159, 1987.

Allen SR, Stahelin HB, Seiler WO, Spiegel R. EEG and sleep in aged hospitalized patients with senile dementia: 24-h recordings. *Experientia* 39:249–255, 1983.

Ancoli-Israel S, Jones D, Hanger M, et al. Sleep in the nursing home. In: Kuna S, Suratt P, Remmers J, eds. *Sleep and Respiration in Aging Adults.* Amsterdam: Elsevier, 1991a.

Ancoli-Israel S, Klauber MR, Butters N, et al. Dementia in institutionalized elderly: Relation to sleep apnea. *J Am Geriatr Soc* 39:258–263, 1991b.

Ancoli-Israel S, Klauber MR, Kripke DF, et al. Sleep apnea in female nursing home patients: Increased risk of mortality. *Chest* 96:1054–1058, 1989a.

Ancoli-Israel S, Kripke DF, Klauber MR, et al. Sleep disordered breathing in community dwelling elderly. *Sleep* 14:486–495, 1991c.

Ancoli-Israel S, Parker L, Sinaee R, et al. Sleep fragmentation in patients from a nursing home. *J Gerontol Med Sci* 44(1):M18–M21, 1989b.

APA. *Diagnostic and Statistical Manual of Mental Disorders,* 4th ed. Revised. Washington, DC: American Psychiatric Association, 1994.

Aurell J, Elmqvist D. Sleep in the surgical intensive care unit: Continuous polygraphic recording of sleep in nine patients receiving postoperative care. *Br Med J* 290:1029–1032, 1985.

Baekeland F. Exercise deprivation: Sleep and psychological reactions. *Arch Gen Psychiatry* 22:365–369, 1970.

Bliwise DL. Neuropsychological function and sleep. *Clin Geriatr Med* 5:381–394, 1989.

Bliwise DL. Cognitive function and SDB in aging adults. In: Kuna ST, Suratt PM, Remmers JE, eds. *Sleep and Respiration in Aging Adults.* Amsterdam: Elsevier, 1991:237–245.

Bliwise DL. Sleep in normal aging and dementia. *Sleep* 16:40–81, 1993.

Bliwise DL. Sleep in dementing illness. In: Oldham JM, Riba MB, eds. *Annual Review of Psychiatry.* Vol 13. Washington, DC: American Psychiatric Press, 1994.

Bliwise DL, Bevier WC, Bliwise NG, et al. Systematic 24-hr behavioral observations of sleep and wakefulness in a skilled care nursing facility. *Psychol Aging* 5:16–24, 1990a.

Bliwise DL, Carroll JS, Dement WC. Predictors of observed sleep/wakefulness in residents in long-term care. *J Gerontol Med Sci* 45:M126–M130, 1990b.

Bliwise DL, Nino-Murcia G, Forno LS, Visekul C. Abundant REM sleep in a patient with Alzheimer's disease. *Neurology* 40:1281–1284, 1990c.

Bliwise DL, Carroll JS, Lee KA, et al. Sleep and sundowning in nursing home patients. *Psychiatry Res* 48:277–292, 1993.

Bliwise DL, Pascualy RA, Dement WC. Sleep disorders. In: Evans JG, Williams TF, eds. *Oxford Textbook of Geriatric Medicine.* New York: Oxford University Press, 1992:507–521.

Bliwise DL, Yesavage JA, Tinklenberg J, Dement WC. Sleep apnea in Alzheimer's disease. *Neurobiol Aging* 10:343–346, 1989.

Cameron DE. Studies in senile nocturnal delirium. *Psychiatr Q* 5:47–53, 1941.

Campbell S. Duration and placement of sleep in a "disentrained" environment. *Psychophysiology* 21:106–113, 1984.

Campbell SS, Dawson D, Anderson MW. Alleviation of sleep maintenance insomnia with timed exposure to bright light. *J Am Geriatr Soc* 41:829–836, 1993.

Campbell SS, Kripke DF, Gillin JC, Hrubovcak JC. Exposure to light in healthy elderly subjects and Alzheimer's patients. *Physiol Behav* 42:141–144, 1988.

Carroll JS, Bliwise DL, Dement WC. A method for checking interobserver reliability in observational sleep studies. *Sleep* 12:363–367, 1989.

Carskadon MA, Seidel WF, Greenblatt DJ, Dement WC. Daytime carryover of triazolam and flurazepam in elderly insomniacs. *Sleep* 5:361–371, 1982.

Castor D, Woods D, Pigott L, Hemmes R. Effect of sunlight on sleep patterns of the elderly. *J Am Acad Phys Assist* 4:321–326, 1991.

Clapin-French E. Sleep patterns of aged persons in long-term care facilities. *J Adv Nurs* 11:57–66, 1986.

Cohen D, Eisdorfer C, Prinz P, et al. Sleep disturbances in the institutionalized aged. *J Am Geriatr Soc* 31:79–82, 1983.

Cohen-Mansfield J, Marx MS. The relationship between sleep disturbances and agitation in a nursing home. *Int J Aging Health* 2:42–57, 1990a.

Cohen-Mansfield J, Waldhorn R, Werner P, Billig N. Validation of sleep observations in a nursing home. *Sleep* 13:512–525, 1990b.

Cohen-Mansfield J, Marx MS, Rosenthal AS. A descritpion of agitation in a nursing home. *J Gerontol Med Sci* 32:M77–M84, 1988.

Cohen-Mansfield J, Marx MS, Werner P, Freeman L. Temporal patterns of agitated nursing home residents. *Int Psychogeriatr* 4:197–206, 1992.

Cohen-Mansfield J, Watson V, Meade W, et al. Does sundowning occur in residents of an Alzheimer's unit? *Int J Geriatr Psychiatry* 4:293–298, 1989.

Czeisler CA, Kronauer RF, Allan JS, et al. Bright light induction of strong (type O) resetting of the human circadian pacemaker. *Science* 244:1328–1333, 1989.

Douglas NJ, Thomas S, Jan MA. Clinical value of polysomnography. *Lancet* 339:347–350, 1992.

Edgar DM, Dement WC. Regularly scheduled voluntary exercise synchronizes the mouse circadian clock. *Am J Physiol* 261:R928–R933, 1991.

Evans LK. Sundown syndrome in institutionalized elderly. *J Am Geriatr Soc* 35:101–108, 1987.

Exum ME, Phelps BJ, Nabers KE, Osborne JG. Sundown syndrome: Is it reflected in the use of PRN medications for nursing home residents? *Gerontologist* 33:756–761, 1993.

Ferini-Strambi L, Franceschi M, Pinto P, et al. Respiration and heart rate variability during sleep in untreated Parkinson patients. *Gerontology* 38:92–98, 1992.

Ferm L. Behavioural activities in demented geriatric patients. *Gerontol Clin* 16:185–194, 1974.

Friedman L, Bliwise DL, Yesavage JA, Salom SR. A preliminary study comparing sleep restriction and relaxation treatments for insomnia in older adults. *J Gerontol Psychol Sci* 46:1–8, 1991.

Gall K, Petersen T, Riesch S. Night life: Nocturnal behavior patterns among hospitalized elderly. *J Gerontol Nurs* 16(10):31–35, 1990.

Gallagher-Thompson D, Brooks JO, Bliwise D, et al. The relations among caregiver stress, "sundowning" symptoms and cognitive decline in Alzheimer's disease. *J Am Geriatr Soc* 40:807–810, 1992.

Granek E, Baker SP, Abbey H, et al. Medications and diagnoses in relation to falls in a long-term care facility. *J Am Geriatr Soc* 35:503–511, 1987.

Gress L, Bahr R, Hassanein R. Nocturnal behavior of selected institutionalized adults. *J Gerontol Nurs* 7(2):86–92, 1981.

Haponik EF, Smith PL, Meyers DA, Bleecker ER. Evaluation of sleep-disordered breathing: Is polysomnography necessary? *Am J Med* 77:671–677, 1984.

Hoch CC, Reynolds CF III, Kupfer DJ, et al. Sleep disordered breathing in normal and pathologic aging. *J Clin Psychiatry* 47:499–503, 1986.

Jacobs D, Ancoli-Israel S, Parker L, Kripke DF. 24-hour sleep/wake patterns in a nursing home population. *Psychol Aging* 4:352–356, 1989.

Kane RL, Ouslander JG, Abrass IB. *Essentials of Clinical Geriatrics.* New York: McGraw-Hill, 1984.

Lipowski ZJ. *Delirium: Acute Brain Failure in Man.* Springfield, IL: Charles C Thomas, 1980.

Lipowski ZJ. Delirium in the elderly patient. *N Engl J Med* 320:578–582, 1989.

Liptzin B, Levkoff SE, Cleary PD, et al. An empirical study of diagnostic criteria for delirium. *Am J Psychiatry* 148:454–457, 1991.

Lugaresi E, Cirignotta F, Coccagna F, Piana C. Some epidemiological data on snoring and cardiocirculatory disturbances. *Sleep* 3:221–224, 1980.

Martino-Saltzman D, Blasch BB, Morris RD, McNeal LW. Travel behavior of nursing home residents perceived as wanderers and nonwanderers. *Gerontologist* 31:666–672, 1991.

McFadden E, Giblin E. Sleep deprivation in patients having open-heart surgery. *Nurs Res* 20:249–254, 1971.

Meguro K, Ueda M, Yamaguchi T, et al. Disturbance in daily sleep/wake patterns in patients with cognitive impairment and decreased daily activity. *J Am Geriatr Soc* 38:1176–1182, 1990.

Morgan K. Sleep and aging: A research-based guide to sleep in later life. Baltimore: The Johns Hopkins University Press, 1987.

Okawa M, Mishima K, Hishikawa Y, et al. Circadian rhythm disorders in sleep-waking and body temperature in elderly patients with dementia and their treatment. *Sleep* 14:478–485, 1991.

O'Leary PA, Haley WE, Paul PB. Behavioral assessment in Alzheimer's disease: Use of a 24-hr log. *Psychol Aging* 8:139–143, 1993.

Orr WC, Shamma-Othman Z, Levin D, et al. Persistent hypoxemia and excessive daytime sleepiness in chronic obstructive pulmonary disease (COPD). *Chest* 97:583–585, 1990.

Pack AI. Simplifying the diagnosis of obstructive sleep apnea. *Ann Intern Med* 119:528–529, 1993.

Paiva Z. Sundown syndrome: Calming the agitated patient. *RN* 53:46–51, 1990.

Pollak CP, Perlick D. Sleep problems and institutionalization of the elderly. *J Geriatr Psychiatry Neurol* 4:204–210, 1991.

Pollak CP, Perlick D, Lonsner JP, et al. Sleep problems in the community elderly as predictors of death and nursing home placement. *J Commun Health* 15:123–135, 1990.

Prinz PN, Peskind ER, Vitaliano PP, et al. Changes in the sleep and waking EEGs of nondemented and demented elderly subjects. *J Am Geriatr Soc* 30:86–93, 1982a.

Prinz PN, Vitaliano PP, Vitiello MV, et al. Sleep, EEG and mental function changes in senile dementia of the Alzheimer type. *Neurobiol Aging* 3:361–370, 1982b.

Regestein QR, Morris J. Daily sleep patterns observed among institutionalized elderly residents. *J Am Geriatr Soc* 35:767–772, 1987.

Reynolds CF, Hoch CC, Kupfer DJ, et al. Bedside differentiation of depressive pseudodementia from dementia. *Am J Psychiatry* 145:1099–1103, 1988a.

Reynolds CF, Kupfer DJ, Houck PR, et al. Reliable discrimination of elderly depressed and demented patients by electroencephalographic sleep data. *Arch Gen Psychiatry* 45:258–264, 1988b.

Satlin A, Volicer L, Ross V, et al. Bright light treatment of behavioral and sleep disturbances in patients with Alzheimer's disease. *Am J Psychiatry* 149:1028–1032, 1992.

Scheving L, Roig R III, Halberg F, et al. Circadian variations in residents of a "senior citizens" home. In: Scheving L, Halberg F, Pauly J, eds. *Chronobiology.* Tokyo: Igaku Shoin, 1974:353–357.

Schnelle JF, Ouslander JG, Simmons SF, et al. Nighttime sleep and bed mobility among incontinent nursing home residents. *J Am Geriatr Soc* 41:903–909, 1993a.

Schnelle JF, Ouslander JG, Simmons SF, et al. The nighttime environment, incontinence care, and sleep disruption in nursing homes. *J Am Geriatr Soc* 41:910–914, 1993b.

Seidel WF, Ball S, Cohen S, et al. Daytime alertness in relation to mood, performance, and nocturnal sleep in chronic insomniacs and noncomplaining sleepers. *Sleep* 7:230–238, 1984.

Series F, Marc I, Cormier Y, La Forge J. Utility of nocturnal home oximetry for case finding in patients with suspected sleep apnea hypopnea syndrome. *Ann Intern Med* 119:449–453, 1993.

Smallwood RG, Vitiello MV, Giblin EC, Prinz PN. Sleep apnea: Relationship to age, sex and Alzheimer's dementia. *Sleep* 6:16–22, 1983.

Touitou Y. Some aspects of the circadian time structure in the elderly. *Gerontology* 28(suppl 1):53–67, 1982.

Vitiello MV, Prinz PN, Williams DE, et al. Sleep disturbances in patients with mild-stage Alzheimer's disease. *J Gerontol Med Sci* 45:M131–M138, 1990.

Webb W, Swinburne H. An observational study of sleep of the aged. *Percept Motor Skills* 32:895–898, 1971.

Winget C, Vernikos-Danellis J, Cronin S, et al. Circadian rhythm asynchrony in man during hypokinesis. *J Appl Psychol* 33:640–643, 1972.

10

Sexuality

Ilana P. Spector, Raymond C. Rosen, and
Sandra R. Leiblum

Older people are living longer. According to the 1990 United States census (U.S. Bureau of the Census, 1992), there are approximately 30 million people over the age of 65, which represents 12.5% of the U.S. population. Estimates indicate that this percentage will continue to rise. The number of people using long-term-care facilities is also increasing; currently, 5% of those over age 65 live in nursing homes, and each person who reaches age 65 has a 25% chance of residing in a nursing home before he or she dies (Kane, 1990). At the same time, medical research on chronic illness has proliferated, so that currently there are a number of more efficacious treatment options available for the chronically ill. With longevity increasing so that a greater percentage of our population may become disabled elderly, concerns about quality of life have heightened.

Quality of life is an elusive construct. Many definitions are available in the literature, usually involving both objective and subjective dimensions. Most researchers agree that physical, emotional, intellectual, and social functioning— along with life satisfaction, perceived health, financial security, ability to pursue recreation, energy, and sexual functioning—should be included in a comprehensive definition (Arnold, 1991). There is little agreement on the relative weighting of each of these components.

In reviewing the literature on quality of life in the elderly, it is noteworthy that much attention has been directed to mood state, cognitive function, health beliefs, and stress. However, sexuality in the elderly patient has been largely neglected; even fewer studies examine the sexual needs of the nursing home patient. What is it about elderly patients or the institutionalized elderly that discourages the study of sexual behavior in these groups?

Ageism, defined as a societal pattern of devaluative attitudes and stereotypes about the elderly (Gatz and Pearson, 1988) is widespread. Whereas the elderly are often seen as fragile and incompetent (Leiblum and Segraves, 1989), one of the most devaluative and unfounded notions about the elderly is that they are asexual (Leiblum and Segraves, 1989; Libman, 1989). Because older people are no longer interested in sex for procreative purposes and are not perceived as physically attractive in our culture, it is either assumed that they are sexually disinterested or that their interest in sex is "inappropriate" or "perverse." This latter belief often leads to the use of pejorative labels for sexually active older persons, such as "dirty old man." Because sexuality is often a difficult topic for clinicians to address with patients of any age, these myths about the elderly often serve to rationalize the avoidance of sexual topics in clinical evaluations of older patients (Poggi and Berland, 1985).

Although there are physiological changes in sexual function that predictably accompany normal aging, it is likely that negative biases and attitudes contribute more to observed changes in sexual behavior (Schover and Jensen, 1988). Sexuality has been recognized as an aspect of quality of life because it is a source of psychological reinforcement (Libman, 1989), and it contributes in an important way to one's self-concept (McCarthy et al., 1987). In fact, it has been noted that difficulties in sexual function that are not addressed can lead to depression, loss of self-esteem, and marital discord. Thus, to avoid addressing the sexual needs of aging populations and nursing home residents is to neglect an important aspect of emotional health and well-being.

The purpose of this chapter is to address problems related to sexuality in long-term-care facilities. Although there are important clinical concerns relevant to this population, limited factual information is available on the sexual needs and attitudes of residents of long-term-care facilities. Given the marked paucity of research and clinical literature, we begin by reviewing what is known about normal aging and sexual function. Next, we discuss the sexual behavior patterns of the cognitively intact and nonintact elderly, residing both in and outside long-term-care facilities. We also consider why aging individuals may be more susceptible to sexual difficulties and offer clinical recommendations on the evaluation and treatment of sexual concerns within the nursing home environment. Finally, the implications for further research are discussed.

Sexual Changes Associated with Aging

Sexual Changes in the Male

The sexual function of the elderly male can best be characterized as involving a lengthening of each stage of the sexual response cycle. Men take longer to achieve an erection and require more tactile stimulation; psychic stimulation may not be sufficient (Bancroft, 1989). There is a decrease in the ability of the erectile smooth muscle tissue to relax, a decline in blood flow to the penis, and reduced capacity for engorgement (Goldstein and Rothstein, 1990). The maximum penile rigidity that older men can attain is reduced, and erection is more difficult to regain following detumescence (Schover and Jensen, 1988). Older men also have more difficulty sustaining erections during intercourse. The refractory period, during which the man is unresponsive to further sexual stimulation, lengthens. More stimulation is required for men to ejaculate as they age, and ejaculations of the older male are generally less forceful than those of younger males (Bancroft, 1989).

It is important to note that these physiological changes usually occur gradually over time. Unlike the female menopause, there is no clear marker for the sexual changes in the aging male. For each individual man, the timing and extent of these changes may vary considerably. Also, changes in physiological capacity need not diminish the older man's enjoyment of sexual activity or his ability to provide pleasure to a partner.

Sexual Changes in the Female

In the female, specific changes in sexual function are associated with menopause, which occurs around age 50. Due to a lowered level of estrogen, most women experience a reduced vascular supply to the pelvic region (Leiblum and Segraves, 1989). Vaginal lubrication is slower and reduced in quantity (Bancroft, 1989), and the vaginal mucosa become thinner and drier (Leiblum and Segraves, 1989). The aging female may take longer to become aroused and require more stimulation than her younger counterparts (Schover and Jensen, 1988). Although most women report little change in orgasm with aging (Leiblum and Segraves, 1989), there is a gradual decrease in the amount and strength of vaginal contractions that occur during orgasm. The most common sexual complaint in the postmenopausal women is dyspareunia (or pain during intercourse) due to vaginal atrophy and decreased lubrication.

It is important to note that, for the female, many of the physiological changes are reversible when hormone replacement therapy is instituted perimenopausally. Estrogen replacement will prevent vaginal atrophy and the reduction in vaginal lubrication. Some women may also benefit from the use of small doses of testosterone to maintain premenopausal levels of desire. For a detailed review of the effects of hormone therapy on postmenopausal women, see Sherwin (1985). For those women who cannot receive hormone therapy for medical reasons, a nonhormonal vaginal lubricant (e.g., K-Y jelly) is recommended during sexual activity to reduce friction and prevent dyspareunia.

Despite the decrease in intensity of sexual response, older women are fully capable of sexual arousal and orgasm. In fact, regular sexual activity (either masturbation or intercourse) may mitigate the physiological effects of aging.

Changes in the Sexual Behavior of Cognitively Intact Aging Adults

In reviewing the literature on aging and sexual health, it can be seen that the elderly are neither asexual nor sexually uninterested and inactive. However, there are several problems that impede interpretation of the available literature on aging and sexuality.

First, there are few methodologically sound studies that adequately describe the sexual behaviors of aging men and women. Some predictors of sexual behavior that might be useful to study in an aging population include attitudes toward sexuality, physical and marital health, previous levels of sexual function, partner availability, and partner health. As well, longitudinal research would yield interesting findings with respect to how sexual desire and behavior change over the life cycle.

Second, there are few studies examining sexual behavior in aging females (Brecher, 1984; Bretschneider and McCoy, 1988; Weinstein and Rosen, 1988; Bachmann and Leiblum, 1991; Leiblum et al., 1994). This is surprising and unfortunate, because there are more aging women than men. It is inappropriate to generalize from what is known about male sexual behavior, so that increased study of the sexual health of aging females is essential in order to better understand this population.

Third, there is a paucity of research on the effects of long-term care on sexual behavior. In fact, only one empirical study to date (Mulligan and Palguta, 1991) has examined this specific issue. Given that nursing home populations are increasing, it is important that information in this area be made available to better plan for the optimal quality-of-life conditions of the residents. In order to better understand the needs of nursing home residents, to establish policies, and to budget for treatment options, more data are needed on the incidence of sexual needs, behaviors, and attitudes of elderly nursing home residents.

Fourth, the studies that have been conducted generally assume that the elderly are a homogeneous group; no distinctions are made in terms of specific subsamples. Among nursing home residents, the reasons for stay may include functional disabilities, chronic illness, and cognitive disabilities. It is likely that the sexual desires, activities, and treatment needs of these subsamples are quite different, and it would serve researchers well to distinguish these groups from one another.

Finally, the methods of assessment used to examine sexual behaviors and experimental designs employed in these studies are often limited. Psychometrically sound instruments are available for these purposes and should be used wherever possible (see Conte, 1983; Davis et al., 1988). Additionally, there is a reliance on self-report data and a neglect of psychophysiological data.

Thus, in terms of understanding the sexual function of the elderly, further investigation is needed before clearer statements can be made about the needs and behaviors of the nursing home resident. However, the following section reviews the available literature on sexual behavior in aging adults, with the caveat that the generalizability of the findings to the long-term-care population may be limited.

Twelve studies review the sexual behavior of aging individuals. In the largest study to date, Brecher (1984) surveyed 4246 adults over the age of 50. He noted that the majority of respondents rated the sexual aspects of their relationship as very important and engaged in regular intercourse. Those who had more frequent intercourse also rated their relationships as more satisfactory. Some 75% of respondents experienced sex as enjoyable. Thus, Brecher (1984) concluded that older individuals are sexually active and received a high level of satisfaction from their activity. It is important to note that Brecher's study evaluated community-living adults rather than nursing home residents. Also, Brecher's sample were all volunteers; thus sampling biases are likely.

Weinstein and Rosen (1988) conducted a study comparing elderly people ages 60 to 80 who lived either in age-segregated communities (e.g., leisure and retirement communities) with those who lived in age-integrated housing communities. There were no differences between groups in age, marital status, health status, education, income, or religiosity. These authors found that age-segregated elderly men and women expressed more interest in sexual activity and were more sexually active than a comparable group of age-integrated elderly. They suggest that one potential reason for the differences noted is that in main-stream society, sexual behavior and desirability are associated with youth, while sexuality in elderly people is often censored. It is possible that when the elderly remove themselves from the mainstream and live in age-matched communities, they can begin to develop new standards of attractiveness and self-esteem and feel more free to express sexuality without risking disapproval. Therefore, this study highlights the important influence of environment on sexual function in the elderly.

Studies Reviewing Male Sexual Behavior

Seven studies were found that assessed the sexual behaviors, attitudes, level of interest, and difficulties of aging men. With respect to behavior, current sexual frequency was found to correlate with past sexual frequency; men who were sexually active in their youth continued to be sexually active in their later years (Martin, 1981). Sexual activity was maintained in 39% of those under age 75 and 25% of those over age 75 (Mulligan et al., 1988). Regular sexual intercourse (more than four times per month) was reported by 54% of aging men (Weizman and Hart, 1987), and masturbation rates ranged from 41 to 72% (Weizman and Hart, 1987; Bretschneider and McCoy, 1988). Although sexual activity has been negatively correlated with age (Schiavi et al., 1990), many healthy aging men continue to be sexually active.

Elderly men not only continue to engage in sexual activity but they also continue to value sex and maintain an interest in fulfilling their sexual needs. Some 40 to 70% of aging men reported that sex is an important aspect of their health (Martin, 1981; Bretschneider and McCoy, 1988; Thomas, 1991). Among those surveyed, 63% stated that masturbation is an acceptable means of sexual gratification (Martin, 1981). Some 40% claimed that they had observed no changes in their levels of sexual desire (Weizman and Hart, 1987), and 60% reported continued levels of sexual interest (Mulligan et al., 1988). Most men reported that sex continued to be important and enjoyable even if they were experiencing sexual difficulties (Bretschneider and McCoy, 1988).

With respect to sexual difficulties, 35% of healthy older men reported erectile dysfunction and 14% reported absence of sexual desire (Weizman and Hart, 1987). Difficulties with erections was predicted by degree of chronic illness and by poor self-reported health (Mulligan et al., 1988). Men who continued to be sexually active reported less problems with erections than did abstinent men (Martin, 1981). With regard to episodes of nocturnal penile tumescence, older men displayed fewer episodes of nocturnal erection, which also did not last as long as those of their younger counterparts (Schiavi et al., 1990).

Only one study has been published in the past 10 years that examined sexual behavior in the nursing home setting. Mulligan and Palguta (1991) conducted a study of males ages 42 to 100 in a nursing home associated with a Veterans Affairs Medical Center. To participate, subjects had to score above 15/30 on the Folstein Mini-Mental State Exam (a measure of cognitive function), and be willing to answer questions about sexual function. Using an interview format, residents were asked to rate their level of sexual interest, activity preference, partner availability, sexual activity level, satisfaction, and distress. Results indicated that there was a low level of sexual activity in the nursing home; however, those who currently had sexual partners and an interest in sex were most distressed because sexual activity with a partner was unavailable to them in the nursing home setting. These authors concluded that nursing home residents who have sexual desire and partners should not be restricted from interacting sexually.

Therefore, to summarize the findings about male sexual behavior, although it is true that there are decreases in erectile function and desire, older men may continue to express an interest in sexual behavior, to value this behavior as important, to act on their desires, and to receive satisfaction from their activity. As well, men become distressed when they experience sexual desire and are denied sexual outlets.

Studies Reviewing Female Sexual Behavior

Four studies have evaluated the sexual behaviors, attitudes, level of interest, and difficulties of aging women. With respect to sexual interest and behavior, Bretschneider and McCoy (1988) found that 14% of healthy aging women fantasize about sex and that 36% rate sex as an important part of their lives. These authors reported that 40% of their sample were currently still masturbating. Brecher (1984) compared postmenopausal women who were taking estrogen with those who were not and found that 93% of those taking estrogen were sexually active, as were 80% of those who did not take estrogen. Those taking estrogen also rated their sexual enjoyment as higher, had sex more frequently, and experienced more adequate lubrication (Brecher, 1984). Bachmann and Leiblum (1991) examined healthy women between the ages of 60 and 70 and found that 66% of them were sexually active. In comparing those who were sexually active with those who were not, the authors found the active women described higher levels of sexual desire and satisfaction. Leiblum et al. (1993) also compared sexually active women with abstinent women. They found that the sexually abstinent women were slightly older and had lower income levels than those who were active. Active women had significantly higher levels of sexual interest than those who were abstinent. The groups were not significantly different with respect to levels of anxiety or depression. The three factors that significantly discriminated between the groups were that the sexually abstinent women were more likely to report poor health of their sexual partner, lower desire on the part of their sexual partner, and lack of privacy. This study shows the significant effect of the male partners' function on sexuality in the elderly female.

With respect to sexual difficulties in aging women, Bachmann and Leiblum (1991) reported the following rates of sexual difficulties in a group aged 60 to 70 years: 61% reported decreased lubrication, 56% lowered sexual interest, 49% lowered arousal, 32% difficulties with orgasm, and 17% dyspareunia. These percentages are slightly higher than those cited in the general population (Spector and Carey, 1990). Half the women noted that their male sexual partners were experiencing sexual difficulties. Of those women who were not sexually active, 60% reported that this was due to difficulties that their partners were experiencing, while 40% described their inactivity as due to their own sexual problems. This study also highlights the importance of examining both members of the couple to better understand the sexual functioning of the female partner; sexual abstinence is not necessarily due to lack of interest on the part of the inactive female partner, but may reflect dysfunction in the male partner.

In summary, although women appear to be less desirous and active than do men of this age, they continue to think about and engage in sexual activity. As well, with the exception of decreased lubrication, dysfunction rates in aging women do not appear to be significantly higher than they are in younger women.

Factors That Contribute to Sexual Difficulties in the Elderly

As we have noted, physiological changes associated with normal aging often do not provide a sufficient explanation for the degree of sexual dysfunction sometimes seen in elderly persons. There are several causes for sexual difficulties in the general population, and elderly persons may be especially vulnerable to them. These risk factors include chronic illness, medication effects, depression, and attitudes toward sexuality. Certain characteristics of the nursing home environment may also affect the sexual satisfaction of residents.

Medical Factors

Increases in age are often accompanied by a higher prevalence of chronic disease states. Several illnesses, surgeries, and medications are associated with sexual difficulties. Disorders that involve pain often lead to sexual disturbances—for example, angina pectoris, arthritis, and cancer pain (Schover and Jensen, 1988). Pain can interfere with both desire and arousal. The risk of cardiovascular disease increases with age and may be associated with reduced vascular supply to the penis, leading to erectile difficulties. Diabetes is associated with both neuropathy and vascular damage, which may impair sexual arousal (Meisler et al., 1989; Spector et al., 1993). Cancer may require surgery leading to neurological impairment (e.g., prostate cancer) or difficulties involving body-image concerns (e.g., mastectomy), and chemotherapy has been associated with decreased sexual desire (Carey, 1990). Any illness, surgical procedure or treatment that can lead to vascular, neurological, or endocrine dysfunction can cause sexual difficulties as well. Thus, it can be seen that the elderly are susceptible to disease states that can lead to sexual difficulties.

Many medications are responsible for changes in sexual function. Antihypertensives are among the most commonly prescribed medications in our society (Rosen, 1991), and several (i.e., beta blockers, diuretics) have been noted to precipitate erectile dysfunction in men and decreased desire in both genders. Several psychiatric drugs have been associated with lower sexual desire, inhibited orgasm and ejaculation, and erectile difficulties. For example, phenothiazines have been associated with delayed ejaculation and erectile problems in men and decreased desire and arousal in women. Several antidepressants (i.e., imipramine, clomipramine) have been noted to lead to delayed ejaculation and erectile problems in men and inhibited orgasm in women. Other prescription medications that have been found to precipitate sexual difficulties include digoxin, cholesterol-lowering agents, anticonvulsant drugs, and cimetidine. Thus, a thorough evaluation of the nursing home resident's medication use is necessary to determine whether his or her sexual difficulty may have been precipitated or is currently being maintained by a prescription drug. For a more detailed review of the effects of medication on sexual function, see Rosen (1991). See Table 10.1 for a list of common medications associated with sexual problems.

As can be seen from the previous review, much more is known about the effects of disease states, medications, and surgeries on the sexual function of men than on that of women. Further research is required to better elucidate the relationship between these factors and female sexual function.

Psychosocial Factors

Depression and dysphoria have been associated with sexual difficulties, including reduced desire in both genders (Schreiner-Engel and Schiavi, 1986), decreased nocturnal penile tumescence (Thase et al., 1987), and subjective arousal in men (Meisler and Carey, 1991). The elderly may be at increased risk for depressive

TABLE 10.1. Medications Associated with Sexual Dysfunction

Medication Name	Use (Class)
Chlorthalidone	Antihypertensive (diuretic)
Spironolactone	Antihypertensive (diuretic)
Methyldopa	Antihypertensive (central antiadrenergic)
Clonidine	Antihypertensive (central antiadrenergic)
Reserpine	Antihypertensive (central antiadrenergic)
Guanethidine	Antihypertensive (peripheral antiadrenergic)
Propranolol	Antihypertensive (beta blocker)
Verapamil	Antihypertensive (calcium channel blocker)
Disopyramide	Antiarrhythmic
Cimetidine	Antiulcer
Clofibrate	Hypolipidemic
Digitalis	Cardiac drug
Acetazolamide	Glaucoma drug (carbonic anhydrase inhibitor)
Ethoxzolamide	Glaucoma drug (carbonic anhydrase inhibitor)
Dichlorphenamide	Glaucoma drug (carbonic anhydrase inhibitor)
Methazolamide	Glaucoma drug (carbonic anhydrase inhibitor)
Disulfiram	Alcohol treatment
Chlorpromazine	Psychiatric drug (phenothiazine antipsychotic)
Pimozide	Psychiatric drug (diphenylbutyl antipsychotic)
Thioridazine	Psychiatric drug (phenothiazine antipsychotic)
Haloperidol	Psychiatric drug (butyrophenone antipsychotic)
Fluphenazine	Psychiatric drug (phenothiazine antipsychotic)
Lithium	Psychiatric drug (mood stabilizer)
Clomipramine	Psychiatric drug (tricyclic antidepressant)
Imipramine	Psychiatric drug (tricyclic antidepressant)
Amitriptyline	Psychiatric drug (tricyclic antidepressant)
Desipramine	Psychiatric drug (tricyclic antidepressant)
Fluoxetine	Psychiatric drug (selective serotonergic reuptake inhibitor)

Source: Adapted from Segraves and Segraves (1989) and Schover and Jensen (1988).

episodes due to failing health, changes in work status, and loss of life partners and friends. Thus, depression may be one precipitant of sexual difficulties in this group.

Another precipitant of sexual difficulties in both men and women is performance anxiety (Wincze and Carey, 1991). Anxiety about whether one will be able to attain an erection or become lubricated can lead to decreased arousal. The elderly may be particularly susceptible to sexual performance anxiety for several reasons. First, as previously noted, sexual function changes as people age, in terms of a slowing of the arousal response and decreased intensity of arousal. As these changes occur, especially in men and women who are not informed about the nature of these changes, some individuals may become concerned about their reduced functioning and the associated reasons. Second, nursing home residents may become preoccupied with their ability to function independently in nonsexual areas, which may lead to loss of self-esteem and self-doubt. As they approach sexual interactions, they may experience anticipatory anxiety with respect to their ability to function appropriately. This anticipatory anxiety and negative attributional state will serve to decrease arousal and increase the likelihood that further difficulties will occur. As well, concern about the ability to function sexually can lead to a secondary loss of desire. Thus, normal aging changes may increase sexual anxiety in the elderly and lead to more pervasive difficulties in sexual function.

Body-image concerns can also affect sexual function. For example, as a person ages, changes occur in body shape, skin, and hair. To the extent that individuals are concerned about their physical attractiveness, they may avoid sexual situations out of concern that their partners may not find them arousing or that they may be rejected and humiliated (Zilbergeld, 1978).

Finally, our society is notorious for discouraging sexual expression in the elderly. Our view of what is attractive involves youth; one has only to examine portrayals in the media to note what and whom we view as sexually attractive. Although it is unclear whether attitudes are changing with respect to sexuality and aging, many of today's elderly developed their sexual attitudes and values during a more conservative era. To the extent that the elderly individual subscribes to these beliefs and attitudes, and to the extent that his or her family or caretakers subscribe to these beliefs, aging individuals may be ashamed to express sexual interest, fear condemnation, and engage in sexual avoidance. In a study of 106 other cultures, Winn and Newton (1982) found that many people of both genders were sexually active well into their eighth and ninth decades, and that in these societies there was no mention of devaluative attitudes about sexuality and aging. In fact, the elderly were sometimes seen as sexually attractive partners. Thus, it is clear that the attitudes of society can have a profound impact on the ability of aging individuals to feel accepted and affirmed as sexual beings.

Clearly, psychosocial factors as well as medical factors can affect the sexual function of aging individuals negatively. Depression, anxiety, body-image concerns, and societal attitudes can all serve to decrease the potential sexual function of men and women over and above the physical changes associated with normal aging.

The Nursing Home Environment

Aside from the factors delineated above, there are variables specific to the nursing home environment that may lead to increased risk for sexual difficulties. These factors include lack of privacy and negative attitudes of nursing home staff and administrators toward sexual expression in residents.

One of the unfortunate elements of most nursing home settings is that residents often lack privacy. Many residents are forced to share rooms either because of a shortage of space or an inability to afford private rooms. The lack of privacy has special impact on expressions of sexual behavior. Residents may not have access to a private room in order to engage in sexual activity with a partner. If they do attempt to have sex, fear of discovery may inhibit arousal. Masturbation may also be avoided because of fear of discovery. In fact, as the residents try to maneuver some private moments for sexual activity, they may decide that the end result (rushing through sex to avoid being caught) is just not worth the trouble. Leiblum et al. (1993) reported that lack of privacy differentiated sexually active from abstinent women in community samples. Thus, both masturbation and dyadic sexual activities may be inhibited because of difficulty in securing private time and space.

A more fundamental concern is whether nursing home residents have a right to behave sexually at all, and if so, whether they have a right to select their sexual partners. No moral issue has received as much attention as individuals' rights as sexual beings (Gorovitz, 1982). One might assume that this right of the elderly should not be debatable because it is not debatable for younger individuals; however, this is unfortunately sometimes not the cse.

With respect to partner status, residents may be divided into three categories: those who have partners who live outside the nursing home, those whose partners live within the same nursing home, and those who are single. Arrangements enabling residents to engage in sexual activity with a visiting partner are rarely provided. Also, nursing homes may not be set up for residents to share rooms with their partners; double beds are often not available. Therefore, partnered residents may experience difficulties with respect to maintaining intimacy in the nursing home environment. Single residents experience another type of difficulty. They must not only combat negative attitudes and myths about aging and sex but also deal with prevailing beliefs—among the staff and other residents—about both heterosexual and homosexual experiences outside of marriage (Striar and Hoffman, 1984).

Sexuality in aging individuals can create anxiety and discomfort in nursing home employees. It would be beneficial if the staff could conceptualize the residents' sexual behaviors as meeting important needs for intimacy, comfort, the physical contact rather than expecting them to inhibit or eliminate the sexual part of themselves that may have been vibrant and necessary throughout their lives. This can be a painful process for the resident and can create unnecessary feelings of sadness and loss.

Improving Sexuality as an Aspect of Quality of Life in the Nursing Home

It is apparent that there is considerable variability in the elderly with respect to sexual interest and function. Although data on nursing home residents are largely unavailable, we can predict that this variability may be even greater in the nursing home population. Thus, we advocate an *individualized approach* to evaluating sexual needs and structuring interventions. As indicated earlier, these interventions might occur on two levels: (1) structuring the nursing home environment so that sexual behavior is possible and (2) addressing the individual sexual concerns of residents as they arise.

Structuring the Nursing Home Environment

Lack of privacy in the nursing home is a likely inhibitor of sexual behavior. This problem could be addressed in several ways. First, wherever possible, married couples or other sexual partners should be allowed to share private rooms. Second, for residents whose partners do not live in the nursing home or who wish to behave sexually either with other residents or to masturbate, privacy should be provided by placing locks on the doors or signs indicating that the resident is not to be disturbed by staff or other residents. Staff should be encouraged to respect this privacy by either obeying the signs or by knocking and not entering the resident's room without permission. Staff should be reminded that according to federal regulations, as stated in The Patient's Bill of Rights (Federal Regulations, 1990), the resident has the right to "associate and communicate privately with persons of his or her choice, including other patients." This is true even if the staff does not approve of the patients' choices in partners or activities (e.g., homosexual or extramarital encounters).

A more difficult problem to address is that of attitudes toward sexuality and aging, especially with respect to the nursing home setting. We recommend that health care workers (i.e., doctors, nurses, mental health professionals) be educated while in training that sexuality is an important aspect of quality of life, and that many older people value their sexuality and may wish to continue to be sexually active late in life. Quinn-Krach and Van Hoozer (1988) noted that nurses may not facilitate sexual expression in the elderly because they lack knowledge of how to do so; sexual concerns are often neglected in medical education (Wallace, 1992). Health care professionals must recognize that sexual behavior in older adults is not abnormal or harmful, and they should be taught how to communicate to patients and residents that sexual interest is normal and appropriate in individuals of all ages.

As residents enter the nursing home, discussion of sexuality should be included in their orientation to this setting. Whatever provisions are made for privacy should be offered to the resident. It should be communicated that the staff are comfortable addressing sexual matters, so that the resident can later approach the staff should he or she have any concerns. This creates an environment that informs the resident that sexuality is a valued aspect of the individual's health, and that guidance will be provided should problems arise.

Addressing Individual Sexual Concerns

Ideally, the resident will feel comfortable approaching one of the staff involved in his or her care should sexual difficulties occur. At least one staff member should be comfortable and skilled in evaluating sexual difficulties and deciding whether more in-depth assessment and treatment is necessary.

A first step in evaluating the sexual problem involves clinical formulation. Special attention should be devoted to examining medical and psychosocial precipitants as well as interpersonal consequences. As noted earlier, there are several illnesses, surgeries, and medications that can lead to sexual difficulties, and these should be evaluated as causes. Next, psychosocial variables such as anxiety and depression should be considered. The resident's attitudes and values regarding sex should be discussed. Finally, the resident should be asked whether the difficulty predated his or her move to the nursing home or whether there is some aspect about the move that may have contributed to the sexual problem. Once this information is obtained, the evaluator should make some attempt to formulate a treatment plan for the sexual difficulty.

At the very least, the staff should be able to reassure the resident that his or her sexual concerns are valid and important. Education should be provided about normal aging changes, as this may help alleviate the residents' anxiety. Residents who experience difficulties with arousal should be encouraged to decrease the focus on intercourse and attempt to meet their needs for intimacy and sexual pleasure through other forms of sexual behavior, such as manual and oral stimulation. Should the resident's needs involve desire for physical contact more than for sexual outlet, perhaps massages either by the partner or by a professional can be offered. Helping the residents to realize that these other sexual and sensual activities are acceptable and valued will increase their repertoire of sexual behaviors, decrease performance anxiety, and help improve sexual communication.

If the staff member decides that further professional involvement is required, the patient can be referred for medical or psychological evaluation. Currently, there are a number of treatment options available to improve sexual difficulties of both organic and psychogenic etiology, and the full range of treatment alternatives should be available to the residents.

Finally, a trained staff member should be able to meet with family members who are uncomfortable with their parent's or relative's sexual activity. Reassurance and education should be provided as necessary.

Sexual Behaviors and Concerns of Patients with Dementia

The previous sections of this chapter have focused primarily on the sexual needs of the cognitively intact resident. Although the predictors of dysfunction and recommendations for evaluating residents' sexual concerns may also be valid for residents with Alzheimer's disease (AD), it seems likely that this population will have additional needs and concerns. Clinical lore about patients with AD suggests that this population tends to be more sexually impulsive. Examples of such behaviors might include masturbating either excessively or in public and making inappropriate sexual gestures or invitations. However, in a study of 178 patients with probable AD, only 12% displayed sexual disinhibition, which was described as using obscene sexual language, exposing themselves publicly, masturbating excessively, and propositioning others (Burns et al., 1990). This sexual disinhibition was uncorrelated with measures obtained by computed tomography (CT). In a second study of 80 patients living in the community with probable AD, even lower rates of inappropriate sexual behavior were noted (3.8%) (Bozzola et al., 1992). In fact, the most common personality change noted by these authors was apathy and low initiative (61.3%), which would not be compatible with increased sexual desire. Together, these studies suggest that the rates of sexual misbehavior observed in patients with AD have been clinically overestimated. However, it is obvious why these behaviors would be troubling to nursing home staff, caregivers, and family members when they do occur.

Three studies have examined the sexual relationships between AD patients living in the community and their spousal caregivers. Wright (1991) found that male AD patients tend to overestimate the frequency of sexual activity. Eighty two percent of intact couples versus 27% of couples with an AD partner describe regular sexual activity. Wright (1991) also noted that couples who had lower levels of sexual activity but maintained high levels of affection were satisfied with their interactions. Also, female caregivers reported feeling exploited by the frequent sexual demands of their afflicted male partners. In a second study, Davies et al. (1992) described the most frequent concerns of spousal caregivers as follows: (1) too frequent initiation of sex by the afflicted partner because he or she forgets when the last sexual interaction occurred and (2) having sex with a partner who may not recognize them. Inappropriate sexual behavior was reported to be infrequent. Finally, Zeiss et al. (1990) noted that 53% of their sample of AD patients experienced erectile dysfunction. These authors were unable to determine whether the erectile dysfunction was caused directly by disease-related effects on nervous system pathways mediating arousal or whether the causes were psychological due to the effects of AD on mood and self-worth.

There are several methodological difficulties with the studies on AD and sexual function. First, only one of the studies used a control group to examine whether Alzheimer's patients differ from age-matched peers (Wright, 1991). Second, not all of the studies differentiated between male and female AD patients in terms of the probability of inappropriate sexual behavior or other sexual difficulties. Third, again, only self-report measures were used; these are subject to biased reporting, poor recall of the patients, and discrepancy in reports between spouses. Finally, the studies were primarily conducted in community-living patients rather than in nursing home residents; it is unclear what the sexual needs and difficulties of nursing home residents with AD and their spouses are and whether these may differ from the needs and difficulties of cognitively intact nursing home residents.

Despite the lack of research available on the sexual concerns of AD patients living in long-term-care facilities, it is clear that nursing home staff and families do need to address sexual issues. In terms of inappropriate sexual behavior, although the empirical data suggests that these behaviors are rare, nursing home staff frequently raise this type of behavior as a management issue. We advocate a thorough assessment of the problem before proceeding. First, it is important, through psychiatric evaluation, to determine whether the inappropriate behavior is a sexual problem per se or symptomatic of an underlying psychiatric disorder such as psychotic thought process. If so, it may be that the sexual behavior does not represent a sexual disorder but rather a behavioral problem that requires management over and above the sexual symptom. Second, it is important to evaluate the circumstances involved in the sexual behavior to determine whether, in fact, the behavior is inappropriate or whether the staff's reactions are inappropriate. For example, if the patient is masturbating in private, the staff may feel that this is age-inappropriate, whereas it is the staff's attitudes and reactions that are more detrimental than the patient's actual behavior. Third, if the sexual behavior is an isolated problem and the staff does not seem to be overreacting, a qualified staff member should meet with the patients involved and review their needs and the reasons for their behavior. It may be possible to meet these needs in a more appropriate fashion. With respect to masturbating in public, for example, the patient should be encouraged to initiate this behavior only when he or she is alone and a private location is available. Partners of patients with AD should be encouraged to discuss their sexual needs and concerns with appropriate staff members, and guidance and support should be provided if possible. Although AD patients have cognitive deficits, the available research indicates that they may continue to have sexual needs and concerns, and that these should be addressed in a professional and respectful manner. Finally, if the inappropriate sexual behavior persists despite discussion of alternative options, a medication consultation can be requested with the goal of decreasing libido or sexual behavior. We stress that this option should be considered only as a last resort, after the previous recommendations have proved unsuccessful.

Other concerns that staff members may have about residents with AD being sexually active is the fear that one of the residents may be taking advantage of a less functional resident. If there is reason to suspect that one of the partners may not be consenting or is not competent to give consent to sexual activity, appropriate professionals should meet with the residents in questions and evaluate whether the concern is valid. Lichtenberg and Strzepek (1990) offer guidelines on conducting such an assessment, including the following: the patient's awareness of the sexual relationship should be evaluated by asking whether the patient knows *who* is initiating sexual contact, whether he or she is cognizant of the identity of the initiator or is acquiescing under the delusional belief that the initiator is a spouse or significant other, and whether the patient can state what level of intimacy he or she would be most comfortable with. Second, the patient's ability to avoid exploitation is evaluated by asking whether his or her current behavior is consistent with former values and behaviors and determining whether the patient has the capacity to refuse undesired sexual contacts. Finally, the patient's ability to avoid potential risks is ascertained by asking whether the patient realizes that the relationship may be time-limited, and how he or she might react when the relationship ends. These authors recommend that the results of this evaluation be shared with concerned family members, and that the patients' ethical rights to autonomy be protected wherever possible.

Conclusions

The lack of empirical data on sexual behavior in the nursing home population necessitates extrapolation of data from other populations (i.e., healthy aged and community-dwelling AD patients). Although existing research suggests that the elderly are both sexually interested and active, not all nursing home residents will wish to engage in sexual activity, and one should not advocate that they should. Instead, it is suggested that there are a substantial number of elderly persons who are interested in being sexually active, and that they should be encouraged to interact as long as they are able or willing. It can only be disruptive and distressing to expect an individual who has been sexually active throughout his or her lifetime to eliminate that aspect of self-expression upon entering a nursing home environment. Many individuals receive great personal gratification from sexual activity and fulfil important intimacy needs through sexual interaction. The basic right of residents to pursue sexual expression should not be questioned unless it is clearly disruptive or harmful to one of the partners.

Ideally, an environment can be created that allows opportunity for residents to express their sexuality, and to interact with staff regarding sexual issues and problems, just as with other medical or psychological difficulties. Some sexual concerns can be addressed by the staff with minimal specialty training, while others may require referral to appropriate specialists.

Because so little research is available on the sexual needs and concerns of nursing home residents, it is difficult to specify what resources are presently needed in this area. Geriatric researchers and those evaluating the nursing home environment must understand that sexuality is an essential element of quality of life and is worthy of continued investigation. Through further study, it is hoped that nursing home staff will come to better understand the sexual needs and concerns of residents and attempt to address these needs with enhanced empathy for the individual, improved communication about sexual concerns, and greater therapeutic skill in the management of sexual difficulties among the elderly.

References

Arnold SB. The measurement of quality of life in the frail elderly. In: Birren JE, Lubben JE, Rower JC, Deutchman DE, eds. *The Concept and Measurement of Quality of Life in the Frail Elderly.* San Diego, CA: Academic Press, 1991.

Bachmann GA, Leiblum SR. Sexuality in sexagenarian women. *Maturitas* 13:43–50, 1991.

Bancroft, J. *Human Sexuality and Its Problems.* Edinburgh: Churchill Livingstone, 1989.

Bozzola FG, Gorelick PB, Freels S. Personality changes in Alzheimer's disease. *Arch Neurol* 49:297–300, 1992.

Brecher E. *Love, Sex and Aging: A Consumer's Union Survey.* Boston: Little, Brown, 1984.

Bretschneider JG, McCoy NL. Sexual interest and behavior in healthy 80- to 102-year-olds. *Arch Sex Behav* 17:109–129, 1988.

Burns A, Jacoby R, Levy R. Psychiatric phenomena in Alzheimer's disease: IV. Disorders of behavior. *Br J Psychiatry* 157:86–94, 1990.

Carey MP. Sexual adjustment among cancer survivors: Research findings and therapeutic suggestions. *Cancer J* 3:310–314, 1990.

Census of Population. Washington, D.C.: U.S. Department of Commerce, Economics and Statistics Administration, Bureau of the Census, 1992.

Cohn J, Sugar JA. Determinants of quality of life in institutions: Perceptions of frail older residents, staff, and families. In: Birren JE, Lubben JE, Rower JC, Deutchman DE, eds. *The Concept and Measurement of Quality of Life in the Frail Elderly.* San Diego, CA: Academic Press, 1991.

Conte HR. Development and use of self-report techniques for assessing sexual functioning: A review and critique. *Arch Sex Behav* 21:555–576, 1983.

Davies HD, Zeiss A, Tinklenberg JR. 'Til death do us part: Intimacy and sexuality in the marriages of Alzheimer's patients. *J Psychosoc Nurs* 30:5–10, 1992.

Davis CM, Yarber WL, Davis SL. *Sexuality-Related Measures: A Compendium.* Lake Mills, IA: Graphic Publishing, 1988.

Federal Regulations. Code 42. *The Patient's Bill of Rights.* Chapter 4, Section 483, 1990.

Gatz M, Pearson CG. Ageism revised and the provision of psychological services. *Am Psychol* 43:184–188, 1988.

Goldstein I, Rothstein L. *The Potent Male: Facts, Fiction, Future.* Los Angeles: Price, Stern, Sloan, 1990.

Gorovitz S. *Doctor's Dilemmas: Moral Conflict and Medical Care.* New York: Macmillan, 1982.

Kane RA. Everyday life in nursing homes: "The way things are." In: Kane RA, Caplan AL, eds. *Everyday Ethics: Resolving Dilemmas in Nursing Home Life.* New York: Springer-Verlag, 1990.

Kass MJ. Sexual expression of the elderly in nursing homes. *Gerontologist* 18:372–377, 1978.

Leiblum SR, Baume RM, Croog S. The sexual functioning of elderly hypertensive women. *J Sex Marital Therapy* 20:259–270, 1994.

Leiblum SR, Segraves RT. Sex therapy and aging adults. In: Leiblum SR, Rosen RC, eds. *Principles and Practice of Sex Therapy: Update of the 1990s.* New York: Guilford, 1989.

Libman E. Sociocultural and cognitive factors in aging and sexual expression: Conceptual and research issues. *Can Psychol* 30:560–567, 1989.

Lichtenberg PA, Strzepek DM. Assessments of institutionalized dementia patients' competencies to participate in intimate relationships. *Gerontologist* 30:117–120, 1990.

Martin CE. Factors affecting sexual functioning in 60–79 year old married men. *Arch Sex Behav* 10:399–420, 1981.

McCarthy JR, Izeman H, Rogers D, Cohen N. Sexuality and the institutionalized elderly. *J Am Geriatr Soc* 35:331–333, 1987.

Meisler AW, Carey MP. Depressed affects and male sexual arousal. *Arch Sex Behav* 20:541–554, 1989.

Meisler AW, Carey MP, Lantinga LJ, Krauss DJ. Erectile dysfunction in diabetes mellitus: A biopsychosocial approach to etiology and assessment. *Ann Behav Med* 11:18–27, 1989.

Mulligan T, Palguta R. Sexual interest, activity, and satisfaction among male nursing home residents. *Arch Sex Behav* 20:199–204, 1991.

Mulligan T, Retchin SM, Chinchilli VM, Bettinger CB. The role of aging and chronic disease in sexual dysfunction. *J Am Geriatr Soc* 36:520–524, 1988.

Poggi RG, Berland DI. The therapist's reactions to the elderly. *Gerontologist* 25:508–513, 1985.

Quinn-Krach P, Van Hoozer H. Sexuality of the aged and the attitudes and knowledge of nursing students. *J Nurs Educ* 27:359–363, 1988.

Rosen RC. Alcohol and drug effects on sexual response: Human experimental and clinical studies. *Annu Rev Sex Res* 2:119–180, 1991.

Schiavi RC, Schreiner-Engel P, Mandeli J, et al. Healthy aging and male sexual function. *Am J Psychiatry* 147:766–771, 1990.

Schover LR, Jensen SB. *Sexuality and Chronic Illness: A Comprehensive Approach.* New York: Guilford, 1988.

Schreiner-Engel P, Schiavi RC. Life psychopathology in individuals with low sexual desire. *J Nerv Ment Dis* 174:646–651, 1986.

Segraves RT, Segraves KB. Aging and drug effects on male sexuality. In: Leiblum SR, Rosen RC, eds. *Principles and Practice of Sex Therapy: Update of the 1990s.* New York: Guilford, 1989.

Sherwin BB. Changes in sexual behavior as a function of plasma sex steroid levels in post-menopausal women. *Maturitas* 4:231–237, 1985.

Spector IP, Carey MP. Incidence an prevalence of the sexual dysfunctions: A critical review of the empirical literature. *Arch Sex Behav* 19:389–408, 1990.

Spector IP, Leiblum SR, Carey MP, Rosen RC. Diabetes and female sexual function: A critical review. *Ann Behav Med* 15:257–264, 1993.

Striar SL, Hoffman KS. Advocating for the socio-sexual rights of the single elderly: A six-step intervention strategy. *J Soc Work Hum Sex* 3:71–83, 1984.

Thase ME, Reynolds CF, Glanz LM, et al. Nocturnal penile tumescence in depressed men. *Am J Psychiatry* 144:89–92, 1987.

Thomas LE. Correlates of sexual interest among elderly men. *Psychol Rep* 68:620–622, 1991.

Wallace M. Management of sexual relationships among elderly residents of long-term care facilities. *Ger Nurs* 13:308–311, 1992.

Weinstein S, Rosen E. Senior adult sexuality in age segregated and age integrated communities. *Int J Aging Hum Devel* 27:261–270, 1988.

Weizman R, Hart J. Sexual behavior in healthy married elderly men. *Arch Sex Behav* 16:39–44, 1987.

Wincze JP, Carey MP. *Sexual Dysfunction: A Guide for Assessment and Treatment.* New York: Guilford, 1991.

Winn RL, Newton N. Sexuality in aging: A study of 106 cultures. *Arch Sex Behav* 11:283–298, 1982.

Wright LK. The impact of Alzheimer's disease on the marital relationship. *Gerontologist* 31:224–237, 1991.

Zeiss AM, Davies HD, Wood M, Tinklenberg JR. The incidence and correlates of erectile problems in patients with Alzheimer's disease. *Arch Sex Behav* 19:325–332, 1990.

Zilbergeld B. *Male Sexuality.* New York: Bantam, 1978.

11

Mental Retardation

Mary C. Howell-Raugust

Although there is general formal consensus that a nursing home is rarely an optimal living situation for a person with mental retardation, a large number of people with mental retardation do, in fact, live in nursing homes that are not specialized for their care. As for all nursing home residents, this placement can provide security and nurturance. But there is also a risk of failure to meet the particular needs of the individual resident. For the caregiving staff, there are likely to be both satisfactions and problems associated with residents who are mentally retarded.

This chapter addresses the question of nursing home placement of persons with mental retardation from a variety of perspectives. First, we consider the nature of the aging process for people with mental retardation. Next, we look at general recommendations, policies, and regulations intended to guarantee the appropriateness of admission and care of individuals with mental retardation in general nursing homes. In addition, we observe the broad picture of this population painted by statistical survey research. Finally, we present a set of clinical vignettes chosen to illustrate the experience of individual placements of persons with mental retardation into nursing homes. Finally, some general recommendations for the provision of service are drawn from these illustrations.

Only nursing homes designed, programmed, and staffed for general admissions are considered here. Those facilities that provide services especially tailored for persons with mental retardation, designated as Intermediate Care Facilities/Mental Retardation (ICF/MRs) and Special Needs Facilities/Mental Retardation (SNF/MRs), are excluded from this review.

Mental Retardation and the Aging Process

Like every other population subgroup, persons with mental retardation have become increasingly likely to live into old age—the eighth and ninth decades and beyond (Janicki and Wisniewski, 1985). This fact surprises some, as our cultural stereotype of mental retardation has focused on young children.

The standard contemporary definition of mental retardation refers to significantly subaverage intellectual function resulting in or associated with impairments in adaptive behavior manifested during the developmental period. In terms of standardized intelligence testing, "significantly subaverage" is usually interpreted to mean an IQ score of less than 70. According to the statistical conventions of the tests, 3% of the population is mentally retarded. It should also be noted that standardized IQ testing is probably not valid for adults past middle age with lifelong histories of impairments in adaptive behavior. As an exception to this proposition, testing administered by professionals with special training and experience in working with this group can sometimes give general information as to cognitive capacity and learning style.

Approximately 75% of persons with mental retardation have no known or detectable cause for their retardation. For the remaining 25%, more than two hundred causes have been described, of which 90% occur prenatally and/or are present at birth (Matson and Mulick, 1983).

The single most frequent known cause of mental retardation is Down's syndrome, or trisomy 21. But, in fact, it is probable that Down's syndrome need not inevitably be associated with "retardation." The tested IQ of persons with Down's syndrome who have not had special education is usually in the range of 55 to 75. But special education has been demonstrated to be beneficial to the intellectual development of those with this syndrome; with such education, their tested IQ has been shown to increase by 10 to 15 points. Therefore, it is probable that many persons with Down's syndrome who are exposed to early special education may not develop the disabilities associated with mental retardation.

The second most frequent known cause of mental retardation is fragile X syndrome. Like Down's syndrome, this malady is genetically determined although variably inherited. It is expressed only in males, who tend to have characteristically enlarged testicles. As with Down's syndrome, the conclusive diagnosis is made by laboratory procedures in genetics.

Not all persons with the same IQ test scores have equivalent disabilities, nor do they have the same functional capabilities. Assessment according to function is an essential component of the definition of developmental disabilities used to fund services in accordance with Public Law 95-602. The elements of the definition are that the disability occurs before the age of 22, is chronic, involves functional limitations in three or more major life areas (of a specific list of areas), and requires an array of long-term services. "Developmental disability" and "mental retardation" are used interchangeably by some (as here); others argue that the label "mental retardation" has so denigrating a stigma that the expression should not be used at all.

Functional assessment of persons with mental retardation is usually accomplished by interview or direct observation. The Adaptive Behavior Scale, a commonly used rating scale for function devised by the American Association of Mental Retardation (1981), examines a variety of domains of independent functioning. These domains include physical functioning, communication, social functioning, economic activity, occupation, and self-direction. To be of maximum usefulness, a functional assessment should designate the individual's strengths as well as areas of impairment, disability, and handicap (Seltzer and Seltzer, 1984).

Of the 3% of the population who are labeled as retarded on the basis of IQ test scores, approximately 95% live in noninstitutional settings. More than 90% of all persons with mental retardation are in the mild to moderate categories; functionally, they may be disabled or retarded in some settings (such as schools or banks) and not in others (such as grocery stores or buses). The 0.3% of the population who are severely or profoundly retarded are not the subject of this chapter, as they are rarely considered for admission to a general nursing home.

It is important to observe that virtually every person who is both old and mentally retarded is capable of some new learning. As with the non-retarded population, this capacity for new learning may be impaired by senile dementia of the Alzheimer's type (or a similar dementia) that destroys short-term memory and, therefore, learning capacity, but this handicap is specific and can be diagnosed. In all other cases, a residential and social setting which assumes that the resident with mental retardation is capable of learning can draw new and adaptive behaviors from that resident (Talkington, 1969; Anderson and Sinclair, 1992). Historically, institutional care for persons with mental retardation improved markedly when the underlying professional and philosophical orientation of these residential institutions shifted from a "medical model" to an "educational model."

Although the proportion of those with mental retardation who live to old age is lower than that for the population as a whole, life expectancies for persons in this group—excluding those with severe physically disabling conditions—approach those of the nondisabled population. Longevity is likely to be highest for women, persons who do not have disabilities of mobility, and those who have been able to live in the community (Anderson, 1989).

It should be noted that a higher proportion of those with Down's syndrome than that of the "normal" population appear to develop a dementia syndrome that is very like the cluster of behaviors labeled as senile dementia of the Alzheimer's type. In some studies, the incidence approaches 100% by age 50, as compared with an incidence of 55% by age 85 for persons who do not have Down's syndrome (Howell et al., 1989).

Service needs for persons who survive into old age with and without mental retardation are likely to converge. With increasing age, a larger and larger proportion of the general population needs assistance with activities of daily living, some level of ongoing medical and nursing attention, provision for recreational and spiritual needs, and safe and secure housing. These requirements are not very different from those of persons with mental retardation who are also old (Howell et al., 1989).

It is important to state affirmatively that, as a group, those who are mentally retarded and also old have no special needs. Their individual needs range widely, but are not predetermined and cannot be assumed by the mere fact of mental retardation. Needs assessment must be based on functional assessment. Provision of services will, in the ideal case, be designed in light of the functional assessment and be intended to preserve function, continue the best of past relationships and opportunities, and offer correctives to past restrictions and deprivations. By this prescription, persons who are mentally retarded are no different in their needs for service than any other nursing home residents.

Admission to the Nursing Home: Social and Public Policy

There are three common circumstances in which an adult with mental retardation—who may be middle-aged or old—is proposed for admission to a nursing home. In the first scenario, the person with retardation has been living with his or her parents or perhaps with another relative such as a sibling or cousin. Often the family has had little or no connection to the formal bureaucracy of caregiving for persons with mental retardation, a system that is regulated and funded primarily by the state government. Typically, the impetus to the request for nursing home placement in these cases is some additional stress on the caregiving household—a death, a financial strain or reversal, or the illness of a family member. The person with mental retardation, who has for some time needed a relatively high level of care, is proposed for nursing home admission much as any other household member with similar service needs.

In the second scenario, the person with mental retardation who is proposed for nursing home admission has been living in a state-run residential institution that has specialized mental retardation expertise but is now slated for downsizing or perhaps for closing altogether. When such wholesale deinstitutionalization occurs, some residents will be moved to small community residences with various capacities for provision of services, but others will appear to be most suited for nursing home placement (Mueller, 1969; Pothier, 1989).

In the third scenario, the person with mental retardation has been living in a small community residence, state regulated and funded, but he or she has progressed through a normal aging process to a point where the rules and regulations of the community residence prohibit his or her continued care. Often this occurs because failing hearing or eyesight prevents ''self-preservation'' (self-guided exit at the time of a fire or a fire drill), or because self-feeding skills are deteriorating and staffing limitations make it impossible to assign a staff member to assist the resident at mealtimes.

In all three of these circumstances, the reasons for nursing home admission are not very dissimilar from reasons that might be put forward for a proposed resident who is not mentally retarded. There are, however, two very different perspectives on whether nursing home placement is appropriate for these persons with mental retardation.

From the first perspective, some would argue that nursing home residence is never "normalization," and that the goal with regard to the living circumstances of persons with mental retardation must be that they are enabled to live as much as possible as members of a diverse community, with the provision of whatever assistance is needed to make that community placement possible. This view is usually based on a political philosophy that gauges the rights of persons with mental retardation to be nearly inviolable—perhaps because of past injustices, the history of inadequate if not frankly cruel care, and the vulnerability of impairment. In this perspective, funds should be prioritized for the honoring of the right to normalization.

The second perspective reflects the observation that, with advancing age and infirmity, *many* otherwise healthy members of a community will have to move to nursing homes as the only placement in the community where their needs can be met economically. From this perspective, such a placement is indeed a "normalized" living situation for a person with mental retardation who is also old. This view accepts the abrogation of individual rights (in this case, of people who are old, with or without mental retardation) as inevitable in a culture of scarce resources—resources inadequate to satisfy the needs of all members of society.

There are three categories of objection to the placement of persons with mental retardation, in need of institutional services, in nursing homes not specialized for their care. Least persuasive and most easily overcome is the argument that such individuals would not "fit in"—would disrupt the living circumstances of other residents or could not receive appropriate everyday services from the facility staff.

It is also argued that it would be impossible for a general nursing home facility to provide the special, corrective, normalizing services that a person with mental retardation who is also old is likely to need; this argument is especially persuasive when the person with mental retardation has lived for many decades in a large public institution, the sort of institution that was likely—some decades past—to have been neglectful or even abusive to residents.

Finally, and most pointed in today's economy, is the argument that if the person with mental retardation were to receive all the services that are mandated (explicitly or by implication) by current law, and the facility, in order to be evenhanded, would have to provide an equal quality and quantity of individualized services for all residents, then the resulting cost would be prohibitive.

These latter two arguments are confounded by the present complex of federal and state regulations. Often, for the individual nursing home, a decision about admission of a person with mental retardation is indeterminate and extremely difficult because of the lack of clarity of these regulations and also because of current funding problems.

The intersection of regulations and funding for the care of people with mental retardation has been called a ''Catch-22.'' On the one hand, standards for care—as promulgated by the U.S. Department of Health and Human Services and by parallel agencies in the individual states—have become markedly elevated over the past several decades, as a consequence, in part, of vigorous lobbying efforts by organizations composed of families and friends of persons with mental retardation. On the other hand, Medicaid expenditures to fund the provision of services to meet these standards of care are a favorite target for those wishing to contain costs, including Congress and the Office of Management and Budget and their parallel agencies in the states. Education and vocational costs are especially likely to be targeted for disallowance (Mayer et al., 1992).

A dispute emerges centering on the concept of ''active treatment,'' often defined as ''services to help recipients function at the greatest physical, intellectual, social, or vocational level they can reach now or in the future.'' One device to limit expenditures for recipients who are mentally retarded and also old is to assert that in old age, no improvement in function can be anticipated.

At the same time that there are moves to limit Medicaid's liability for certain services mandated in the care of persons with mental retardation, the Health Care Financing Administration has continued to allow grave uncertainties in the standards used to survey institutional adequacy of care. As a result, a nursing home might be cited for failing to provide adequate services to a resident who is mentally retarded or disallowed for the costs of providing those very services (Anonymous, 1989; Wagner, 1989).

Current regulations under the Omnibus Budget Reconciliation Act (OBRA, P.L. 100.203) require that every proposed resident be considered for the possibility of mental retardation and screened by appropriate assessment procedures. Such procedures are not fully spelled out (Anonymous, 1992). Clearly, if the proposed resident had undergone IQ testing at an earlier time and the results had been recorded and these records preserved, that information could be used as part of the assessment. Because of validity problems, discussed above, IQ testing not performed until the person is in midlife or old age is generally less useful for persons with mental retardation.

On the other hand, a functional assessment of contemporaneous behaviors, along with a detailed history taken from someone who has known the proposed resident for some years, will usually yield useful information. Such an assessment may have to be accompanied by a clinical summary to justify the diagnosis of mental retardation. Aside from compliance with OBRA regulations, though, a functional assessment—as described above—is always necessary for provision of appropriate services.

It should be noted that long-term residence in an institution ''for the mentally retarded'' or the receipt of services from the state bureaucracy ''for the mentally retarded'' does not necessarily constitute firm evidence that the individual does, in fact, have mental retardation. On the other hand, ''institutional retardation''—the long-term effects of years or even decades of residence in an institution in which one has been treated as a person who is mentally retarded—is real and has behavioral consequences.

In 1965, the U.S. Congress established the Intermediate Care Facility (ICF) Program under Medical Assistance within the Social Security Program, or Medicaid. The intention was to provide long-term care in nursing homes to needy individuals. As a consequence, the number of general nursing home beds nearly tripled in the years from 1963 to 1971 (National Center for Health Care Statistics, 1970, 1974).

In 1971, Medicaid reimbursement was authorized for care of people with mental retardation in public institutions classified as ICF/MRs. Congress's intention apparently was to help states pay for this care, to guarantee minimally adequate residential and habilitative programs in public institutions, and to counteract the growing tendency to place people with mental retardation in general nursing homes (Mitchell and Braddock, 1990).

Beginning at about the same time, there was a strong movement for the deinstitutionalization of adults with mental retardation; as a result, placements in large state institutions decreased by approximately 34% (Lakin et al., 1982). A significant number of those who left the large institutions, however, were actually placed in general nursing homes. In addition, as admissions to the large state residential institutions were severely curtailed, many persons who were requesting state services for the first time (having previously lived, for instance, in their own family homes with family members) were placed directly into general nursing homes. This is often described as a "back door" placement option (Gettings et al., 1988).

Because nursing homes are generally regulated by state departments of public aid or welfare, their residents may be removed from the rolls and from the oversight of a state department of mental health, mental retardation, and/or developmental disabilities and may thus lose safeguards for ensuring appropriate placement and active treatment.

Taken together, these myriad factors point to a direct conflict between the federal policy of reimbursing care in ICF/MRs and the policy of the caregiving establishment of placing persons with mental retardation in community settings. For the most part, the ICF/MRs that meet federal standards for Medicaid reimbursement are large, state-supported residential facilities. But other, smaller institutions, including general nursing homes, can apply for ICF/MR status.

Survey Research Results: Persons with Mental Retardation in General Nursing Homes

In the view of many, the reinstitutionalization of persons with mental retardation into general nursing homes frustrates the reasons for the shift in public policy toward placement in communities. These reasons include a mixture of legal and fiscal principles, advocacy for the rights of persons with mental retardation and a growing understanding of their needs, and the emergence of a new group of professionals prepared to support, deliver, and administer community-based services. As a consequence, a variety of survey-research projects considering the welfare of adults with mental retardation placed in general nursing homes were undertaken. The results of these research projects continue to be reported (Sirrocco, 1989).

In a survey of general nursing homes in Illinois (Uehara, 1991), it was determined that only 10% of the residents with mental retardation were appropriately placed "in medical settings," and that only 27% were enrolled in "developmental training programs." Only one-fifth of those originally studied in the general nursing home placements were deemed to be appropriately placed.

However, some of these residents in general nursing homes had significantly more intense needs than do typical residents in residential facilities for persons with developmental disabilities. These needs were noted to be in the areas of medical care, adaptive behavior, self-care, and self-preservation.

As a result of the reported study, the state of Illinois made plans to remove two-thirds of the nursing home residents with mental retardation to family or small group homes as true "community placements." An additional number, less than 10%, were to be moved to ICF/MRs because their medical needs exceeded the capacity of the general nursing homes. These plans were made in the face of known difficulties in siting, the training of personnel, and funding of family and small group community homes.

A parallel report on residents in general nursing homes in New England (primarily Massachusetts) concluded that, on a variety of measures and as a group, persons with mental retardation living in nursing homes are at least as competent as those who live in community-based programs. It was concluded that initial placements were made for reasons other than the goodness of fit between the residents' needs and the services provided in the nursing homes (Seltzer et al., 1988).

Surveys conducted in 1977 and 1985 demonstrated that, with respect to residents with mental retardation in general nursing homes, the size of the population essentially did not change over the 12-year study period (an estimated 40,500 nationally in 1985), and the services received by these residents remained at "essentially the same low level," as measured against the level and variety of services mandated by law for persons with mental retardation (Schmidt et al., 1977; Mitchell and Braddock, 1990; Lakin, 1991). Although the people with mental retardation placed in general nursing homes were older, on average, than people with mental retardation placed in other types of residential care, they tended to be much younger than other residents of general nursing homes; an estimated 68% of nursing home residents with mental retardation were below the age of 65 years in 1985 as compared with 12% of the overall nursing home population.

In addition, there was a relatively low prevalence of substantial physical and sensory limitations in nursing home residents with mental retardation; an extremely limited involvement in therapeutic services, and a very high reported level of resident "need for assistance" with basic activities of daily living. These findings suggest that insufficient effort has been made to increase the independence of these residents with mental retardation (Schmidt, 1977; Benz et al., 1986).

Public Law 100-203, passed in part with the direct intention of ameliorating the situation described above, requires not only preadmission assessment of mental retardation but the provision of "active treatment" for residents with mental retardation. Those residents who had been placed in a general nursing home more than 30 months prior to enactment of the law in 1989 were given the option of remaining in their present placement, but now with required (and, presumably, enforced) provision of adequate "active treatment" services.

One method of providing some of the active treatment services required is to make use of day programs in the community. Residents might be sent out during the day to existing day programs. Alternatively, day programs specifically designed to accommodate the residents of general nursing homes who are in need of these services might be instituted.

There is general agreement that small community residences are almost always more appropriate placements for adults of middle to old age with mental retardation than are general nursing homes. Still, there is an impressive shortage of such community residences. Two noteworthy problems with their establishment and maintenance are (1) siting difficulties—the resistance of neighborhoods to having such residences in their midst—and (2) the inevitable gradual increase in staffing and service needs as residents progress into old age, an increase that so far has not been well addressed by regulations or funding.

Clinical Vignettes

Until more appropriate residential placements are established, it is likely that there will continue to be residents with mental retardation in general nursing homes. The clinical vignettes that follow are illustrative of the service needs, problems, and satisfactions experienced with these residents.

1. One nursing home was asked in 1972, by the social work department of a large state residential institution for adults with mental retardation, to accept a group of five persons between the ages of 65 and 75. One had Down's syndrome but none of the behavioral characteristics of senile dementia of the Alzheimer's type. All had only mild to moderate levels of retardation. They were accepted for admission.

The five were observed to act like a sibling group with an internal order of hierarchy, referred to by the staff as a "pecking order." In the nursing home, they were housed in adjacent rooms. None had disturbing or acting-out behaviors, and they all seemed relatively content with their new home. They demonstrated, as one aftermath of years of institutional living, extreme tidiness and attachment to predictable routines.

Of the five, initially only the person with Down's syndrome had a family member, a sister, who visited. That sister, however, in collaboration with the social work department of the nursing home, was able to locate and make contact with a sister of one of the other former state institutional residents.

None of the five had any particular need for ongoing medical care and skilled nursing services. Of the other services that would at the present time be mandated by law—such as access to recreational and spiritual communities and activities, encouragement and training in self-care, and possibly vocational training and opportunities to earn money—the nursing home had no means for provision.

Socially, the five presented no problems to the staff or to the other residents. They were, however, treated somewhat as "pets," spoken to as children, offered childlike objects for amusement, and in general infantilized in ways that were quite inappropriate but not unusual in the early 1970s.

All five died of "old age" (chronic congestive heart failure, small recurrent strokes, rampant urinary tract infections, and the like) and not of acute treatable disease. The nursing home, in conjunction with a local funeral establishment and a local cemetery, arranged that all five would be buried in the same plot.

2. Another nursing home has had three admissions, separate in time, from a small, private "community residence" that is geographically isolated in a rural area near the town in which the nursing home is located. All three of these admitted residents has Down's syndrome: their ages at the time of admission to the general nursing home ranged from 49 to 68 years. In each case the resident had suffered some physical deterioration and thus required increasing assistance with activities of daily living; two were also unable to walk and needed wheelchairs.

One of the residents appeared to have senile dementia of the Alzheimer's type at the time of admission. The other two, although considered to have mental retardation on the basis of their characteristic facies, seemed to function in a low-normal range of intelligence. They, too, however, were infantilized—both on the basis of assumptions about persons with Down's syndrome and assumptions derived from their prior residence.

3. In 1982, a nursing home in an urban working-class neighborhood admitted Dora, a 45-year-old woman with Down's syndrome. She had always lived at home with her family of origin and had never been enrolled with or received services from the state department of mental retardation.

In the year before her admission, Dora's father died and her mother, age 87, fell at home and broke her hip. An older sister moved into the house to care for the convalescing mother and the handicapped sibling, who had always before been cared for by the mother. As the mother regained her strength and some degree of mobility, it was clear that she could not continue to be the primary caretaker for her daughter with Down's syndrome.

Because the family knew nothing about access to services provided by the state department of mental retardation and had no reason to trust that bureaucracy, they applied directly for nursing home admission for Dora. Dora was accepted.

Dora adapted easily to the routines of the nursing home but was obviously mourning her dead father as well as the separation from her mother and from her lifelong home. Although her mother and sister visited Dora often, she often said "I have no family" and "I have no home."

Within weeks after admission, Dora began to develop symptoms of progressive dementia, including failure of short-term memory and judgment, with rapid progression to seizures and loss of mobility. She died of pneumonia 3 years later, having displayed the rapid course of dementia that is often seen when it begins at a young age. Dora's mother and sister had asked that she not be resuscitated in the event of cardiorespiratory failure.

4. Carl, a man of 82, had lived with his unmarried sister for the previous 30 years, following the death of his parents in an auto accident. He had never attended school past the second grade, worked at a job, prepared his own meals, or taken care of his own laundry—though the nursing home staff reported that they believed he could have done all of these things. Although his IQ had never been tested, in early grade school it had been decided that he was "strange" and "ineducable," and his parents had kept him at home and cared for him on their farm.

When his sister became too crippled with arthritis to continue to keep her own home and care for her brother, they were both admitted to the same general nursing home. They each had their own roommates, but their rooms were near each other in the same unit. The staff remembers that Carl took a major role in attending to his sister after their admission to the nursing home.

When the sister died of a myocardial infarction 3 years after her admission, Carl became very depressed. Four months later he himself died when a urinary tract infection rapidly developed into a sepsis.

5. Two sisters, Edith and Ethyl, who were deaf and communicated only with a rudimentary sign language, were admitted to a general nursing home when the large state-run institution, where they had lived for more than sixty years, began to downsize. They shared a room and initially their social interactions were primarily with each other.

An aide, who happened to know modified sign language because her older sister had worked at the state-run institution for the mentally retarded, took an interest in the sisters and began to teach them a more extensive sign-language vocabulary. At the same time, she instructed several other staff members in this modified sign language.

Within a year of their admission to the nursing home, the sisters, then 65 and 68, blossomed both socially and in their capacity for self-care. Efforts were made to enroll them in a local "sheltered workshop" employment program, but no places were available to them because of their age. It was likewise not possible, because of nursing home regulations, for the sisters to have responsible tasks assigned to them in the nursing home.

They lived on at the nursing home for 10 and 12 more years, respectively, both ultimately dying of pneumonia.

Conclusion: Recommendations for the Provision of Service

These vignettes describing the placement of persons with mental retardation into nursing homes that are not specialized for their care raise several issues related to the needs of this population. It should be emphasized, however, that their needs are not essentially different from the needs of other persons who are institutionalized because they are old and/or infirm.

Dignity

Adults who have lost or never developed some of the competencies that we think of as defining maturity may appear to us to be "childlike." Sometimes it is tempting to treat them like children. Such treatment is not compatible with a demonstration of respect for their essential dignity.

A Stable, Concerned, and Affectionate Cadre of Caregivers

Residents in nursing homes sometimes have no known close kin or simply no visitors; people who have spent much of their lives in residential institutions may be especially likely to be without a network of caring family members. While the nursing home staff cannot "replace" or simulate family, staff stability and availability to show concern and affection can contribute to the resident's sense of well-being.

A Learning-Focused Environment

The assumption that a resident is "past change" or "past learning" condemns that person to a static and probably boring existence. The contrary assumption, that learning is possible and desirable, generates an environment that provides excitement, challenge, and the pleasure of mastery.

A "good" outcome for any one individual still ultimately depends on the availability of some one service provider who cares. Regulations can go a long way toward preventing abuse but probably cannot foresee how to enable an institution to encourage growth-promoting care. It is important that regulations, in their detailed complexity, do not foreclose the possibilities of inventive, nurturing, and idiosyncratic circumstances of caregiving.

References

American Association of Mental Retardation. *Adaptive Behavior Scale.* Austin, TX: Pro-Ed, 1981.

Anderson DJ. Healthy and institutionalized: health and related conditions among older persons with developmental disabilities. *J Appl Gerontol* 8:228–241, 1989.

Anderson L, Sinclair SV. Program to enhance ADL skills improves resident self esteem. *Provider* 18(2):33–34, 1992.

Anonymous. New nursing home law creates confusion. *Wis Med J* 88(4):44, 1989.

Anonymous. Medicare and Medicaid programs: Preadmission screening and annual resident review—HCFA. Final rule with comment period. *Federal Register* 57:56450–56514, 1992.

Benz MR, Halpern AS, Close DW. Access to day programs and leisure activities by nursing home residents with mental retardation. *Ment Retard* 24:147–152, 1986.

Gettings R, Smith G, Katz R. *Nursing Home Reform: Implications for Services to Persons with Developmental Disabilities.* Alexandria VA: National Association of State Mental Retardation Program Directors, 1988.

Howell MC, Gavin DG, Cabrerra GA, Beyer HA, eds. *Serving the Underserved.* Boston: Exceptional Parent Press, 1989.

Janicki MP, Wisniewski HM. *Aging and Developmental Disabilities: Issues and Approaches.* Baltimore: Brookes, 1985.

Lakin KC, Hill BK, Anderson DJ. Persons with mental retardation in nursing homes in 1977 and 1985. *Ment Retard* 29:25–33, 1991.

Lakin KC, Krantz G, Bruininks RA, et al. *One Hundred Years of Data on Populations of Public Residential Facilities for Mentally Retarded People.* Minneapolis: University of Minnesota Department of Psychoeducational Studies, 1982.

Matson JL, Mulick JA, eds. *Handbook of Mental Retardation.* New York: Pergamon, 1983.

Mayer JA, Heal LW, Trach JS. Income allowance policies of state Medicaid agencies as work incentives or disincentives for ICF/MR residents. *Ment Retard* 30:215–219, 1992.

Mitchell D, Braddock D. Historical and contemporary issues in nursing home reform. *Ment Retard* 28:201–210, 1990.

Mueller BJ, Porter R. Placement of adult retardates from state institutions in community care facilities. *Commun Ment Health J* 5:289–294, 1969.

National Center for Health Care Statistics. *Health Resources Statistics, PHS #70-1509.* Washington DC: Vital and Health Statistics, 1970.

National Center for Health Care Statistics. *Health Resources Statistics, PHS #74-1509.* Washington DC: Vital and Health Statistics, 1974.

Pothier PC. Yet another form of deinstitutionalization. *Arch Psychiatr Nurs* 3:251–253, 1989.

Schmidt LJ, Reinhardt AM, Kane RL, Olsen DM. The mentally ill in nursing homes: New back wards in the community. *Arch Gen Psychiatry* 34:687–691, 1977.

Seltzer GB, Finaly E, Howell M. Functional characteristics of elderly persons with mental retardation in community settings and nursing homes. *Ment Retard* 26:213–217, 1988.

Seltzer GB, Seltzer MM. Functional assessment of persons with mental retardation. In: Granger CV, Gresham GE, eds. *Functional Assessment in Rehabilitation Medicine.* Baltimore: Williams & Wilkins, 1984.

Sirrocco A. *Characteristics of Facilities for the Mentally Retarded, 1986.* Vital & Health
    Statistics. Series 14, Data from the National Health Survey. Washington, DC: Vital
    and Health Statistics, 1989.
Talkington LW, Chiovaro SJ. An approach to programming for aged MR. *Ment Retard*
    7:29–30, 1969.
Uehara ES, Silverstein BJ, Davis R, Geron S. Assessment of needs of adults with develop-
    mental disabilities in skilled nursing and intermediate care facilities in Illinois.
    Ment Retard 29:223–231, 1991.
Wagner L. Nursing home groups join assault on directive. *Mod Healthcare* 19(156):20,
    1989.

12

Substance Abuse Disorders

Kenneth Solomon and James B. Shackson

The substance abuse disorders (SADs), or alcohol and chemical dependency, are probably underdiagnosed in the elderly. The effects of this underdiagnosis are magnified in the nursing home setting, with potentially disastrous results. Like syphilis and tuberculosis, the manifest morbidity from these disorders may be protean. Subtle and not-so-subtle cognitive deficits, affective changes, anxiety, agitation, sleep disturbances, withdrawal symptoms, and falls are among the many manifestations of SADs.

The causes for the underdiagnosis of these disorders are many. A major one is that the criteria of the *Diagnostic and Statistical Manual,* 4th ed. (DSM-IV) (APA, 1994), for SADs are heavily biased toward functional disturbances that are most likely to occur to younger people (Solomon et al., 1993). According to these criteria, the frequent use of an addictive compound must be coupled with academic, occupational, marital, legal, and/or social dysfunctions if a diagnosis of SAD is to be made. Solomon and Stark (1993) have demonstrated that there are significant differences between elderly and young addicts living in the community, and that many of the dysfunctions noted in younger addicts (and required by the diagnostic criteria) do not occur in elderly addicts. This is especially truer of the nursing home population, but appropriate diagnostic criteria for SADs in this population do not exist. In addition, the DSM-IV criteria assume that substance abuse must precede substance dependence. This is not usually the case with elderly addicts (Solomon, 1993).

Another factor in underdiagnosis is that most nursing home patients with a SAD take on legal medications prescribed by their physicians. While some of these patients may have had a previous diagnosis of SAD, many develop a psychological dependence on these medications only after they are admitted to the nursing home. Thus, the physicians who prescribe these medications with the laudable intention of helping relieve patients' symptoms and discomforts are likely to develop diagnostic blind spots and subsequently miss an iatrogenic diagnosis.

A third factor that leads to the underdiagnosis of SADs in nursing home patients is the widespread denial among health and mental health professionals that SADs are a significant problem in the elderly. Negative stereotypes of older people and of addicts are common among health professionals (Solomon and Vickers, 1979); the nursing home patient is usually perceived to fit into the former but not the latter stereotype. Thus, the diagnosis is unlikely to be made unless the older addict manifests drug-seeking behaviors that are clearly dysfunctional.

The final factors that interfere with the accurate diagnosis of SADs in nursing home patients are the educational lacunae among health and mental health professionals regarding SADs. Few professionals have had the opportunity to learn more than the most basic information about these disorders, and fewer still have had any significant clinical experience with patients with these disorders.

This chapter reviews SADs in elderly patients residing in nursing homes. It discusses the epidemiology of and risk factors for developing these disorders. The clinical presentation and evaluation of these disorders are covered. Treatment options and preventive strategies are also reviewed.

To adequately discuss SADs in the long-term-care setting, we feel that it is necessary to offer a heuristic definition of SADs in the elderly. This definition is much broader than the DSM-IV criteria. However, this breadth is necessary to include most, if not all, elderly patients with SADs. The definition is derived in part from the DSM-IV and the National Council on Alcoholism and Drug Dependence (Morse and Flavin, 1992) definitions, modified by years of clinical experience working with elderly addicts. According to these, a SAD is a primary, chronic, progressive, treatable disorder with a complex, multifactorial etiology that is manifested by the regular but not necessarily daily use of a potentially addictive compound to the degree that the individual (1) manifests biological, psychological, or social sequelae of the drug use or (2) is at risk for the development of symptoms of withdrawal if use of the drug is suddenly curtailed or significantly diminished.

Epidemiology

There have been few studies of the prevalence of SADs in nursing homes. This is surprising, as many nursing homes offer ''happy hours'' or use small ''doses'' of wine or beer as appetite stimulants. In addition, as benzodiazepines and other potentially addictive medications are amongst the most frequently prescribed medications in this setting (Ingman et al., 1975; Kalchthaler et al., 1977; Segal et al., 1979; Ray et al., 1980; Morgan and Gilleard, 1981; Reynolds, 1984; Buck, 1988; Morriss et al., 1990), one would expect that data about the misuse of these medications would be available. Finally, with patterns of illegal drug use changing among all age groups in the community and with AIDS becoming a disease that affects all population groups, data on illegal substance abuse would be helpful in planning services to this segment of the elderly population.

The few studies that have been published are fraught with methodological difficulties. Most epidemiological studies of psychiatric or cognitive disorders in the elderly do not ask questions relevant to the prevalence of SADs. Studies of the epidemiology of dementia in nursing homes rarely identify patients with alcohol- or drug-related cognitive changes, although these disorders are usually included in similar studies of hospitalized or community-dwelling elderly. Those studies that note the presence or absence of SADs usually do not clarify the diagnostic criteria used in the study. Some studies use data based on chart diagnosis; others are based on structured interviews. The reported prevalence of these disorders in the nursing home is significantly lower than that in the community, which is probably an artifact of the study methodology and is related to the underdiagnosis of these disorders. In addition, the presence of alcohol- or drug-related physical problems, which may be a factor in admission to the nursing home, have rarely been examined in these studies.

The pioneering work of Stotsky and his colleagues (Chien, 1971; Chien et al., 1973) demonstrated that small doses of alcohol, usually in the form of beer, when added to a specific activity such as watching a baseball game, can enhance socialization of patients in the nursing home. After those initial studies were published, many nursing homes added a "happy hour," wine with meals, or other forms of social activity that added beverage alcohol to their programs. Unfortunately, many programs included patients in an indiscriminate manner, and many nursing homes allowed patients with SADs, including alcoholics, to join in and drink during these programs.

It is surprising, therefore, that there has been only one study examining current alcohol use and abuse in a nursing home setting. Jensen and Bellecci (1987) compared 33 men aged 90 to 99 with 32 men aged 65 to 75. All resided in a veterans home in California that allowed unrestricted alcohol intake by residents. The subjects were those who were able to live "independently" within the home and who required a minimum of nursing care. Thus, the sample was neither representative of the residents of this home nor of most nursing homes in the United States. Diagnostic criteria were not described in their paper. A history of alcoholism was present in 14 (44%) of the younger subjects and 5 (15%) of the older subjects. Of the younger group, 9 (28%) continued to drink more than 2 oz of alcohol daily, but none of the subjects in the older group drank that much. Because of the peculiarities of the sampling technique and the uniqueness of the setting, it is difficult to extrapolate any implications of these data to the nursing home population in general.

There has been only one large study of psychiatric disorders in nursing homes that included the diagnoses of alcoholism and other SADs. Kramer (1986) performed a secondary analysis of the data from the National Nursing Home Survey of 1977 (National Center for Health Statistics, 1977). Of 1,303,100 patients residing in nursing homes, 36,900 (2.8%) were given a diagnosis of alcoholism as their primary diagnosis at their most recent medical examination prior to the survey. In 6800 additional patients (0.5%), this condition was noted as chronic, although it was not considered a primary diagnosis.

In another study, German et al., (1986) interviewed 386 patients in 21 nursing homes in Baltimore. All patients had been given a psychiatric diagnosis prior to the interview. They found that 0.6% of the patients who had been in the nursing home for less than 1 year and none of the patients who had been in the nursing home for more than 1 year had a diagnosis of "substance abuse or dependence." Although it is unclear if the authors included alcoholism in this diagnostic category, their data suggest that alcoholism was the primary form of SAD in their study sample.

Chandler and Chandler (1988) examined 65 patients in a nursing home in Iowa City, using the Association for Gerontopsychiatry semistructured interview system. Diagnoses were made using DSM-IIIR criteria. They found that three patients (4.6%) had alcoholic dementia and another two patients (3.1%) had Wernicke-Korsakoff syndrome. One of the three patients with alcoholic dementia also suffered from organic hallucinosis. They also delineated a group of 14 patients (21.5%) with previous psychiatric treatment unrelated to their nursing home admission. Alcoholism was noted to be the most frequent diagnosis in this group, although the exact prevalence of alcoholism was not noted by the authors.

Teeter et al. (1976) evaluated 74 patients from a representative sample of patients in two midwestern nursing homes. Almost all were at least 65 years old. The authors used a semistructured interview. None of the patients were given a primary diagnosis of "chronic alcoholism." However, five patients (6.8%) received this diagnosis as a secondary diagnosis.

In a study of 257 nursing home patients in New York with "serious" behavioral problems (Zimmer et al., 1984), only 4 (1.6%) had a diagnosis of alcoholism in their charts. Graux (1969) and Lugand (1969) suggest that the prevalence of alcoholism in a nursing home population is approximately 20%, which would be similar to the prevalence in the general elderly population. However, these authors do not present their substantiating data in enough detail to allow for the critical evaluation of their statements. This prevalence rate is also noted by Abrams and Alexopoulos (1991) without citing source data. A slightly lower prevalence, 12%, was noted by Douglass (1980); however, this study included only women nursing home admissions that were paid by Medicare. Blose (1978) has suggested that 40 to 60% of Caucasian men residing in nursing homes had "alcohol-related problems," also without presenting substantiating data.

Data from the Department of Veterans Affairs (1991) support the commonly held belief that patients treated in Veterans Administration (VA) facilities are more likely to have diagnoses of SADs than patients treated elsewhere. Based on diagnoses documented in patients' charts, approximately 16% of patients residing in VA nursing homes have a diagnosis of alcoholism and approximately 1% have a diagnosis of drug dependence. Several other VA studies have yielded a wide range of prevalence rates. For example, Linn et al. (1972) reported a prevalence of 12%, and Joseph (unpublished communication) reported a lifetime prevalence of 47%, with a prevalence of active drinking present in 33% of nursing home admissions from a VA hospital in Oregon.

There have been many studies in the United States and elsewhere in the world demonstrating that approximately 25% of nursing home patients are prescribed a potentially addictive psychotropic medication (Ingman et al., 1975; Kalchthaler et al., 1977; Segal et al., 1979; Ray et al., 1980; Morgan and Gilleard, 1981; Reynolds, 1984; Buck, 1988; Morriss et al., 1990). The most common of these medications are the benzodiazepines, but barbiturates continue to be prescribed more frequently than one would expect. Oral narcotics, especially propoxyphene, are also prescribed quite frequently. These studies document an inappropriately high frequency of the concomitant prescription of multiple benzodiazepines or combinations of benzodiazepines with other sedative/hypnotics or oral narcotics. The misguided use of these medications has been noted quite often, most recently in several studies by Rovner and his associates (Rovner et al., 1986; Morriss et al., 1990).

These studies suffer from a variety of methodological flaws. Foremost among these is the lack of awareness that a physician's order for a medication is not identical to the ingestion of the medication by the patient. These studies also do not differentiate between the "as needed" (prn) use of the medication from regular use. Nor do these studies differentiate appropriate use of these medications from inappropriate use.

To date, there has been only one study of the epidemiology of psychotropic drug dependence in nursing home patients. Solomon and colleagues (1993, unpublished), using a chart review, studied the actual use (not prescription) of potentially addictive medications in nursing home patients in Baltimore. They noted that the group of nursing home patients who received prn doses of potentially addictive drugs received these drugs on a routine basis, and often as frequently as those patients who had these medications prescribed on a regular basis. The authors noted that 84 of 251 patients (33.5%) received potentially addictive drugs on a regular basis. The distribution of the drug use is noted in Table 12.1. The most frequently prescribed potentially addictive psychotropic drug group comprised the benzodiazepines, particularly the long-acting benzodiazepines. The mean daily dose of benzodiazepines was 39.72 mg chlordiazepoxide equivalents—a rather high dose for this age group.

There are no known data on the use of illegal drugs in nursing home patients. Kramer (1986) reported that drug addiction was not the primary diagnosis for any patient and the diagnosis as a chronic condition was recorded so rarely as to make statistical analysis impossible. However, we are aware of at least one nursing home that had to fire one of its employees because the employee was caught selling marijuana and crack cocaine to some of the more cognitively intact residents of the home when he worked during the night (11:00 P.M. to 7:30 A.M.) shift. In addition, the increase in the number of individuals with AIDS who are being admitted to nursing homes in one of the results of the increasing numbers of people of all ages with SADs in the community.

TABLE 12.1.   Distribution of Potentially Addictive Psychotropic Medications
in Nursing Home Patients ($N = 84$)

Benzodiazepines	76 (90.5%)
Alprazolam	8 (9.5%)
Chlordiazepoxide	2 (2.4%)
Clorazepate	6 (7.1%)
Diazepam	15 (17.9%)
Flurazepam	24 (28.6%)
Lorazepam	9 (10.7%)
Oxazepam	2 (2.4%)
Prazepam	1 (1.2%)
Temazepam	6 (7.1%)
Triazolam	10 (11.9%)
Sedative/Hypnotics	11 (13.1%)
Alcohol	1 (1.2%)
Chloral hydrate	6 (7.1%)
Glutethemide	1 (1.2%)
Amobarbital	1 (1.2%)
Butalbital	3 (3.6%)
Phenobarbital	2 (2.4%)
Pentobarbital	1 (1.2%)
Secobarbital	1 (1.2%)
Narcotics	9 (10.7%)
Codeine	1 (1.2%)
Meperidine	1 (1.2%)
Oxycodone	1 (1.2%)
Pentazocine	1 (1.2%)
Propoxyphene	7 (8.3%)

Source: Solomon et al. (1993, unpublished).

In summary, more research is clearly necessary. The need for valid and operational diagnostic criteria must be met if these studies are to have any value. In addition, screening for these disorders in nursing homes will lead to more valid diagnoses and better epidemiological studies.

Risk Factors for Substance Abuse in Nursing Home Patients

There are several risk factors that put elderly nursing home patients at risk for developing a SAD. Some of these risk factors are identical to the risk factors for all individuals with SADs. Others are unique to this population.

Some of these nonspecific risk factors are biological. For example, the type II alcoholic (Cloninger et al., 1981; Cloninger, 1987) seems to have a strong genetic predisposition for the development of a fulminant form of this disorder early in life. Very few type II alcoholics survive into old age without an abstinence-producing intervention; however, many of those who do survive end up in nursing homes because of the medical, neurological or cognitive sequelae of their disorder.

Although a genetic predisposition may be present for type I alcoholics and for nonalcoholic drug abusers, the exact nature of this predisposition has not been clarified (Solomon et al., 1990; Anthenelli and Schuckit, 1992). Another biological factor associated with risk of developing a SAD is the addictive potential of the drug (Solomon et al., 1990). The final biological factors associated with the development of a SAD in the elderly are the increased sensitivity of the older neuron to the effects of potentially addictive compounds, the increased permeability of the blood-brain barrier in the elderly, and the slower metabolism and subsequent longer half-life of these drugs in the elderly (Friedel, 1977; Kruse, 1990; Greenblatt et al., 1991; Abernethy, 1992; Solomon et al., 1993).

Sociological factors may play a role in the development of SADs in the elderly. It has frequently been documented that the prevalence rates of SADs in younger populations differ dramatically among the different countries of the world (Winick, 1992). Similarly, there are data demonstrating that different ethnic groups in the United States have different preferences for the various potentially addictive drugs. These findings must be examined in elderly populations (Johnson and Muffler, 1992; Winick, 1992).

Other nonbiological risk factors include the psychological state of the individual when that individual starts taking the drug (Solomon et al., 1990). There have been several studies suggesting that stress (a nonspecific variable) (Clipp and George, 1990), anxiety (Patterson et al., 1980), depression (Dupree, 1990), or loneliness (Dupree, 1990) may increase the risk that an elderly person will develop a SAD. Other studies have questioned these findings (Atkinson et al., 1990; Adams and Waskel, 1991; Schoenfeld and Dupree, 1991). However, one psychological constant may be a cognitive set that creates denial; in other words, the individual believes that although the drug is potentially dangerous, he or she cannot become addicted to the drug.

Khantzian and his associates (Khantzian, 1974, 1978, 1985, 1990; Brehm and Khantzian, 1992) and Wurmser (1974) have described the role of specific deficits in personality development (specifically, the development of ego lacunae and excessive grandiosity) and dysphoria in the development SADs. Solomon et al. (1990) have described, although in less detail, a similar process in late-onset addicts. Although these factors are nonspecific for all elderly addicts, they may also occur in nursing home patients. Specifically, Solomon et al. (1990) have noted that older men who develop late-onset SADs often demonstrated a significant dependence on a love object. Although these men were able to function fairly well when younger, they had poorly developed ego structures. Their addictions seemed to be triggered by a specific sequence of events, involving the loss of an overinvested love object (e.g., spouse or job), followed by the development of feelings of dysphoria. At times, overt major depression may develop in such individuals. These men, experiencing a loss of mastery and increasing feelings of helplessness, turn to a form of self-medication, often alcohol, but also other prescription or illegal drugs, in an attempt to rid themselves of these dysphoric feelings. In vulnerable individuals, the biological, psychological, and social factors noted above may then combine and rapidly create a cycle of tolerance, withdrawal, and continued drug-seeking and drug-using behaviors, with the result being the rapid onset of a SAD.

For elderly women, a similar sequence of events seem to occur. However, instead of being overly dependent on a love object, the woman's feelings about the love object are quite ambivalent, with repressed anger being a prominent affect. This ambivalence occurs against a backdrop of a poor ego structure that may not have been manifested by poor personal functioning earlier in life. This ambivalence leads to a depression of these feelings of anger and a sense of helplessness against a potentially overpowering and overwhelming rage. This helplessness and subsequent dysphoria triggers the process of self-medication, similar to that seen in men. Further clarification of this psychological process is important, as Atkinson (1990) has noted that women are more likely to develop late-onset alcoholism than are men.

The American Psychiatric Association Task Force *Report on Benzodiazepine Dependency, Toxicity and Abuse* identified several groups of patients who used benzodiazepines chronically (APA, 1990). Although this task force did not examine the literature on nursing home patients, most of those who were identified to be at risk were also patients who were commonly living in nursing homes. Specifically these were patients with chronic insomnia, older medically ill patients, and psychiatric patients with depressive symptoms.

As noted above, depression may be a risk factor for the development of late-life alcoholism. As depression is a common disorder in nursing home residents (Rovner et al., 1986), one can probably extrapolate these data to the nursing home resident, who may be at risk for developing alcoholism or relapsing into alcoholic symptoms after admission to the nursing home.

Solomon et al. (1993) extrapolated these data to investigate risk factors for prescription drug dependence in nursing home patients. Based on a study of 253 such patients, these authors have recently delineated three factors that may put elderly nursing home patients at risk for developing prescription drug dependence. The first of these is a biological risk factor. In their study, they noted that nursing home patients who were receiving regular doses of potentially addictive prescription drugs, when compared to nursing home patients who did not receive these drugs, were more likely to have a family history of alcoholism or other substance use disorder, to have a family history of psychiatric disorder, and to have been diagnosed with a SAD prior to admission to the nursing home. The second risk factor noted by these authors was the severity of the comorbid psychiatric disorder. The group of nursing home patients who were receiving potentially addictive medications were more likely to have had a past psychiatric treatment. They were also more likely to have been given multiple psychiatric diagnoses. They received a mean dose of neuroleptic medication that was significantly higher than that of the group that did not receive potentially addictive medications. The patients receiving potentially addictive drugs were also receiving a greater number of psychotropic medications, even after detoxification from these medications. Finally, this group was more likely to display overt psychotic symptoms than the group that did not receive potentially addictive drugs. The third factor was the presence of depression. Finlayson and his colleagues (Finlayson et al., 1988) have noted the high incidence of depression (as well as alcoholism) in hospitalized elderly patients with prescription drug dependence. This was also noted in these authors' sample of nursing home patients. Not only did the group receiving potentially addictive drugs have a higher incidence of major depression, they also had a higher incidence of many of the individual signs and symptoms associated with depression.

Clinical Presentation

The clinical presentation of SADs in nursing home patients, as in other settings, varies greatly. Evidence of addiction can be obvious, as in the case of dramatic withdrawal phenomena, or it can be relatively inconspicuous, as with the subtle cognitive changes associated with hypnotics. Since denial by the patient, family, and caretakers and professional staff is part of the disorder (Solomon et al., 1990, 1993; Miller, 1991; Solomon, 1993), the clinician must learn to use subtle clues and hints in order to adequately diagnose and treat SADs in the nursing home population.

The sources of drugs are multiple. Both beverage and nonbeverage alcohol is readily available in most nursing homes. Beverage alcohol may be available on a physician's orders, during "happy hour," at mealtimes, or upon request by the patient. Beverage alcohol may be consumed when the patient is out of the facility, or it may be smuggled into the facility in a variety of ways. It is not unusual for a patient to have a bottle of beverage alcohol hidden under the bed so that it is available for an occasional nip. Finally, nonbeverage alcohol is readily available, as most liquid medications are dissolved in alcohol, and many of these contain as much alcohol as a fine liqueur.

However, the most likely source of the addictive compound is the physician's order for prescription medications. Since the physician is the most common supplier of medications of abuse (Beardsley et al., 1988), a well-educated physician is the best protection against the development of iatrogenic drug dependence. Medicine had for many years ignored the plight of nursing home residents who were subjected to the administration of various psychotropic medications, many of which caused addiction. The adverse effects of these practices resulted in the federal legislation and regulations (the Omnibus Budget Reconciliation Acts of 1987, 1989, and 1991, or OBRA) that have forced the medical community to look at chemical dependence in the nursing home.

Substance abuse disorders may present with various medical scenarios in the nursing home patient. It is not uncommon for the first manifestation of a SAD to be withdrawal symptoms during the first few days of admission as the patient suddenly must go without the addicting drug. Another common time to see withdrawal reactions is after the physician has discontinued medications felt to be unnecessary or harmful. This has happened frequently in the last few years, as many American nursing homes have interpreted the OBRA regulations to require discontinuation of nearly all psychotropic drugs. A simple review of the patient's chart will reveal the temporal relationship of the medication discontinuation to the appearance of withdrawal.

The classic presentation of acute alcohol or drug withdrawal should be familiar to all staff (Victor and Adams, 1953; Tavel, 1962). In the case of alcohol withdrawal, signs and symptoms will usually occur 8 to 72 hours after the last drink, although symptoms may not become manifest for more than a week. In the case of dependence on benzodiazepines, barbiturates, other sedative/hypnotics, or other oral narcotics, symptoms may occur anywhere from a few hours after the last dose or dosage reduction up until a week later, depending on the half-life of the agent being withdrawn. The specific withdrawal symptoms and their severity will vary considerably from patient to patient. The patient's own reported history of withdrawal reactions is often an excellent predictor of future withdrawal reactions. For example, if someone reports a classic history of delirium tremens, that patient should be watched particularly closely during detoxification. The clinical staff must keep in mind, however, that a patient may exaggerate the past history of withdrawal in the hope of receiving more medications during detoxification. Another frequent risk factor for severe withdrawal reactions is the presence of an underlying medical disorder such as infection, electrolyte disturbance, or malnutrition.

In the early stages of a severe withdrawal syndrome, the patient may complain of general discomfort, malaise, and "sickness." He or she may develop a tremor or "the shakes." The patient also may complain of "inner" shakiness. Diaphoresis may be marked to the point of soaking clothing or bedclothes. The patient may experience insomnia that can last weeks or even months. Grand mal seizures and cardiovascular collapse may occur. The most accurate and reliable signs of a true withdrawal reaction are those of the autonomic instability that is part of withdrawal. This takes the form of changes in vital signs, most notably elevations in systolic and diastolic blood pressures, pulse rate, and temperature. Delirium tremens and similar withdrawal syndromes are life-threatening emergencies, with a 20% mortality if not treated (Tavel, 1962).

For many drugs, particularly benzodiazepines, the withdrawal syndrome may be misdiagnosed as an anxiety, panic, or sleep disorder. The severe withdrawal syndromes usually occur if the patient has been dependent upon alcohol, barbiturates or other nonbenzodiazepine sedative/hypnotics, or meprobamate. Milder withdrawal syndromes are usually seen in patients who have been dependent upon benzodiazepines, although significant withdrawal symptoms including seizures may occur, particularly if the patient has used short-half-life benzodiazepines. In addition, a postwithdrawal syndrome or protracted withdrawal syndrome may occur, especially in patients who have been dependent upon long-half-life benzodiazepines. These symptoms are usually psychiatric in nature and include anxiety, insomnia, depression, and episodes of panic (Ashton, 1991; Tyrer, 1991).

The presence of certain medical conditions should alert the treating physician to the possibility of a SAD. Since a geriatric patient may have a number of coexisting medical problems that may all be variously exacerbated by a SAD, the overall medical picture of the elderly patient with a SAD is not easily described; i.e., there are no typical cases (Atkinson, 1990). As there are many excellent reviews of the medical and neurological complications of SADs in the elderly (i.e., Victor and Adams, 1953; Gambert et al., 1984; Benzer, 1991; Engel and Benzer, 1991; Geller, 1991; Solomon et al., 1993), only a brief review is offered in this chapter.

A relatively common effect of long-term alcohol abuse is cirrhosis. Alcoholism can lead to gastritis and associated upper gastrointestinal bleeding. Pancreatitis is also more common in someone with a significant history of alcohol abuse. Alcohol abuse damages the heart muscle, causing alcohol-related cardiomyopathy. Long-term alcohol abuse leads to decreased absorption of vitamin B_{12} and folate, both of which are vital to cognitive and hematological functioning in the elderly patient. General malnutrition is extremely common. Protein intake is often low in alcoholics, causing protein-calorie malnutrition, which is manifest by muscle wasting, hypoproteinemia, and edema. Anemia and susceptibility to infection are also more likely to occur in someone having a history of addiction. Hypertension and an exacerbation of diabetes, hypercortisolism, and hypomagnesemia are other common medical sequelae of alcohol dependence. Elderly persons who are taking benzodiazepines or alcohol are at an increased risk of falls (Macdonald, 1985; Sorock and Shimkin, 1988), which represent a significant part of nursing home morbidity. The above-mentioned medical presentations, occurring singly or especially in combinations, should cause the treating physician to suspect a SAD.

The nursing home patient with a SAD may demonstrate cognitive disturbances, ataxia, dizziness, or impaired motor coordination. Behavioral symptoms include sedation, reduced coordination, and the emergence of hostility. The acute use of these drugs, particularly benzodiazepines, may cause loss of recent memory or other cognitive deficits, even after a single dose. When benzodiazepines are used more chronically, they can cause subtle but progressive impairments of attention and recall (Kales, 1991; Salzman, 1992). Chronic constipation is a common problem in patients dependent upon oral narcotics. Finally drug-drug interactions and the effects of the effects of the ingestion of multiple central nervous system drugs can further complicate the medical picture.

Psychiatric and neurological symptoms are the most common presentation for addictions in the elderly. Solomon and Stark (1993) noted that elderly addicts are more likely to demonstrate neurological symptoms (gait disturbance, cognitive deficits, or peripheral neuropathy), psychotic symptoms (delusions or hallucinations), self-care deficits (diminished ability to perform activities of daily living), and behavioral problems (threatening violence and being noncompliant with medical care) than younger addicts. Thus, the patient with a SAD in a nursing home setting may present with psychiatric symptoms such as anxiety or depression. Often, the anxiety has been treated with a benzodiazepine, when, in actuality, an affective disorder is the cause of the anxiety. This is especially true when the patient has an agitated major depression, where the most prominent symptoms are anxiety and psychomotor agitation. These patients look and feel anxious or ''nervous,'' but if the clinician persists, he or she will find an underlying constellation of depressive symptoms. When the physician merely prescribes an antianxiety medication, the patient's true pathology is disguised, and the intervention may merely have added another problem in the form of benzodiazepine dependence.

Another common type of anxiety seen in patients with a SAD is end-of-dose anxiety or the "clock-watching syndrome." This is seen more frequently since clinicians have begun to prescribe benzodiazepines with short half-lives to the elderly in order to minimize drug accumulation. Insomnia is a common complaint of addicts. This can be a form of medication-seeking behavior or a result of reliance on a hypnotic agent for an extended period of time.

The cognitive effects of addictive medications are often the presenting symptom in nursing homes. Poor concentration, poor short-term and recent memory, and decreased problem-solving skills have been shown to occur in elderly patients taking even single doses of benzodiazepines (Curran et al., 1987; Hinrichs and Ghoneim, 1987). A severe consequence of a SAD that is frequently seen in the nursing home is dementia. Alcohol use, as well as other drug use, can cause irreversible dementias and may also exacerbate other forms of dementia.

A common presentation of substance abuse and dependence in the nursing home is depression. Often, the patient's symptoms are severe enough that they meet the DSM-IV criteria for major depressive disorder. However, if this same patient is concurrently on one or more benzodiazepines or opiate analgesics, it is possible that the medication is causing an organic mood syndrome, and this must be investigated by gradual detoxification.

Regardless of other signs or symptoms, several symptoms are always present in the nondemented or mildly demented patient with a SAD (Solomon et al., 1990, 1993; Solomon, 1993). The most prominent of these symptoms is denial. This allows the patient to deny that he or she even drinks or uses a drug, even in the face of irrefutable evidence to the contrary. Most often, the patient denies that he or she has a problem because of the drug use, although the patient will generally admit to some drug use. Closely related to denial is minimization, in which the patient minimizes the amount of drug used or the severity or presence of consequences of this drug use. Rationalization is also extremely common. This symptom allows the patient to "explain," in a rational way, the necessity or appropriateness of the drug use. Finally, the patient may demonstrate defocusing, which is an attempt to get the clinician to discuss or examine any other aspect of the patient's life or medical complaints so as to avoid a discussion of the SAD.

Significant others may also demonstrate any or all of these symptoms. In addition, they may demonstrate enabling behaviors, by which they attempt to bring some semblance of control to the patient's symptoms and behaviors, when in reality they are only allowing the addiction and its consequences to continue unchecked.

Clinical Evaluation

Before attempting to treat the elderly patient with a SAD, the clinician should examine his or her own biases about SADs in the elderly. Many health care clinicians believe that substance abuse in old age is rare and inconsequential. In general, clinicians fail to recognize drug and alcohol problems in the elderly, especially as compared to younger persons (Curtis et al., 1989). It is difficult to quantify and accurately judge what constitutes "problem drinking" or drug use in the elderly (Graham, 1986). The accurate diagnosis of a SAD in the nursing home resident relies on a complete clinical evaluation, including medical history, physical exam, mental status assessment, and the gathering of corroborating data from family or significant others (Solomon et al., 1993).

History taking is often overlooked in the nursing home, as databases obtained by physicians are often brief and perfunctory or even photocopied from a recent hospital admission or office visit. A thorough initial history, however, is vital, since it is often within the first few days after admission to a nursing home that SADs may become manifest via dangerous withdrawal symptoms.

In obtaining a history of possible alcohol or drug abuse, not only the specific content of questioning but also the manner of the patient's response is important. An addict will often answer questions in such a way as to attempt to convince the physician that there is no problem. When questioning the patient about the use of potentially addictive drugs, the physician should maintain an attitude of nonjudgmental acceptance, realizing that part of the addiction is the combination of denial and distortions of behavior and motives that make this kind of history taking so frustrating. The clinician should be direct and firm, and use only highly specific and factual questions that make it difficult to answer evasively. Persistence is also extremely important, since the addict may hope that the clinician will tire of discussing the addiction and move on to other subjects. The interviewer should avoid getting into lengthy discussions regarding the addict's excuses for the addictive behaviors, since these are often counterproductive and confusing.

In the elderly, special attention should be directed toward the medical, psychological, and social consequences of alcohol or drug use in the context of the elderly person's life. For example, elderly addicts usually have negative histories of arrests for driving under the influence because they no longer drive. However, the social deterioration in an addict's life may manifest itself through separation or divorce, along with estrangement from adult children. A history of medication-seeking behavior or "doctor shopping" should alert the clinician to the possibility of addiction. A history of any falls, recent change in mental status, recent onset of anxiety or depression, poor self-care skills, or recent development of threatening, violent, or psychotic behaviors should raise the clinician's level of suspicion (Solomon and Stark, 1993). Finally, an adequate history for addiction includes questioning significant others to obtain more objective and accurate information and to corroborate the patient's history.

A thorough physical exam can be helpful in identifying signs of a SAD. The characteristic smell of alcohol or the fruity odor of acetaldehyde should prompt the physician to ask about recent drinking. Signs of alcoholism include evidence of liver disease or cardiomyopathy. More subtle clues to the existence of alcoholism can be found in the ataxia caused by Wernicke-Korsakoff syndrome, cerebellar degeneration, or vitamin B_{12} deficiency. Peripheral and autonomic neuropathies—as well as muscle weakness, orthostatic hypotension, and dehydration—may result from alcoholism. Any patient with a SAD may demonstrate evidence of head trauma or other injuries due to falls, gait disturbances, or the physical sequelae of poor self-care, including cutaneous infections, tuberculosis, decubiti, or malnutrition.

The mental status examination of nursing home patients can identify signs of drug dependence and toxicity. Intoxicated patients may appear drowsy; their concentration will be poor. Hallucinations, especially visual ones, may be present in states of intoxication and withdrawal. Paranoid delusions may also develop. Signs of anxiety or agitation, irritability, suicidal ideation, or depressed affect and mood are common.

The use of structured rating scales may be helpful in screening and helping to identify the nursing home patient with a SAD. Although convenient and easily administered by support staff or even self-administered, most of these scales have been developed using general populations and may not be particularly valid when used with the elderly (Graham, 1986; Moran et al., 1991; Tabisz et al., 1991; Widner and Zeichner, 1991). This is especially true of the popular CAGE (Mayfield et al., 1974) questionnaire and of the Michigan Alcoholism Screening Test (MAST) (Selzer, 1971). Recently, the Michigan Alcohol Screening Test— Geriatric (MAST-G) (Table 12.2) has been introduced (Blow, 1993). A survey of 24 questions that focus on the consequences of drinking or addictive behavior in an age-appropriate context, this instrument has been shown to be highly sensitive and specific for alcoholism in the elderly. Although the MAST-G has yet to be validated in a nursing home population, the authors recommend its use as a screening tool in this setting, as it remains a superior instrument when compared with the other available screening tools.

The routine laboratory examination is rarely helpful in making a diagnosis of a SAD. However, abnormalities in laboratory values (e.g., elevations in SGOT, GGT, LDH, and bilirubin) or an electrocardiogram or chest radiograph can aid in establishing proof of organ damage secondary to drugs or alcohol. Serum electrolytes are often abnormal and should be closely monitored. Magnesium levels are often decreased, possibly affecting mental status. Elevations of serum amylase and lipase suggest chronic pancreatitis.

However, nonroutine laboratory studies can aid the diagnosis. The authors recommend that a urine drug screen be obtained on all elderly patients seen for the first time, and that a blood alcohol level be obtained on any patient who demonstrates signs or symptoms of alcoholism or who has a history of alcoholism, even if other signs or symptoms are absent.

A dementia workup, including magnetic resonance imaging of the brain, should be performed to ascertain the accurate diagnosis of any dementia that is present and to rule out any treatable causes of dementia, particularly subdural hematomata or other evidence of head trauma. This test is mandatory in any patient with a SAD who has a history of falls, head trauma, or cognitive deficits. An elderly patient who has used intravenous drugs should also have an HIV titer obtained.

TABLE 12.2. Michigan Alcoholism Screening Test—Geriatric Version

	Yes (1)	No (0)
1. After drinking, have you ever noticed an increase in your heart rate or beating in your chest?	1. ____	____
2. When talking with others, do you ever underestimate how much you actually drink?	2. ____	____
3. Does alcohol make you sleepy, so that you often fall asleep in your chair?	3. ____	____
4. After a few drinks, have you sometimes not eaten or been able to skip a meal because you didn't feel hungry?	4. ____	____
5. Does having a few drinks help decrease your shakiness or tremors?	5. ____	____
6. Does alcohol sometimes make it hard for you to remember parts of the day or night?	6. ____	____
7. Do you have rules for yourself that you won't drink before a certain time of the day or night?	7. ____	____
8. Have you lost interest in hobbies or activities you used to enjoy?	8. ____	____
9. When you wake up in the morning, do you ever have trouble remembering part of the night before?	9. ____	____
10. Does having a drink help you sleep?	10. ____	____
11. Do you hide your alcohol bottles from family members?	11. ____	____
12. After a social gathering, have you ever felt embarrassed because you drank too much?	12. ____	____
13. Have you ever been concerned that drinking might be harmful to your health?	13. ____	____
14. Do you like to end an evening with a nightcap?	14. ____	____
15. Did you find your drinking increased after someone close to you died?	15. ____	____
16. In general, would you prefer to have a few drinks at home rather than go out to social events?	16. ____	____
17. Are you drinking more now than in the past?	17. ____	____
18. Do you usually take a drink to relax or calm your nerves?	18. ____	____
19. Do you drink to take your mind off your problems?	19. ____	____
20. Have you ever increased your drinking after experiencing a loss in life?	20. ____	____
21. Do you sometimes drive when you have had too much to drink?	21. ____	____
22. Has a doctor or nurse ever said they were worried or concerned about your drinking?	22. ____	____
23. Have you ever made rules to manage your drinking?	23. ____	____
24. When you feel lonely, does having a drink help?	24. ____	____

Treatment

For elderly outpatients with a SAD, treatment within the context of a 12-step program has been demonstrated to be effective and is probably necessary if the patient is to maintain abstinence (Janik and Dunham, 1983; Dupree et al., 1984). However, the population in a nursing home is significantly different from outpatients with SADs. As noted above, the frequency of comorbid and severe psychiatric disturbances such as depression and the high frequency of dementia in nursing home patients make the use of a 12-step program unfeasible for the large majority of elderly in the nursing home. However, the principles of a 12-step program (Alcoholics Anonymous, 1976; Nace, 1987) and of medical detoxification are no different in a nursing home than in any other setting.

The first step in the treatment of any patient with a SAD is medical stabilization and detoxification (Solomon et al. 1990, 1993; Solomon, 1993). Patients admitted to a nursing home with a history of active alcohol dependence within the previous 2 years should be treated with thiamine. There are no data supporting or refuting the value of the many proposed regimens of thiamine. We prefer to use high doses of thiamine, usually 200 mg twice daily, in the hope of reversing any neurological (both peripheral and central) changes that have occurred. In addition, a medical evaluation to rule out any medical sequelae of drug use is also necessary. As individuals with SADs are frequently malnourished or suffer from hypovitaminoses, appropriate nutritional stabilization is important.

Detoxification should proceed slowly and with close attention paid to the physiological aspects of withdrawal. If the patient has used only alcohol and has done so within the last several weeks, the only pharmacological intervention that may be necessary is the short-term use of "as needed" (prn) chlordiazepoxide. If the individual has been drinking regularly just prior to admission to the nursing home, the following conversion between alcohol and chlordiazepoxide can be made. Chlordiazepoxide 5 mg is equivalent to 12 oz of beer, 4.5 oz of wine, or 1.5 oz of hard liquor. If the individual is taking a benzodiazepine, the total dose of the drug should be converted to chlordiazepoxide equivalents (Table 12.3). Once chlordiazepoxide is started, the total daily dosage should be given in equally divided doses. It is important to assess the patient's vital signs, particularly pulse and blood pressure, every 4 hours while the patient is awake. Chlordiazepoxide should be available as additional medication on a prn basis if the patient begins to demonstrate objective signs or symptoms of alcohol or benzodiazepine withdrawal. Because some individuals with a SAD complain of poor sleep, anxiety, or inner tremulousness in an attempt to get more medication, the prn chlordiazepoxide should be given only if objective changes consistent with withdrawal are present. Specific and fairly high vital-sign parameters should be chosen for the use of prn medication. Once the chlordiazepoxide is started, the daily dose should be decreased by 5 mg every other day until the patient is completely detoxified. At that time, the prn medication should be made available for an additional week. At the end of that period, if prn medication has not been necessary, we discontinue

TABLE 12.3. Benzodiazepine Dosage Equivalents in Milligrams

Halazepam	40.00
Chlordiazepoxide	25.00
Flurazepam	15.00
Oxazepam	15.00
Clorazepate	10.00
Prazepam	10.00
Temazepam	10.00
Quazepam	7.50
Diazepam	5.00
Estazolam	1.00
Lorazepam	1.00
Alprazolam	0.50
Clonazepam	0.25
Triazolam	0.25

Source: Adapted from Bezchlibnyk-Butler and Jeffries (1989).

the prn chlordiazepoxide and measure that patient's vital signs according to the nursing home routine.

Detoxification from barbiturates and meprobamate can be done in two different ways. The barbiturate dose can be converted to the equivalent dose of either phenobarbital or chlordiazepoxide. Patients with meprobamate dependence can be detoxified with either meprobamate or equivalent doses of chlordiazepoxide.

Patients who are dependent on oral narcotics can be detoxified using that oral narcotic. Severe withdrawal symptoms can be treated with clonidine 0.1 to 0.3 mg daily. Careful attention must be paid to the patient's blood pressure so that orthostatic hypotension does not occur. A true withdrawal does not occur with the use of cocaine in any of its forms. However, the craving for the drug can be reduced with the use of desipramine 50 mg daily.

While medical stabilization and detoxification are proceeding, it is important to start to educate the patient's family about the nature of addictions and the risks of the continuation of the potentially addictive medications or alcohol. A detailed history should be obtained from the patient's family or significant others and, if possible, also from the patient.

For patients with a significant degree of cognitive impairment, treatment of the SAD is essentially complete at this time. If depression, an agitated dementia, or a psychotic process is present, appropriate psychopharmacological interventions can be started after it is determined that these psychiatric problems are not the result of the use, abuse, or withdrawal from potentially addictive medications or alcohol.

For the patient who is cognitively intact, more comprehensive treatment is necessary. A complete and detailed history must be obtained. Psychological interventions should focus on the use of a 12-step paradigm and other supportive psychotherapeutic measures. The ''Twelve Steps'' of Alcoholics Anonymous (Alcoholics Anonymous, 1976; Nace, 1987) are used to break down the patient's denial, minimization, defocusing, and rationalization and the family's enabling behavior. Individual psychotherapy can be modified to include such a program, as is it unlikely that the nursing home would host AA meetings. If possible, the patient should be transported to community-based AA meetings to participate in their program. If Pills Anonymous groups are available in the community, these should be utilized in a similar manner. Psychotherapy based on a 12-step model does not proceed in a clean, stepwise manner. However, the detailed biographical information from the patient and family can be used to help the patient with the "first step." Family members should be referred to Al-Anon, Ala-Teen, or Pills Anonymous to help them deal with issues of enabling, guilt, and addiction-related matters. Of course, the appropriate psychopharmacological and psychotherapeutic treatment of any comorbid psychiatric disorders should be included as part of treatment.

Prevention

The prevention of new cases or relapses of SADs in elderly nursing home patients requires an awareness of the risk factors noted above. Although the interpersonal benefits of "happy hours" or the appetitive benefits of allowing nursing home residents to partake of a small amount of beer or wine before or during a meal are great, many institutions have been indiscriminate in deciding which patients to allow to participate in those programs. It is imperative that patients with a history of a SAD be excluded from the intake of any alcohol or potentially addictive prescription drug. These patients can be allowed to participate in "happy hours," but they should be offered coffee, soda, lemonade, or other nonalcoholic beverages. The social value of these programs is great and the presence of a history of a SAD should not be a barrier to a patient's involvement in such a program.

As noted above, another source of alcohol is liquid medications, which many patients in nursing homes are given. The liquid used in most such medication is alcohol, and it is important for pharmacists, physicians, and nursing staff to be aware that patients with SADs may be receiving a significant amount of alcohol during the day and actually be maintaining a low level of inebriation by doing so. Alternatives to these medications should be actively sought.

As depression is a major risk factor for the development of SADs in nursing homes, it is important for physicians and nursing staff to be aware of the signs and symptoms of depression, especially in patients with a concurrent dementia. Treatment of the agitation, anxiety, or insomnia associated with depression should exclude benzodiazepines and other potentially addictive drugs. The appropriate use of antidepressants or buspirone, along with cognitive therapy or other psycho-therapeutic interventions, will go far to prevent the development of SADs in nursing home patients.

Similarly, agitation in demented patients should not be treated with benzodiaze-pines or barbiturates. The same is true for the sleep disturbances associated with dementias. A diagnostic assessment to rule out a concurrent delirium or other causes of agitation—such as medication side effects, urinary tract infections, fever, pain, and other medical problems—is necessary. If a specific and treatable cause for these symptoms cannot be found, treatment with antipsychotic medications, buspirone, trazodone, anticonvulsants, or lithium is preferable to treatment with benzodiazepines or barbiturates. (The reader is referred to Chapters 2, 3, 4, and 9 for more complete discussions of behavioral problems associated with dementia and their treatment.) A glass of warm milk, or, if medication is necessary, the use of zolpidem, may aid in relieving the sleep disturbance. Similarly, pain should not be treated symptomatically until a thorough evaluation of the possible source of pain has been completed. If pain occurs, treatment with nonnarcotic analgesics such as nonsteroidal anti-inflammatory drugs, aspirin or acetaminophen is preferred to the use of narcotics. Finally, educational interventions to help nursing staff, families, and physicians become aware of the dangers and risks of using narcotic medications, a familiarity with alternatives, both medical and nonmedical, and the use of these alternatives will also help prevent the development or maintenance of SADs in nursing homes.

References

Abernethy DR. Psychotropic drugs and the aging process: Pharmacokinetics and pharmacodynamics. In: Salzman C, ed. *Clinical Geriatric Psychopharmacology,* 2nd ed. Baltimore: Williams & Wilkins, 1992:61–76.

Abrams RC, Alexopoulos G. Geriatric addictions. In: Frances RJ, Miller SI, eds. *Clinical Textbook of Addictive Disorders.* New York: Guilford Press, New York, 1991:347–364.

Adams SL, Waskel SA. Late onset of alcoholism among older midwestern men in treatment. *Psychol Rep* 68:432–434, 1991.

Alcoholics Anonymous. *Alcoholics Anonymous,* 3rd ed. New York: Alcoholics Anonymous World Service, 1976.

Anthenelli RM, Schuckit MA. Genetics. In: Lowinson JH, Ruiz P, Millman RB, eds. *Substance Abuse. A Comprehensive Textbook,* 2nd ed. Baltimore: Williams & Wilkins, 1992:39–50.

APA. Substance-related disorders. In: *Diagnostic and Statistical Manual,* 4th ed. Washington, DC: American Psychiatric Association, 1994:175–272.

APA. Patterns of benzodiazepine use. In: *Benzodiazepine Dependence, Toxicity and Abuse.* Washington, DC: American Psychiatric Association, 1990:7–13.

Ashton H. Protracted withdrawal syndromes from benzodiazepines. In: Miller NS, ed. *Comprehensive Handbook of Drug and Alcohol Addiction.* New York: Marcel Dekker, 1991:915–929.

Atkinson RM. Aging and alcohol use disorders: Diagnostic issues in the elderly. *Int Psychogeriatr* 2:55–72, 1990.

Atkinson RM, Tolson RL, Turner JA. Late versus early onset problem drinking in older men. *Alcohol Clin Exp Res* 14:574–579, 1990.

Beardsley RS, Gardocki GJ, Larson DB, Hidalgo J. Prescribing of psychotropic medication by primary care physicians and psychiatrists. *Arch Gen Psychiatry* 45:1117–1119, 1988.

Benzer DG. Medical consequences of alcohol addiction. In: Miller NS, ed. *Comprehensive Handbook of Drug and Alcohol Addiction,* New York: Marcel Dekker, 1991: 551–571.

Bezchlibnyk-Butler KZ, Jeffries JJ. *Clinical Handbook of Psychotropic Drugs.* Toronto: Hogrefe & Huber, 1989:37–41.

Blose IL. The relationship of alcohol and the elderly. *Alcoholism* 2:17–21, 1978.

Brehm NM, Khantzian EJ. A psychodynamic perspective. In: Lowinson JH, Ruiz P, Millman RB, eds. *Substance Abuse. A Comprehensive Textbook,* 2nd ed. Baltimore: Williams & Wilkins, 1992:106–117.

Buck JA. Psychotropic drug practice in nursing homes. *J Am Geriatr Soc* 36:409–418, 1988.

Chandler JD, Chandler JE. The prevalence of neuropsychiatric disorders in a nursing home population. *J Geriat Psychiatry Neurol* 1:71–76, 1988.

Chien C-P. Psychiatric treatment for geriatric patients: "Pub" or drug? *Am J Psychiatry* 127:1070–1075, 1971.

Chien C-P, Stotsky BA, Cole JO. Psychiatric treatment for nursing home patients: Drug, alcohol, and milieu. *Am J Psychiatry* 130:543–548, 1973.

Clipp EC, George LK. Psychotropic drug use among caregivers of patients with dementia. *J Am Geriatr Soc* 38:227–235, 1990.

Cloninger CR. Neurogenic adaptive mechanisms in alcoholism. *Science* 236:410–416, 1987.

Cloninger CR, Bohman M, Sigardsson S. Inheritance of alcohol abuse: Cross-fostering analysis of adopted men. *Arch Gen Psychiatry* 38:861–868, 1981.

Curran HV, Allen D, Lader M. The effects of single doses of alpidem and lorazepam on memory and psychomotor performance in normal humans. *J Psychopharmacol* 2:81–89, 1987.

Curtis JR, Geller G, Stokes EJ, et al. Characteristics, diagnosis, and treatment of alcoholism in elderly patients. *J Am Geriatr Soc* 37:310–316, 1989.

Department of Veterans Affairs. *1990 Survey of VA Nursing Homes.* Washington, DC: Department of Veterans Affairs, 1991:B-6.

Douglass R. Aged alcoholic widows in the nursing home. *Focus on Women* 1:258, 1980.

Dupree LW. Older problem drinkers: Long-term and late-life onset abuses: What triggers their drinking. *Aging* 36:5–8, 1990.

Dupree LW, Broskowski H, Schonfeld L. The Gerontology Alcohol Project: A behavioral treatment program for elderly alcohol abusers. *Gerontologist* 24:510–516, 1987.

Engel CJ, Benzer DG. Medical complications of drug addiction. In: Miller NS, ed. *Comprehensive Handbook of Drug and Alcohol Addiction,* New York: Marcel Dekker, 1991:573–598.

Finlayson RE, Davis LJ Jr. Prescription drug dependence in the elderly population: Demographic and clinical features of 100 inpatients. *Mayo Clinic Proceedings* 69:1137–1145, 1994.

Finlayson RE, Hurt RD, Davis LJ Jr, Morse RM. Alcoholism in elderly persons: A Study of the psychiatric and psychosocial features of 216 inpatients. *Mayo Clin Proc* 63:761–768, 1988.

Friedel RO. Pharmacokinetics of psychotherapeutic agents in aged patients. In: Gisdorfer C. Friedel RO, eds. *Cognitive and Emotional Disturbance in the Elderly, Clinical Issues,* Chicago: Year Book Medical Publishers, 1977:139–149.

Gambert SR, Newton EH, Duthie EH JR. Medical issues in alcoholism in the elderly. In: Hartford JT, Samorajski T, eds. *Alcoholism in the Elderly. Social and Biomedical Issues.* New York: Raven Press, 1984:175–191.

Geller A. Neurological effects of drug and alcohol addiction. In: Miller NS, ed. *Comprehensive Handbook of Drug and Alcohol Addiction.* New York: Marcel Dekker, 1991:599–621.

German PS, Shapiro S, Kramer M. Nursing home study of the Eastern Baltimore Epidemiological Catchment Area Study. In: Harper MS, Lebowitz, BD, eds. *Mental Illness in Nursing Homes: Agenda for Research.* Rockville, MD: National Institute of Mental Health, 1986:27–40.

Graham K. Identifying and measuring alcohol abuse among the elderly: Serious problems with existing instrumentation. *J Studies Alcohol* 47:322–326, 1986.

Graux P. Alcoholism of the elderly. *Rev Alcoholism* 15:61–63, 1969.

Greenblatt DJ, Harmatz JS, Shader RI. Clinical pharmacokinetics of anxiolytics and hypnotics in the elderly: Part I. Therapeutic considerations. *Clin Pharmacokinet* 21:165–177, 1991.

Hinrichs JV, Ghoneim MM. Diazepam, behavior, and aging: Increased sensitivity or lower baseline performance? *Psychopharmacology* 92:100–105, 1987.

Ingman SR, Lawson IR, Pierpaoli PG, Blake P. A survey of the prescribing and administration of drugs in a long-term care institution for the elderly. *J Am Geriatr Soc* 23:309–316, 1975.

Janik SW, Dunham RG. A nationwide examination of the need for specific alcoholism treatment programs for the elderly. *J Studies Alcohol* 44:307–317, 1983.

Jensen GD, Bellecci P. Alcohol and the elderly: Relationships to illness and smoking. *Alcohol Alcohol* 22:193–198, 1987.

Johnson BD, Muffler J. Sociocultural aspects of drug use and abuse in the 1990s. In: Lowinson JF, Ruiz P, Millman RB, eds. *Substance Abuse: A Comprehensive Textbook,* 2nd ed. Baltimore: Williams & Wilkins, 1992:118–137.

Kalchthaler T, Coccaro E, Lichtiger S. Incidence of polypharmacy in a long-term care facility. *J Am Geriatr Soc* 25:308–313, 1977.

Kales A. An overview of safety problems of triazolam. *Int Drug Ther Newsl* 26:25–28, 1991.

Khantzian EJ. Opiate addiction: A critique of theory and some implications for treatment. *Am J Psychother* 28:59–74, 1974.

Khantzian EJ. The ego, the self and opiate addiction: Theoretical and treatment considerations. *Int Rev Psychoanal* 5:189–198, 1978.

Khantzian EJ. The self-medication hypothesis of addictive disorders. *Am J Psychiatry* 142:1259–1264, 1985.

Khantzian EJ. Self-regulation and self-medication factors in alcoholism and the addictions: Similarities and differences. In: *Gelanter M, ed. Recent Developments in Alcoholism.* Vol 8. New York: Plenum Press, 1990:255–270.

Kramer M. Trends of institutionalization and prevalence of mental disorders in nursing homes. In: Harper MS, Lebowitz BD, eds. *Mental Illness in Nursing Homes: Agenda for Research.* Rockville, MD: National Institute of Mental Health, 1986: 7–26.

Kruse WH-H. Problems and pitfalls in the use of benzodiazepines in the elderly. *Drug Safety* 5:328–344, 1990.

Linn M, Linn B, Greenwald S. The alcoholic patient in the nursing home. *Int J Aging Hum Dev* 3:273, 1972.

Lugand A. The situation in a hospital in Isere. *Rev Alcohol* 15:61–63, 1969.

Macdonald JB. The role of drugs in falls in the elderly. *Clin Geriatr Med* 1:621–636, 1985.

Mayfield D, McLeod G, Hall P. The CAGE questionnaire: Validation of a new alcoholism screening instrument. *Am J Psychiatry* 131:1121–1123, 1974.

Miller NS. Alcohol and drug dependence. In: Sadavoy J, Lazarus LW, Jarvik LF, eds. *Comprehensive Review of Geriatric Psychiatry.* Washington, DC: American Psychiatric Press, 1991:387–401.

Moran MB, Naughton BJ, Hughes SL. Performance of an alcoholism screening test in elderly men. *Clin Gerontol* 11:86–88, 1991.

Morgan K, Gilleard CJ. Patterns of hypnotic prescribing and usage in residential homes for the elderly. *Neuropsychopharmacology* 20:1355–1356, 1981.

Morriss RK, Rovner BW, Folstein MF, German PS. Delusions in newly admitted residents of nursing homes. *Am J Psychiatry* 147:299–302, 1990.

Morse RM, Flavin DK. The definition of alcoholism. *JAMA* 268:1012–1014, 1992.

Nace EP. Alcoholics Anonymous. In: *The Treatment of Alcoholism,* New York: Brunner/ Mazel, 1987:236–250.

National Center for Health Statistics. *Characteristics, Social Contacts and Activities of Nursing Home Residents.* Washington, DC: Department of Health, Education and Welfare, 1977.

Patterson R, O'Sullivan M, Spielberger CO. Measurement of state trait anxiety in elderly mental health clients. *J Behav Assess* 2:89–97, 1980.

Ray WA, Federspiel CF, Schaffner W. A study of antipsychotic drug use in nursing home: Epidemiologic evidence suggesting misuse. *Am J Public Health* 70:485–491, 1980.

Reynolds MD. Institutional prescribing for the elderly: Patterns of prescribing in a municipal hospital and a municipal nursing home. *J Am Geriatr Soc* 32:640–645, 1984.

Rovner BW, Kafonek S, Fillipp L, et al. Prevalence of mental illness in a community nursing home. *Am J Psychiatry* 143:1446–1449, 1986.

Salzman C. Treatment of anxiety. In: Salzman C, ed. *Clinical Geriatric Psychopharmacology,* 2nd ed. Baltimore: Williams & Wilkins, 1992:189–212.

Schonfeld L, Dupree LW. Antecedents of drinking for early- and late-onset elderly alcohol abusers. *J Studies Alcohol* 52:587–592, 1991.

Segal JL, Thompson JF, Floyd RA. Drug utilization and prescribing patterns in a skilled nursing facility: The need for a rational approach to therapeutics. *J Am Geriatr Soc* 27:117–122, 1979.

Selzer ML. The Michigan Alcoholism Screening Test: The quest for a new diagnostic instrument. *Am J Psychiatry* 127:89–94, 1971.

Solomon K. Alcohol and drug abuse. In: Reuben DB, Yoshikawa TT, Besdine RW, eds. *Geriatrics Review Syllabus Supplement: A Core Curriculum in Geriatric Medicine.* New York: American Geriatrics Society, 1993:113S–116S.

Solomon K, Cutler LH, Pierce E. Alcoholism and drug abuse in the elderly. In: Cornman R, Rogers D, Williams D, eds. *Proceedings of the Seventh Annual Conference of the Maryland Gerontological Association.* Baltimore: Maryland Gerontological Association, 1990:60–63.

Solomon K, Manepalli J, Ireland GA, Mahon GM. Alcoholism and prescription drug abuse in the elderly: St. Louis University Grand Rounds. *J Am Geriatr Soc* 41:57–69, 1993.

Solomon K, Stark S. Comparison of older and younger alcoholics and prescription drug abusers: History and clinical presentation. *Clin Gerontol* 12(3):41–56, 1993.

Solomon K, Vickers R. Attitudes of health workers toward old people. *J Am Geriatr Soc* 27:186–191, 1979.

Sorock GS, Shimkin EE. Benzodiazepine sedative and the risk of falling in a community-dwelling elderly cohort. *Arch Intern Med* 148:2241–2444, 1988.

Tabisz E, Badger M, Meatherall R, et al. Identification of chemical abuse in the elderly admitted to emergency. *Clin Gerontol* 11(2):27–38, 1991.

Tavel ME. A new look at an old syndrome: Delirium tremens. *Arch Intern Med* 109:129–134, 1962.

Teeter RB, Garetz FK, Miller WR, Hailand WF. Psychiatric disturbances of aged patients in skilled nursing homes. *Am J Psychiatry* 133:1430–1434, 1976.

Tyrer P. The benzodiazepine post-withdrawal syndrome. *Stress Med* 7:1–2, 1991.

Victor M, Adams RD. The effect of alcohol on the nervous system. *Assoc Res Nerv Ment Dis* 32:526–573, 1953.

Widner S, Zeichner A. Alcohol abuse in the elderly: Review of epidemiology research and treatment. *Clin Gerontol* 11(1):3–18, 1991.

Winick C. Epidemiology of alcohol and drug abuse. In: Lowinson JF, Ruiz P, Millman RB, eds. *Substance Abuse. A Comprehensive Textbook,* 2nd ed. Baltimore: Williams & Wilkins, 1992:15–29.

Wurmser L. Psychoanalytic considerations of the etiology of compulsive drug use. *J Am Psychoanal Assoc* 22:820–843, 1974.

Zimmer JG, Watson N, Treat A. Behavioral problems among patients in skilled nursing facilities. *Am J Public Health* 74:1118–1121, 1984.

13

Insight-Oriented and Supportive Psychotherapy

Richard A. Zweig and Gregory A. Hinrichsen

For most older adults, nursing home placement represents the culmination of a series of traumatic psychological experiences. Their physical integrity has been undermined by chronic illnesses and decline in physical functioning. Their psychological integrity has been severely challenged by an onslaught of stresses, emotional upheaval, and often impairment of the very cognitive abilities that undergird the experience of selfhood. Their social integrity has been fragmented by dislocation from familiar environments, loss of social networks, and the alienating effects of institutionalization. To nursing home staff, the treatment of these individuals may be overwhelming—all systems appear in decline, yet they are complexly interdependent. Interventions to help these patients seem only partially effective, and outcomes are rarely certain. Not surprisingly, older nursing home residents experience higher levels of psychological distress than any other group of elderly (NIH, 1991). Paradoxically, their psychological treatment is rarely commensurate with their distress. Despite increasing documentation of the efficacy of psychological treatments, particularly psychotherapy, for community-dwelling elderly (Borson et al., 1989; Newton and Lazarus, 1992), these treatments remain underutilized in the nursing home (Herst and Moulton, 1985; Shea et al., 1992).

There are signs, however, that psychological and psychiatric treatments are gradually becoming available to psychologically distressed elderly nursing home residents. Nursing homes are increasingly adopting rehabilitative models of care to maximize residents' functioning. The Omnibus Budget Reconciliation Acts (OBRA) of 1987 and 1989 mandated that nursing homes provide "active treatment'' to mentally ill residents, and they increased the financial incentives for mental health clinicians serving these elderly residents. Research has documented the potentially deleterious effects of prolonged treatment of institutionalized elderly with chemical and physical restraints (German et al., 1992), and recent legislation has both regulated their use and promoted alternate treatments. As standards of care have evolved, nursing home medical personnel have increasingly sought mental health professionals skilled in using psychotherapeutic techniques to better manage the aberrant behaviors of elderly residents and reduce their psychological distress.

This chapter provides an overview of psychotherapy for the mentally ill elderly living in nursing homes. Psychotherapeutic interventions may be broadly defined as ''planned processes of behavioral change that employ a deliberate application of psychological principles and theory to persons experiencing mental dysfunction or distress'' (Smyer et al., 1990). Below, we emphasize insight-oriented and supportive psychotherapy and exclude discussions of cognitive-behavioral psychotherapy (which is covered separately in Chapter 14) or of other psychosocial interventions (for an excellent review of these, see Karuza and Katz, 1991). In addition, while we recognize that individuals of varied ages reside in nursing homes, our focus is on elderly nursing home residents. To provide an overall framework for understanding the utility of psychotherapy in treating nursing home residents, this chapter is divided into four main sections: (1) an overview of the theoretical bases for psychotherapy in institutionalized mentally ill older adults, (2) a review of the prevalence of mental disorders and the availability of psychotherapeutic treatment in nursing homes, (3) a review of models of psychotherapeutic treatment and how they apply to special problems of elderly nursing home residents, and (4) an overview of social and environmental factors that affect the utility of psychotherapy in the nursing home setting.

Theoretical Bases for Psychotherapy

Treatment models for insight-oriented and supportive psychotherapy are derived from theoretical and empirical research in psychology, medicine, and sociology. Psychotherapy in the nursing home setting is specifically based on research in three primary areas briefly reviewed here: (1) developmental psychology and psychodynamic theory; (2) stress and coping research and health psychology; and (3) social and environmental psychology.

Developmental Psychology and Psychodynamic Theory

Early work in the field of developmental psychology held that cognition and personality develop incrementally until the individual reaches early adulthood or maturity. However, other theorists have argued that personality continues to develop throughout the life-span. Erikson (1950) posited that each era of the life-cycle is characterized by developmentally specific intrapsychic tasks. The task of older adulthood is to develop an integrated sense of self and to stave off despair and meaninglessness. Indeed, maintaining an inner sense of self-continuity despite physical and environmental changes is often seen as a central theme in the lives of older adults (Atchley, 1989; Griffin and Grunes, 1990). The mechanisms through which older individuals maintain a sense of self-continuity are varied and complex. For example, Neugarten (1977) has suggested that most middle-aged and older adults view many typically stressful life changes (e.g., launching of children, physical decline, the loss of a spouse) as expectable and normative. When these stressors occur ''on time,'' individuals have often psychologically rehearsed for them and typically cope adequately. It is only when stressors are unrehearsed, unpredictable, or ''off time'' that they present psychological crises.

The psychological impact of an illness for some older individuals may be best understood when viewed within a developmental context. The following case example is illustrative:

> A 55-year-old divorced woman suffered a stroke affecting the right middle cerebral artery, leaving her with left hemiparesis, confining her to a wheelchair, and ultimately prompting a psychotic depression that required hospitalization. Following her stabilization on psychotropic medication and discharge to a nursing home, she was referred for psychotherapy. In the course of her psychological treatment, she said that prior to her stroke and after having launched her children from the home, she had obtained a divorce and had looked forward to establishing her own career. She was in the midst of completing a bachelor's degree when the stroke occurred, which left her disabled, financially destitute, and stripped of the autonomy she had so cherished.

In sum, research in adult development suggests that difficulties in resolving phase-specific developmental tasks, disruptions in self-continuity, and the developmental ''timing'' of life stressors may be determinants of psychopathology in later life.

Psychodynamic theory and research provide a second perspective through which psychopathology may be understood and upon which psychotherapeutic techniques with medically ill older adults may be based. Psychodynamic theory holds that how an individual copes with life stresses is strongly influenced by early life experiences, personality structure, characteristic psychological defenses, and unconscious fears and impulses. Because of the complex interplay of these factors, the conscious and unconscious meaning of life stresses to an individual is highly idiosyncratic. This subjective meaning may determine how the individual reacts emotionally and perceives others. For example, a medical condition may cause one person to reject others' help because such help is perceived as a threat to autonomy. For another individual, the same condition will trigger persistent demands for others' assistance because of fears of being abandoned. A psychodynamic understanding of an individual's modal personality type and characteristic coping styles, defenses, and fears may thus be used as a basis for psychological intervention (Groves and Kucharski, 1987).

Late-life theorists such as Gutmann (1988) have also argued that a physically ill older adult's psychological reactions to expectable physical decline often have their roots in the subjective meaning of that decline. The following vignette illustrates this issue:

> A woman in her early 80s was transferred to a medical rehabilitation unit for muscle weakness, which was attributed to a late-onset postpolio syndrome. While her functioning was only mildly compromised, she felt markedly distraught and humiliated by her condition and the thought of staying on a rehabilitation unit. During the psychological consultation, she reported that as a child with polio, she could not participate in activities with others and had felt deeply ashamed. Once cured of her childhood polio, she had enjoyed robust health and had never spoken again of that time in her life. Now, the return of a milder form of her childhood illness had shattered her view of herself as fiercely independent and caused her to reexperience intense feelings of humiliation and anger more appropriate to her childhood illness than to her current one.

Based on developmental and psychodynamic theory and research, insight-oriented and supportive psychotherapy with older physically ill nursing home residents can have multiple objectives. First, psychotherapy helps identify the predispositions (i.e., personality structure, developmental context) that the older individual brings to his or her experience of the illness and clarifies the subjective meaning of the illness to the individual. In fact, clarifying the subjective meaning may, in itself, have lasting psychotherapeutic benefit to the medically ill (Viederman and Perry, 1980). Second, psychotherapeutic interventions may be utilized to limit maladaptive behaviors and restore an older individual's sense of self-continuity. Third, as nursing home staff come to understand the meaning of an individual's behavior, counterproductive interpersonal interactions may be reduced. Finally, as meanings are clarified and adaptive behaviors are fostered, the individual gains a sense of mastery over the traumatizing illness.

Stress, Coping, and Health Psychology

By definition, almost all residents of nursing homes are experiencing high levels of stress. Most would meet the criteria of the *Diagnostic and Statistical Manual of Mental Disorders,* 4th ed. (APA, 1994) for one or more "extreme psychosocial stressors" by virtue of acute or enduring physical illness. Life in a nursing home confronts residents with an ongoing series of daily stresses—from the interpersonal demands of sharing a room with another person to the incessant screaming of a patient with dementia on the same hallway. A sizable number of studies have generally documented the deleterious mental and physical health effects of stressful life circumstances (Kaplan, 1983) and specifically the negative emotional impact of physical health problems (Moos, 1984). The growing fields of health psychology and behavioral medicine testify to interest in finding ways to understand the mind-body interface better and in developing ways to help patients cope will illness more successfully.

Little research has specifically addressed how nursing home residents cope with these stresses. However, a large body of social and behavioral science literature has documented that different strategies for coping with stressful life circumstances are associated with psychological distress (Snyder and Ford, 1987). Theory suggests that when life experiences "tax or exceed" an individual's available resources, the individual appraises what can be done to cope with them (Lazarus and Folkman, 1984). Coping theory portrays people as active responders to stressful events who engage in problem-focused efforts to change the stressful event, cognitive efforts to change the meaning of the event so that it is less stressful, or emotion-focused efforts to contend with the dysphoric affects aroused by the event. Coping theory also suggests that people draw upon a variety of existing resources to deal with stressful situations, including physical health and energy, positive beliefs, problem-solving skills, social skills, social support, and material resources.

Research has examined how people cope with a variety of chronic medical conditions. The psychological, practical, and interpersonal demands of different chronic medical conditions often vary (Felton et al., 1984; Biegel et al., 1991). The degree to which an individual successfully copes with the demands of a particular illness may partly depend on aspects of the premorbid self. For example, an individual who has a lifelong pattern of conscientiously attending to work- and family-related responsibilities may contend better with the demands of dietary vigilance and daily insulin injections, characteristic of severe diabetes, than someone with a pattern of neglecting responsibility. An individual with rheumatoid arthritis who valued physical attractiveness and independence highly may adapt less successfully to the potentially crippling effects of arthritis than someone for whom these attributes were less valued. Nonetheless, research has indicated that successful adaptation to chronic illness requires acknowledgment of the medical problem only as one aspect of one's identity and a flexible use of internal and external resources to deal with the emotional and practical problems engendered by the condition (Burish and Bradley, 1983).

Studies in psychoimmunology suggest that coping ability, emotional distress, and immune system functioning are interrelated. Individuals who adapt poorly to chronic medical problems often become depressed. Untreated depression has been associated with impaired immune function (Asnis and Miller, 1989), thus increasing the patient's risk for further medical problems. The negative impact of depression on close social relationships (Weissman and Paykel, 1974) may also impede the use of social support as a coping strategy, and poor support has been tied to impaired immune function (Cohen, 1988). Preliminary studies in psychoimmunology suggest that the way in which individuals cope with chronic medical illness may influence both their future mental and physical health.

From a coping perspective, a physically ill individual at a nursing home is confronted with a formidable series of stresses. Serious physical health problems are one of the greatest threats to well-being. Placement in a nursing home may underscore the threat and reduce expectations of functional improvement. Coping resources that might be drawn upon to deal with life stresses prior to nursing home entry may now be unavailable or less useful in the new environment: physical health problems often diminish physical energy; society does not engender a set of positive beliefs about nursing homes but rather the opposite; established problem-solving skills that worked well in the community may not work in an institutional setting; social support in the form of friends or family may not be readily available. As a consequence, the nursing home resident may experience diminished expectations about the utility of engaging in any type of coping and limited resources upon which to draw for coping, thus engendering feelings of helplessness (Seligman, 1975). For residents with cognitive impairments, the process of coping is further compounded by the loss of intellectual skills that are critical to the whole coping enterprise.

Clinical reports suggest that there are nursing home residents who make successful adaptations to the stresses of chronic physical health problems and life in an institutional setting. However, the processes that promote successful coping within the nursing home, for the most part, have not been studied. Facilitating "successful coping" should result in reductions in depression, anxiety, subjective distress, and related psychiatric phenomena. Psychotherapy may facilitate better adaptation by helping the resident to reappraise or reassess the life circumstances that made placement in the nursing home necessary, to take stock of remaining resources and build new resources to facilitate coping, and to learn to utilize existing or new coping strategies to maintain emotional equilibrium.

Social and Environmental Psychology

Efforts by an individual to cope with physical illness and other stresses obviously take place within the physical and interpersonal environment of the nursing home. Specific models have been proposed to account for the interface between individual coping and the institutional environment (Moos and Lemke, 1985). Over the past 30 years, social and behavioral scientists have examined the influence of institutional settings for the elderly (ranging from "senior-citizen housing" to nursing homes) on their residents. Their research has documented that physical and neighborhood characteristics of the setting, social and recreational aspects of the environment, staffing patterns, and other factors directly or indirectly influence the social, physical, and emotional well-being of elderly residents (Moos and Lemke, 1985).

In nursing homes in particular, institutions that facilitate environmental stimulation, interaction with other residents, and greater choice have residents who function better (Moos and Lemke, 1985). A basic theme that runs throughout much of this research is the question of autonomy versus security (Parmelee and Lawton, 1990)—that is, how an institution balances the resident's need to exercise some measure of control over the environment and the institution's mandate to provide a safe structured setting. Concern about the potentially helplessness-engendering aspects of institutions was most forcefully articulated by Goffman (1961) in his treatise on the "total" institution. Researchers such as Langer and Rodin (1975; Rodin and Langer, 1977) have tested interventions designed to increase feelings of control in nursing home residents. In one study, enlarging nursing home residents' decision-making responsibilities was associated not only with enhanced emotional and social well-being but also with dramatically reduced death rates compared with controls. Others have found, however (Schulz and Hanusa, 1979), that raising residents' expectations about control without providing substantive opportunities to exert control may actually be harmful.

Several research studies have suggested that the psychological impact of one's environment is determined by the balance between the functional capacity of the individual and what is available in the environment—or "person-environment fit" (Kahana, 1982). Lawton (1982) has proposed that, for each person, there is a level of demand or "press" from the immediate environment that facilitates maximum performance. He suggests that there are negative consequences for the individual when there is too little or too much demand relative to an individual's capacities. One corollary of this perspective (known as the "environmental docility hypothesis") is that as the mental and physical vigor of an individual diminishes, the well-being of that individual become proportionately more dependent on the immediate environment. Thus there is an ongoing transaction between the individual and the environment.

Efforts to enhance coping and emotional well-being in psychotherapy require a simultaneous accounting for individual capacity and environmental opportunities. A better "fit" between resident and nursing home may be identified by a clearer understanding of the resident's psychological strengths and vulnerabilities and the constraints and resources within the nursing home. The therapist can educate the staff about the resident's unique psychology, which then may guide staff in how to interact optimally with the resident. By helping the resident to reckon more fully with the problems that required nursing home placement, the resident should then be better able to engage in a more realistic discussion of the options that exist within the nursing home that can make daily life more satisfying. Such a process should result in enhanced feelings of control for both the patient and staff—with reductions in patient distress and staff frustration.

Prevalence of Mental Disorders and the Availability of Psychotherapeutic Treatment in Nursing Homes

Epidemiology

As indicated in other chapters of this volume, the prevalence of potentially treatable mental disorders among nursing home residents is strikingly high. As many as 80% of elderly individuals residing in a nursing home suffer from a mental disorder (German et al., 1992). In a recent review, Rovner and Katz (1993) estimated that 40% of nursing home residents with dementia have complicating depressive or delusional symptoms. Further, 6 to 25% of older residents are estimated to suffer from major depression.

Other manifestations of potentially treatable mental disorders, while less well studied, are alarmingly high in nursing home residents. For example, 30 to 50% of elderly residents manifest symptoms of "minor depression," which may predispose to more severe depression (Rovner and Katz, 1993). The rate of life-threatening behaviors (e.g., refusal of food or medications or intentional self-harm) has been conservatively estimated at 95/100,000 in nursing home residents, or almost five times the suicide rate for this age group (Osgood and Theilman, 1990). An estimated 11 to 23% of nursing home residents suffer from personality disorders (Teeter et al., 1976; Hing, 1991) characterized by emotional distress and disturbed interpersonal interactions, and these may predispose to severe mental disorders. Other disorders known to be prevalent in community-dwelling elderly (e.g., anxiety disorders, adjustment disorders, sleep disorders) have been less well researched but are probably present in high rates among nursing home elderly.

Despite the high prevalence of both major and minor mental disorders among elderly nursing home residents, evidence suggests that these disorders frequently are undiagnosed and/or untreated. Teeter et al. (1976) found a missed or incorrect psychiatric diagnosis in 68% of nursing home residents with mental disorders. More recently, using data from the Institutional Population Component of the 1987 National Medical Expenditure Survey, Shea et al. (1992) reported that less than 40% of nursing home residents with mental illness uncomplicated by dementia received any mental health treatment. Those residents who are older and physically ill and are thereby at greater risk for depression (Parmelee et al., 1989) are the least likely to be offered treatment. Lack of effective psychotherapeutic or somatic treatment has been associated with increased morbidity and mortality (Rovner and Katz, 1993), medical rehospitalization (Lipzin, 1992), and increased overall health care utilization (Mumford et al., 1982). The gap between the high prevalence of mental disorders and the minimal mental health services currently delivered in the nursing home setting warrants further explanation. (See Chapter 1 for a more complete discussion of the nursing home as a psychiatric hospital.)

Barriers to Access to Psychotherapeutic Treatment

Gerontological researchers have long argued that few elderly receive mental health services not only because of their own biases against using these services but because of barriers raised by health care providers, institutions, and public policies (Smyer et al., 1990). In the nursing home setting, the complex clinical picture of most older residents, institutional and economic constraints, and staff attitudes and behaviors may all reduce access to appropriate psychotherapeutic treatment (Gunther, 1987; Spayd and Smyer, 1988; Cohen, 1989) (see Table 13.1).

Older mentally ill nursing home residents may go misdiagnosed and untreated due to the problems inherent in diagnosing mental disorder in the context of physical illness. Biological, psychological, and social factors are interdependent; behavior problems may be secondary to physical illness; physical symptoms may mask a psychological disorder. Distinguishing whether behavioral problems evidenced by a resident reflect the resident's poor adaptation, a staff member's mismanagement of the patient, or both is difficult to discern.

Institutional and economic barriers to the delivery of mental health services in the nursing home are declining. By mandating active treatment of mentally

TABLE 13.1.   Barriers to Access to Psychotherapy
in the Nursing Home Setting

Clinical complexity
Economic/institutional constraints
Staff attitudes and behaviors
  Ageist biases
  Biological reductionism
  Countertransference

Sources: Adapted from Smyer et al., 1990; Spayd and Smyer, 1988; Cohen, 1989; and Gunther, 1987.

ill nursing home residents, improving payment and eliminating caps on mental health services under Medicare/Medicaid, and opening the nursing home to qualified psychologist and social work consultants, the 1987 OBRA legislation improved access to psychotherapy services for mentally ill residents. While nursing homes have increasingly contracted with mental health clinicians to provide psychotherapy (Greenwald et al., 1993), the ratio of providers to mentally ill residents remains low.

Staff attitudes often reveal ageist biases: depression in the nursing home is viewed as inevitable; mental health problems are attributed to ''aging''; older individuals are perceived as incapable of change. Referral for psychotherapy may also be constrained by biological reductionism, or an overemphasis on biological factors and an underemphasis on psychosocial factors that contribute to functioning. For example, Cohen (1989) points out that health care providers often assume that depression in an individual with dementia must have a biological etiology; the role of psychosocial factors, especially in early dementia, is underrecognized. Staff countertransference, or the emotional response of staff to older nursing home residents, presents another barrier to access for psychotherapeutic services. For example, Gunther (1987) has argued that institutional staff often avoid close interaction with patients who are emotionally distressed in order to manage their own anxieties. Thus, for a variety of reasons, nursing home staff may underrecognize the presence, source, and psychotherapeutic treatability of mental disorders in elderly nursing home residents.

Indications for Psychotherapy in Nursing Home Residents

Some have sought to clarify guidelines for appropriate psychotherapeutic treatment of problems common to elderly nursing home residents (Goldfarb, 1955; Miller, 1989; Sadavoy and Robinson, 1989; Cohen, 1990; Lewis and Rosenberg, 1990; Smith and Kramer, 1992; Rovner and Katz, 1993). It must be emphasized that these are guidelines regarding the use of insight-oriented and supportive psychotherapy; behavior management or psychosocial interventions would likely require less stringent criteria. These referral guidelines may be grouped into three main criteria (see Table 13.2).

First, for psychotherapy to be warranted, a mental disorder must be present. Signs of mental disorder may be expressed explicitly (through depressive, anxious, or psychotic symptoms or significant behavior problems) or implicitly (e.g.,

TABLE 13.2. Proposed Indications for Psychotherapy
in the Nursing Home Setting

Presence of mental disorder
Depressive, anxious, or psychotic symptoms
Evidence of significant behavior problems
Demanding, disruptive, or dependent behaviors
Interpersonal conflict with staff
Behavior inconsistent with goal of rehabilitation
Capacity to engage in psychotherapy
Some capacity to communicate with others
Some awareness that a problem exists, and motivation toward mastery
Some capacity for retention/carryover
Possible additional factors
Presence of signs of personality disorder
Symptoms subclinical in degree
Somatic treatment only partially effective or contraindicated

Sources: Adapted from Goldfarb, 1954; Miller, 1989; Sadavoy and Robinson, 1989; Cohen, 1990; Lewis and Rosenberg, 1990; Smith and Kramer, 1992; Rovner and Katz, 1993.

interpersonal conflict with staff; behavior inconsistent with goal of rehabilitation). Second, the patient must evidence some capacity to engage in the psychotherapeutic process. This requires at least a limited ability to communicate with others, an understanding that a problem exists, a willingness to remedy the problem, and a capacity to retain some of the products of the therapeutic session. Thus, psychotherapy is indicated for some individuals with dementia. Just as nursing home residents with dementia may retain partial capacity to make decisions about their care, so too may their capacity to engage in psychotherapy be relative rather than absolute. Third, other factors—such as the presence of personality disorder, a subclinical presentation of psychiatric symptoms, and a contraindication for or partial response to somatic treatment—may indicate that an evaluation for psychotherapy is warranted.

Psychotherapeutic Treatment Models

As noted, a large body of research argues for the utility of a psychotherapeutic approach to the problems of elderly nursing home residents. However, what is the efficacy of psychotherapeutic treatments for younger as well as older individuals? Efficacy rates of 60 to 70% have been repeatedly demonstrated in metaanalytic studies of psychotherapy as a treatment for individuals of mixed ages (Smith et al., 1980). More recently, clinical and empirical research has examined the effectiveness of psychotherapy with community-dwelling and institutionalized elderly. This literature may be broadly grouped into five sections: (1) individual psychotherapy, (2) group psychotherapy, (3) specialized techniques for older adults with depression, (4) specialized techniques for older adults with personality disorder, (5) specialized techniques for older adults with dementia.

Individual Psychotherapy

There is general agreement that community-dwelling elderly with mental disorders can be successfully treated with slightly modified forms of insight-oriented and supportive psychotherapy (Myers, 1984; Sadavoy and Lescecz, 1987; Spayd and Smyer, 1988). Similarly, clinical reports have long supported the utility of psychotherapy with institutionalized older adults. Goldfarb (Goldfarb and Sheps, 1954; Goldfarb, 1955) found that older nursing home residents could overcome feelings of helplessness through their alliance with a therapist. Grunes (1984) and others (Ronch and Maizler, 1977; Cohen, 1985; Kahana, 1987; Sadavoy and Robinson, 1989) have suggested that even brief forms of individual psychotherapy can assist institutionalized older adults to cope adaptively with physical illness, adjust to greater dependency on others, and maintain a sense of self-continuity. Psychotherapeutic efforts may also assist staff and family to better understand and manage a resident's behavior (Tobin, 1989).

These clinical reports have been validated by recent empirical research. In a study of brief individual psychotherapy for community-based elderly with major depressive disorder, 70% of subjects evidenced substantial improvement and therapeutic gains that were maintained at a 1-year follow-up (Thompson et al., 1987). Brief insight-oriented individual psychotherapy also reduces symptoms in older adults with mild depression (Lazarus et al., 1987). Early studies of elderly nursing home residents also demonstrated favorable results. Goldfarb and Turner (1952–53) found that even infrequent psychotherapeutic contact improved the symptoms of 49% of mentally ill residents. Power and McCarron (1975) reported that a modified psychotherapeutic approach reduced psychiatric symptoms in withdrawn elderly residents. Frey et al. (1992) demonstrated that brief counseling significantly enhanced nursing home residents' self-esteem and sense of self-continuity. These studies suggest the potential for significant benefit from insight-oriented and supportive psychotherapy.

In sum, a growing body of clinical and empirical evidence supports the rationale for insight-oriented and supportive individual psychotherapy as a treatment for elderly nursing home residents. Further research will be needed to replicate and expand the existing research base on psychotherapy for nursing home residents, examine whether therapeutic gains are maintained over time, and clarify which factors make psychotherapy most efficacious for elders residing in a nursing home.

Group Psychotherapy

Group psychotherapy, an effective alternative to individual psychotherapy, has been used in the elderly to reduce aberrant behavior, dependency, and social withdrawal and to enhance self-esteem, adaptive problem solving, and affiliation with others (Ripeckyj and Lazarus, 1984; Spayd and Smyer, 1988). In institutionalized elderly, it has also been proposed as a means to enhance social skills, communication and memory skills, and emotional self-control (Herst and Moulton, 1985).

Subsequent research has established that group therapy is as effective as individual therapy in treating the elderly. For example, Steurer et al. (1984) found that both insight-oriented psychodynamic and cognitive-behavioral forms of group therapy reduced symptoms of depression and anxiety in clinically depressed community-dwelling elders. In nursing home residents, group approaches have been widely studied, but research regarding insight-oriented and supportive group psychotherapy is less common. Still, preliminary studies suggest that group psychotherapy improves residents' psychological well-being, self-reliance, and sense of personal control (Moran and Gatz, 1987; Christopher et al., 1988; Rattenbury and Stones, 1989). Given the proven utility of group psychotherapy approaches in institutional settings, further research on this modality and use of it are likely.

Specialized Techniques: Older Adults with Depression

Existing models of insight-oriented and supportive psychotherapy have recently been refined in an effort to develop specialized techniques to treat depressive disorders (APA, 1989). The theoretical basis of these models is that depression has both biological and psychosocial etiologies. An individual's personality is held to play a pivotal role in determining how the individual reacts to intrapsychic or interpersonal stressors and regulates self-esteem. In addition, an individual's capacity to relate interpersonally is theorized to mediate the ability to contend successfully with loss, transition, and interpersonal conflicts. Thus, maladaptive personality development or poor interpersonal functioning are viewed as factors contributing to a vulnerability to depression. In order to target these vulnerabilities and better operationalize supportive and insight-oriented psychotherapies, interpersonal psychotherapy (IPT) was developed as a specialized technique to treat depressed adults and has recently been used to treat older adults as well.

Interpersonal psychotherapy has been shown to be effective in studies of depressed younger adults. In the multisite NIMH Treatment of Depression Collaborative Research Program study, IPT was comparable in effectiveness to tricyclic antidepressants and superior to placebo controls in treating severely depressed younger adults (Elkin et al., 1989). Other work has demonstrated that maintenance treatment with IPT significantly prolongs remission in young adults treated for depression (Frank et al., 1990). Preliminary findings in a study of depressed older adults suggest that IPT enhances the overall treatment response rate (Reynolds et al., 1992).

Specialized techniques for the treatment of depression in elderly nursing home residents are based upon an adaptation and integration of models of insight-oriented, supportive, and interpersonal psychotherapy. This proposed integrated model has three basic goals: (1) identification and clarification of the depressive experience and its internal and external precipitants, (2) limitation of maladaptive behavior and facilitation of effective coping, and (3) restoration of emotional self-regulation, effective social functioning, self-continuity, and mastery.

Various specific techniques are utilized to achieve these goals. Symptoms and interpersonal problems are reviewed; education is provided regarding the nature of depression; emotional states and subjective versus objective perceptions of events are identified; premorbid and current strengths and limitations are assessed. The patient-therapist relationship plays a critical role in this form of psychotherapy, both in providing an empathic environment and in enhancing interpersonal learning: self-defeating interpersonal behaviors are confronted and more adaptive mechanisms are supported; verbalization and effective communication are practiced and encouraged; testing of subjective perceptions is fostered; and, when indicated, the therapist may actively advocate on behalf of the resident or assist staff to understand the interpersonal behavior of the resident. Restoration of effective functioning may require various techniques: mourning for internal and external losses is facilitated, strengths and limitations are reappraised, strategies to maintain emotional regulation and resolve interpersonal conflicts are promoted, and self-mastery and a new sense of identity are highlighted and integrated. The following case vignette is illustrative:

> An 83-year-old married woman suffered a right cerebrovascular accident with a dense left hemiplegia, leaving her dependent on others for most activities of daily living (ADLs) and prompting her nursing home admission. Earlier in her life, she had worked as an English teacher, loved to read and to travel, and had prided herself on her ability to manage an array of household and family affairs. In her later years, she served as a caregiver to her ailing husband. Her stroke, while sparing much of her intellect, left her feeling suddenly useless and helpless, "like I'd lost part of myself," with little interest in activities and steady weight loss. In the course of psychotherapy, as she began to survey her remaining attributes, she recognized that her capacity to be opinionated could now be enlisted to control aspects of her care; her ability to call up visual memories of her travels could be used for entertainment and for solace; and her family still valued her advice. She also became reconciled to her limitations, as she realized that she could no longer be a "female Atlas" who takes on the problems of others, and she could no longer control many of her life's circumstances. While she yearned for independence and to return home, she understood that this was not possible. Despite her stroke, she began to again view herself as capable and whole, with accompanying stabilization of her weight and a lifting of her dysphoria.

Specialized Techniques: Older Adults with Personality Disorder

The diagnosis of personality disorder is used to describe individuals who display patterns of maladaptive behaviors or traits that are associated with impaired social or occupational functioning or subjective distress (APA, 1994). These disorders encompass a variety of behavioral characteristics: some individuals with personality disorder may be self-aggrandizing, hypersensitive to criticism, and unable to empathize with others; others may be aloof, solitary, and indifferent; still others may be submissive, uncomfortable when alone, and excessively dependent. Recent research has suggested that personality disorder in the elderly is associated with a vulnerability to developing depression (Abrams, 1987), recurrence of depressive episodes, and a history of suicide attempts (Kunik, 1993). In the nursing home population, as mentioned previously, an estimated 11 to 23% of residents have a diagnosable personality disorder (Teeter et al., 1976; Hing, 1991). Individuals with untreated personality disorder often create havoc for medical personnel by sabotaging treatment efforts, provoking and disturbing other residents, and inciting intrastaff conflict.

Insight-oriented and supportive psychotherapy is widely viewed as the preferred treatment for individuals with personality disorder, yet there are no empirical studies examining its use in treating nursing home residents. Clinical reports suggest that psychotherapy is effective in reducing pathological acting out (e.g., sabotaging of treatment), reducing maladaptive patterns of interaction, and improving the emotional control of personality-disordered elderly nursing home residents (Sadavoy and Dorian, 1983; Sadavoy, 1987).

> A 73-year-old widowed woman was admitted to the nursing home following hemicolectomy for metastatic cancer. She had additional medical problems and was quite debilitated and reliant on others for assistance with ADLs. She was estranged from her children and only rarely in contact with siblings. Her medical prognosis was poor. She alternately denied the seriousness of her condition and tearfully stated that the surgery was unsuccessful and she was "waiting to die." As her medical problems worsened, she became demanding and verbally abusive toward nursing staff, whom she perceived as withholding of the care she required. As conflicts with staff escalated, she threatened to commit suicide and to refuse medications, but she withdrew these threats later. Her psychotherapeutic treatment consisted of setting limits on her manipulative threats, reaching agreement regarding appropriate ways to manage feelings of hopelessness and suicidality, clarifying that anger precipitated by her helpless and painful condition was misdirected at staff, and enlisting staff in efforts to understand and better manage her behavior. The threats and conflicts lessened, her family contacted her more often, and shortly thereafter she died rather quietly.

Specialized Techniques: Older Adults with Dementia

Some of the earliest reports of effective psychotherapeutic treatment of older adults included institutionalized elderly with dementia and behavioral problems (Goldfarb and Turner, 1952; Wolk and Goldfarb, 1967). There is growing clinical evidence that cognitive impairment is not a contraindication for successful psychotherapy. Smith and Kramer (1992) reported that 60% of elderly clinic patients with organic mental disorders were assessed as suitable for psychotherapy, as were 30% of elderly nursing home residents with dementia. Clinical reports suggest that individuals with early dementia often develop depression and can utilize psychotherapy to improve emotional control, maintain self-esteem, adjust to increased reliance on others, and reestablish a sense of identity (Cohen, 1989; Miller, 1989; Lewis and Rosenberg, 1990; Forrest, 1992). Some have suggested that cognitively impaired elderly are particularly sensitive to feeling misunderstood by others and often require psychotherapy (Sadavoy and Robinson, 1989).

In order for psychotherapy to be beneficial, patients with dementia must evidence preservation of some cognitive abilities, such as a capacity to communicate, an understanding that a problem exists, and an ability to retain some of the products of a therapeutic session (Miller, 1989; Sadavoy and Robinson, 1989; Lewis and Rosenberg, 1990; Smith and Kramer, 1992).

> A 90-year-old widowed woman was admitted to the nursing home with crippling arthritis and a mild dementia. While she was partly aware of her cognitive impairment, her depression arose from her loss of autonomy and perception of herself as useless and living a "wasted life." She had been a wife, mother, and grandmother but took less interest in these roles than her peers and rarely saw her only son. She proudly recounted how she had worked in business through the latter half of her life, but she now viewed the nursing home as understimulating. Most notably, she derided herself for "not contributing anything to anybody." She was unable to remember any interactions or conversations with others that might counter this view of herself as worthless. In the course of psychotherapy, she often appeared initially tearful and dysphoric but then would become more animated as she engaged her psychologist in arguing about whether she was still capable of contributing to others. After several such sessions, the psychologist confronted her with the fact that she could probably carry on his side of the "argument" herself. "Yes" she replied. "You'd disagree. . . . You'd say I contribute." To the psychologist's surprise, she proceeded to give examples of how she could be useful to others. She later conceded that she enjoyed her psychotherapy sessions because they offered her a chance to argue with someone; it reminded her of her good-natured arguments with her husband and son and helped lessen her despair.

Impact of Social and Environmental Factors

The impact of social and environmental factors, most notably the institutional environment and staff behaviors, is rarely mentioned in discussions of psychotherapy in the nursing home. Yet, as noted earlier, numerous studies have documented the impact of social and environmental factors on the general emotional well-being of community- and institutionally residing elderly. The older individual's interpersonal environment has also been shown to affect the course of major depression in community-dwelling elderly (Hinrichsen and Hernandez, 1993; Zweig and Hinrichsen, 1993). It therefore seems likely that the effectiveness of psychotherapy for elderly living in the nursing home partly depends upon aspects of the institutional environment and the interpersonal context provided by primary care staff.

Elderly nursing home residents whose physical, psychological, and social integrity have been compromised require a facilitating psychological environment to begin the psychotherapeutic process of self-restoration. Yet certain attributes of the institutional environment militate against this goal. The nursing home environment is often impersonal; staff upon whom residents depend change frequently and unpredictably; privacy and autonomy are compromised; the nature of one's interpersonal relationships is often dictated by one's care needs; rooms and roommates change; if one is medically hospitalized, the security of having a bed and a "home" is often guaranteed only for a limited time. Further, some institutions organize service delivery in a manner that instills dependency in residents and creates a cycle of helplessness, demandingness, and increased staff utilization (Gatz et al., 1985).

As noted, the interpersonal environment created by primary care staff is probably critical to the genesis, course, and treatment outcome of mentally ill nursing home residents. However, caring for community-dwelling depressed elderly patients has in itself been tied to feelings of anger, depression, and anxiety in caregivers (Hinrichsen et al., 1992). While less well studied, similar emotional reactions are probably elicited in nursing home staff caring for residents with these problems. Gunther (1987) has observed that "the price a dedicated and effective rehabilitation staff pays for significant therapeutic involvement with seriously damaged patients is periodic subjective distress and impaired professional behavior" (p. 219). More commonly, he noted, institutional staff respond to physically and psychologically traumatized patients by avoiding true empathic contact with the patient repressing the patients' and their own distress, and failing to attend to behavioral principles in delivering care. Thus, for psychotherapy to be effective, interventions must target the emotional responses and behaviors of primary staff as well as those of the mentally ill resident.

Conclusions

Mental disorders are prevalent in elderly nursing home residents. While mental health treatment is still underutilized in this setting, the provision of psychological treatment is on the rise. Psychotherapy, based on a body of well-developed theory and grounded in research, has been shown to be effective in treating mental illness in community-dwelling elderly and in groups of institutionalized elders. Existing models of psychotherapy are being modified to treat the special clinical problems found in residents of nursing homes; barriers to treatment are being identified, and guidelines for psychotherapeutic treatment are being developed; the social and environmental conditions that enable psychotherapy in the nursing home are being clarified.

However, the delivery of mental health services, including psychotherapy, to elderly nursing home residents is in a nascent stage. Future treatment programs will probably continue to borrow from existing models of psychiatric and rehabilitative care and employ mental health clinicians to further develop methods for the early detection of mental illness, maximize the physical rehabilitation of residents suffering from mental illness, and develop educational programs for primary staff and family members of residents. Therein will the treatment needs of this underserved population be met and the public policy mandate for "active treatment" be realized.

References

Abrams R, Alexopoulos G, Young R. Geriatric depression and the DSM-III-R criteria. *J Am Geriatr Soc* 35:383, 1987.

APA. *Diagnostic and Statistical Manual of Mental Disorders,* 4th ed. Washington DC: American Psychiatric Association, 1994.

APA. *Diagnostic and Statistical Manual of Mental Disorders* (DSM-III-R), 3rd ed. Revised. Washington DC: American Psychiatric Association, 1987.

APA. *Treatments of Psychiatric Disorders: A Task Force Report of the American Psychiatric Association.* Washington DC: American Psychiatric Association, 1989.

Asnis GM, Miller AH. Phenomenology and biology of depression-potential mechanisms for neuromodulation of immunity. In: Miller AH, ed. *Depressive Disorders and Immunity,* American Psychiatric Press, Washington, DC, 1989: 53–63.

Atchley RC. A continuity theory of normal aging. *Gerontologist* 29:183, 1989.

Biegel DE, Sales E, Schulz R, eds. *Family Caregiving in Chronic Illness.* Newbury Park, CA: Sage, 1991.

Borson S, Liptzin B, Nininger J, Rabins P. *A Report of the Task Force on Nursing Homes and the Mentally Ill Elderly: American Psychiatric Association.* Washington DC: American Psychiatric Association, 1989.

Burish TG, Bradley LA, eds. *Coping with Chronic Illness: Research and Applications.* New York: Academic Press, 1983.

Christopher F, Loeb P, Zaretsky H, Jassani A. A group psychotherapy intervention to promote the functional independence of older adults in a long-term rehabilitation hospital: A preliminary study. *Phys Occup Ther Geriatr* 6:51, 1988.

Cohen G. Mental health aspects of nursing home care. In Schneider EL, Wendland CJ, Zimmer AW, et al., eds. *The Teaching Nursing Home.* New York: Raven Press, 1985:157–164.

Cohen G. Psychodynamic perspectives in the clinical approach to brain disease in the elderly. In: Conn DE, Grek A, Sadavoy J, eds. *Psychiatric Consequences of Brain Disease in the Elderly: A Focus on Management.* New York: Plenum Press, 1989:85–99.

Cohen G. Psychopathology of mental health in the mature and elderly adult. In: Birren JE, Schaie KW, eds. *Handbook of the Psychology of Aging.* San Diego, CA: Academic Press, 1990:359–371.

Cohen S. Psychosocial models of the role of social support in the etiology of physical disease. *Health Psychol* 7:269, 1988.

Elkin I, Shea MT, Watkins JT, et al. National Institute of Mental Health Treatment of Depression Collaborative Research Program: General effectiveness of treatments. *Arch Gen Psychiatry,* 46:971, 1989.

Erikson E. *Childhood and Society.* New York: Norton, 1950.

Felton BJ, Revenson TA, Hinrichsen GA. Stress and coping in the explanation of psychological adjustment among chronically ill adults. *Soc Sci Med* 18:889, 1984.

Forrest DV. Psychotherapy of patients with neuropsychiatric disorders. In: Yudofsky SC, Hales RE, eds. *The American Psychiatric Association Press Textbook of*

Neuropsychiatry. Washington DC: American Psychiatric Association, 1992:703–739.

Frank E, Kupfer DJ, Perel JM, et al. Three-year outcomes for maintenance therapies in recurrent depression. *Arch Gen Psychiatry* 47:1093, 1990.

Frey DE, Kelbley TJ, Durham L, James J. Enhancing the self-esteem of selected male nursing home residents. *Gerontologist* 32:552, 1992.

Gatz M, Popkin SJ, Pino CD, VandenBos GR. Psychological interventions with older adults. In: Birren JE, Schaie KW, eds. *Handbook of the Psychology of Aging,* 2nd ed. New York: Van Nostrand Reinhold, 1985:755–785.

German PS, Rovner BW, Burton LL, et al. The role of mental morbidity in the nursing home experience. *Gerontologist* 32:152, 1992.

Goffman E. *Asylums: Essays on the Social Situation of Mental Patients and Other Inmates.* Garden City, NY: Doubleday, 1961.

Goldfarb A. Psychotherapy of aged persons: IV. One aspect of the psychodynamics of the therapeutic situation with aged persons. *Psychoanal Rev* 42:180, 1955.

Goldfarb AI, Sheps J. Psychotherapy of the aged: III. Brief therapy of interrelated psychological and somatic disorders. *Psychosom Med* 16:209, 1954.

Goldfarb A, Turner H. Psychotherapy of aged persons: II. Utilization and effectiveness of brief therapy. *Am J Psychiatry* 109:916, 1952–53.

Griffin BP, Grunes JM. A developmental approach to psychoanalytic psychotherapy with the aged. In: Nemiroff RA, Colarusso CA, eds. *New Dimensions in Adult Development.* New York: Basic Books, 1990:267–283.

Greenwald BS, Gemson DH, Kramer-Ginsberg E. A survey of mental health services in nursing homes. Presented at the 146th Annual Meeting of the American Psychiatric Association, San Francisco, May 1993.

Groves JE, Kucharski A. Brief psychotherapy. In: Hackett TP, Cassem NH, eds. *Massachusetts General Hospital Handbook of General Hospital Psychiatry,* 2nd ed. Littleton, MA: PSG Publishing, 1987:309–331.

Grunes JM. Brief psychotherapy with the aged: A clinical approach. In: Abrahams JP, Crooks VJ, eds. *Geriatric Mental Health.* Orlando, FL: Grune & Stratton, 1984;97–107.

Gunther MS. Catastrophic illness and the caregivers: Real burdens and solutions with respect to the behavioral sciences. In: Caplan B, ed. *Rehabilitation Psychology Desk Reference,* Gaithersburg MD: Aspen Publications, 1987:219–243.

Gutmann DL. Late onset pathogenesis: Dyanamic models. *Topics Geriatr Rehabil* 3:1, 1988.

Herst L, Moulton P. Psychiatry in the nursing home. *Psychiatr Clin North Am* 8:551, 1985.

Hing E. National Center for Health Statistics: Use of nursing homes by the elderly, preliminary data from the 1985 National Nursing Home Survey. In: *Advance Data from Vital and Health Statistics,* No. 135, DHHS Pub. No. ADM 87-1516. Washington, DC: U.S. Government Printing Office, 1987.

Hinrichsen GA, Hernandez N. Factors associated with recovery and relapse from major depressive disorder in the elderly. *Am J Psychiatry* 150:1820, 1993.

Hinrichsen GA, Hernandez N, Pollack S. Difficulties and rewards in family care of the depressed older adult. *Gerontologist* 32:486, 1992.

Kahana E. A congruence model of person-environment interaction. In: Windley PG, Byert TO, eds. *Aging and the Environment: Theoretical Approaches.* New York: Springer-Verlag, 1982:97.

Kahana RJ. Geriatric psychotherapy: Beyond crisis management. In Sadavoy J, Leszcz M, eds. *Treating the Elderly with Psychotherapy: The Scope for Change in Later Life.* Madison, WI: International Universities Press, 1987:233–263.

Kaplan HB, ed. *Psychosocial Stress: Trends in Theory and Research.* New York: Academic Press, 1983.

Karuza J, Katz PR. Psychosocial interventions in long-term care: A critical overview. In: Katz P, Kane R, Mezey M, eds. *Advances in Long Term Care.* Vol I. New York: Springer-Verlag, 1991.

Kunik ME, Mulsant BH, Rifai AH, et al. Personality disorders in elderly inpatients with major depression. *Am J Geriatr Psychiatry* 1:38, 1993.

Langer EJ, Rodin J. The effects of choice and enhanced personal responsibility for the aged: A field experiment in an institutional setting. *J Pers Soc Psychol* 34:191, 1975.

Lawton MP. Competence, environmental press, and the adaptation of older people. In: Lawton MP, Windley PG, Byerts TO, eds. *Aging and the Environment: Theoretical Approaches.* New York: Springer-Verlag, 1982:33.

Lazarus LW, Groves L, Gutmann D, et al. Brief psychotherapy with the elderly: A study of process and outcome: In: Sadavoy J, Leszcz M, eds. *Treating the Elderly with Psychotherapy: The Scope for Change in Later Life.* Madison, WI: International Universities Press, 1987:265–293.

Lazarus RS, Folkman S. *Stress, Appraisal, and Coping.* New York: Springer-Verlag, 1984.

Lewis L, Rosenberg SJ. Psychoanalytic psychotherapy with brain-injured adult psychiatric patients. *J Nerv Ment Dis* 178:69, 1990.

Lipzin B. Nursing home care. In: Birren JE, Sloane RB, Cohen G, eds. *Handbook of Mental Health and Aging,* 2nd ed. San Diego, CA: Academic Press, 1992:833–852.

Miller M. Opportunities for psychotherapy in the management of dementia. *J Geriatr Psychiatry Neurol* 2:11, 1989.

Moos RH, ed. *Coping with Physical Illness: 2. New Perspectives.* New York: Plenum Press, 1984.

Moos RH, Lemke S. Specialized living environments for older people. In: Birren JE, Schaie KW, eds. *The Handbook of the Psychology of Aging,* 2nd ed. New York: Van Nostrand Reinhold, 1985:864.

Moran TA, Gatz M. Group therapies for nursing home adults: An evaluation of two treatment approaches. *Gerontologist* 27:588, 1987.

Mumford E, Schlesinger HJ, Glass G. The effects of psychological intervention on recovery from surgery and heart attacks: An analysis of the literature. *Am J Public Health* 72:141, 1982.

Myers WA. *Dynamic Therapy of the Older Patient.* New York: Jason Aronson, 1984.

Neugarten BL. Time, age, and the life cycle. *Am J Psychiatry* 136:887, 1977.

Newton N, Lazarus L. Behavioral and psychotherapeutic interventions. In: Birren JE, Sloane RB, Cohen G, eds. *Handbook of Mental Health and Aging,* 2nd ed. San Diego, CA: Academic Press, 1992:699–719.

NIH. *Diagnosis and Treatment of Depression in Late Life.* (Reprinted from NIH Consensus Development Conference Consensus Statement 1991, Nov 4–6: 9 (3)). Bethesda MD: National Institutes of Health, 1991.

Osgood N, Theilman S. Geriatric suicidal behavior. In: Blumenthal SJ, Kupfer D, eds. *Suicide Over the Life Cycle.* Washington DC: American Psychiatric Association, 1990:341–379.

Parmelee P, Katz IR, Lawton MP. Depression among institutionalized aged: Assessment and prevalence estimation. *J Gerontol* 44:M22, 1989.

Parmelee PA, Lawton MP. The design of special environments for the aged. In: Birren JE, Schaie KW, eds. *Handbook of the Psychology of Aging,* 3rd ed. San Diego, CA: Academic Press, 1990:465.

Power CA, McCarron LT. Treatment of depression in persons residing in homes for the aged. *Gerontologist* 15:132, 1975.

Rattenbury C, Stones MJ. A controlled evaluation of reminiscence and current topics discussion groups in a nursing home context. *Gerontologist* 29:768, 1989.

Reynolds CF, Frank E, Perel JM, et al. Combined pharmacotherapy and psychotherapy in the acute and continuation treatment of elderly patients with recurrent major depression: A preliminary report. *Am J Psychiatry* 149:1687, 1992.

Ripeckyj AJ, Lazarus LW. Management of old age—Psychotherapy: Individual, group, and family. In: Kay D, Burrows G, eds. *Handbook of Studies on Psychiatry and Old Age.* Amsterdam: Elsevier, 1984:375–388.

Rodin J, Langer E. Long-term effects of a control-relevant intervention. *J Pers Soc Psychol* 35:891, 1977.

Ronch J, Maizler J. Individual psychotherapy with the institutionalized aged. *Am J Orthopsychiatry* 47:275, 1977.

Rovner BW, Katz IR. Psychiatric disorders in the nursing home: A selective review of studies related to clinical care. *Int J Geriatr Psychiatry* 8:75, 1993.

Sadavoy J, Dorian B. Treatment of the elderly characterologically disturbed patient in the chronic care institution. *J Geriatr Psychiatry* 16:223, 1983.

Sadavoy J. Character disorders in the elderly. In: Sadavoy J, Leszcz M, eds. *Treating the Elderly with Psychotherapy: The Scope for Change in Later Life.* Madison, WI: International Universities Press, 1987:175–229.

Sadavoy J, Leszcz M. *Treating the Elderly with Psychotherapy: The Scope for Change in Late Life.* Madison, WI: International Universities Press, 1987.

Sadavoy J, Robinson A. Psychotherapy and the cognitively impaired elderly. In: Conn DE, Grek A, Sadavoy J, eds. *Psychiatric Consequences of Brain Disease in the Elderly: A Focus on Management.* New York: Plenum Press, 1989:101–135.

Schulz R, Hanusa BH. Environmental influences on the effectiveness of control- and competence-enhancing interventions. In: Perlmuter LC, Monty RA, eds. *Choice and Perceived Control.* Hillsdale, NJ: Erlbaum, 1979:315.

Seligman MEP. *Helplessness.* San Francisco: Freeman, 1975.

Shea DG, Smyer MA, Streit A. Receipt of mental health treatment by nursing home residents. Presented at the 45th Annual Meeting of the Gerontological Society of America, Washington DC, November 1992.

Smith MC, Kramer NA. Psychotherapy with persons with dementia. Presented at the 45th Annual Meeting of the Gerontological Society of America, Washington DC, November, 1992.

Smith ML, Glass GV, Miller TI. *The Benefits of Psychotherapy.* Baltimore: Johns Hopkins University Press, 1980.

Smyer MA, Zarit SH, Qualls SH. Psychological intervention in the aging individual. In Birren JE, Schaie KW, eds. *Handbook of the Psychology of Aging,* 3rd ed. San Diego, CA: Academic Press, 1990:375–403.

Snyder CR, Ford CE, eds. *Coping with Negative Life Events.* New York: Plenum Press, 1987.

Spayd CS, Smyer MA. Individual interventions for nursing home residents. In: Smyer M, Cohn M, Brannon D, eds. *Mental Health Consultation in the Nursing Home.* New York: New York University Press, 1988:100–122.

Steurer JL, Mintz J, Hammen CL, et al. Cognitive behavioral and psychodynamic group psychotherapy in the treatment of geriatric depression. *J Consult Clin Psychol* 52:180, 1984.

Teeter RB, Garetz FK, Miller WR, Heiland WF. Psychiatric disturbances of aged patients in skilled nursing homes. *Am J Psychiatry* 133:1430, 1976.

Thompson L, Gallagher D, Breckenridge J. Comparative effectiveness of psychotherapies for depressed elders. *J Consult Clin Psychol* 52:385, 1987.

Tobin S. Issues of care in long term settings. In: Conn DE, Grek A, Sadavoy J, eds. *Psychiatric Consequences of Brain Disease in the Elderly: A Focus on Management.* New York: Plenum Press, 1989:163–187.

Viederman M, Perry SW. Use of a psychodynamic life narrative in the treatment of depression in the physically ill. *Gen Hosp Psychiatry* 2:177, 1980.

Weissman M, Paykel E. *The Depressed Woman.* Chicago: University of Chicago Press, 1974.

Wolk RL, Goldfarb AI. The response to group psychotherapy of aged recent admissions compared with long term mental hospital patients. *Am J Psychiatry* 123:1251, 1967.

Zweig RA, Hinrichsen GA. Factors associated with suicide attempts by depressed older adults: A prospective study. *Am J Psychiatry* 150:1687, 1993.

14

Cognitive and Behavioral Therapy

Deborah J. Ossip-Klein and Jurgis Karuza

This chapter provides an overview of cognitive and behavioral interventions in nursing home settings. The first section defines behavioral and cognitive therapies and discusses their application in frail elderly institutionalized populations. The next section selectively reviews the empirical literature on behavioral and cognitive interventions in nursing homes. The final section deals with special issues in applying these procedures in nursing homes.

Cognitive and Behavioral Therapy—An Overview

Behavioral Therapy

Behavioral therapy represents a collection of interventions that focus on identifying specific behavioral problems associated with clients' presenting complaints and on teaching clients to change these behaviors. Often defined as the application of learning principles to the treatment of maladaptive behavior (e.g., Krasner, 1971), behavioral therapy draws its theoretical roots mainly from operant and classical conditioning (e.g., Watson, 1925; Pavlov, 1927; Skinner, 1974) and social learning theory (Bandura, 1977, 1986). These theories have generated a range of behavioral interventions, such as systematic desensitization, biofeedback, social skills training, and lifestyle modification approaches.

There are two key characteristics of a behavioral approach. The first is reliance on a functional analysis of behavior. Psychological and behavioral dysfunctions are viewed as resulting from learning experiences in which the environment shapes and reinforces maladaptive behavior. Cognitive behavioral therapists also examine cognitive mediators, or how clients perceive environmental prompts and reinforcers. In changing the undesired behaviors, behavioral therapists and clients attempt to identify and alter these environmental factors and to build in new prompts and reinforcements for desired behaviors. Therapists and clients typically work as partners in this effort and use the outcomes of these interventions to guide further treatment efforts.

A second defining characteristic of behavioral interventions is the clear specification of treatment procedures and careful assessment of outcome (e.g., Mahoney, 1974). Thus, priority has been given to controlled outcome studies to evaluate the effectiveness of behavioral interventions. Further, when interventions are shown to be effective, a clear protocol for implementation is typically provided, so that the procedures can be replicated in other settings.

The fields of behavioral gerontology (e.g., Burgio and Burgio, 1986) and behavioral geriatrics (Hussian, 1984) have applied behavioral approaches to older populations. These interventions have been used, in particular, to treat specific response deficits, such as appropriate voiding, good hygiene, self-care, ambulation, and social interaction. Such behaviors are often amenable to specific behavioral therapy techniques and do not require more lengthy and costly psychotherapies that focus on large-scale personality modifications (Hussian, 1984).

Cognitive Therapy

From the perspective of cognitive-based therapeutic approaches, people's underlying cognitions influence their mental health problems. Simply put, it is assumed that negative emotions and maladaptive behaviors result from maladaptive thoughts. It follows, then, that the treatment of mental health problems requires modification of the patient's cognitions. A variety of approaches have been developed to directly or indirectly restructure the ways patients think about themselves, their problems, and their lives. One example is Ellis's (1962) rational emotive therapy, which views negative emotions and inappropriate behavior as resulting from illogical thinking. Another is Meichenbaum's self-instructional therapy, which seeks to change patients' thoughts about themselves by teaching patients to talk to themselves in more positive and constructive ways (Meichenbaum, 1975). This approach has been used with some success in helping older adults develop better problem-solving skills (Labouvie-Vief and Gonda, 1976). A third example is Beck's cognitive therapy, which seeks to identify, challenge, and reinterpret the illogical and negative thoughts and self-perceptions that underlie depression (Beck and Young, 1985).

A common theme running through these approaches is that patients can be made aware of their thought patterns and that there is little need for the analytic interpretation that is typically used in traditional psychotherapeutic approaches. While the directiveness of the therapist varies, the relationship between therapist and patient is, at its roots, a collaborative one, with the patient playing a major role in the therapeutic effort. While behavioral- and cognitive-based approaches both employ behavioral change methods, cognitive approaches see behavioral change as a means to achieve cognitive change rather than an end "in and of" itself.

Rationale for Cognitive and Behavioral Therapies in Nursing Homes

Cognitive and behavioral therapies are useful for dealing with at least two general types of disorders. First, they can address a host of functional issues and include interventions to enhance autonomy, functional level, and activities of daily living. Second, they can target the usual range of psychiatric disorders such as depression and dementia. The availability of cognitive and behavioral interventions is particularly relevant to nursing homes, because the very mental health problems that are the most prevalent in residents are the ones that are effectively treated by behavioral and cognitive therapies. A random sampling of elderly residents in Medicare facilities showed that 79.6% of residents had moderate to severe mental health needs (APA, 1993). Notable among psychiatric disorders is depression, affecting about 30% of elderly in medical settings (Phan and Reifler, 1988). Further, a survey of skilled nursing facilities conducted by Zimmer et al. (1984) found that 64% of residents had significant behavioral problems, and 23% were described as having serious behavioral problems. A similar high frequency of behavioral problems—such as incontinence, ambulation difficulties, and others—was reported by Burgio and Burgio (1986). These authors note that all of the identified behavior problems have been treated with some success in younger populations and some in elderly groups. Thus, cognitive and behavioral approaches can offer a means of effectively dealing with clinically significant psychiatric and behavioral disorders that affect care and quality of life in nursing homes. In addition, research suggests that these procedures are acceptable to nursing home residents and, in some cases, are rated more highly than pharmacotherapy (Burgio and Sinnott, 1990). Despite the evidence on effectiveness and acceptability, only moderate usage of these interventions has been found in nursing homes (Guy and Morice, 1985).

Studies of Behavioral and Cognitive Therapies in Nursing Homes

The sections below provide a selected review of behavioral and cognitive therapies in nursing homes. Although the literature on cognitive and behavioral therapies in the nursing home setting is limited, existing research supports the viability of a number of specific approaches. To identify empirical work in these areas, literature searches were conducted through Medline and Psychological Abstracts for the 10-year period from 1983 to 1993 (for reviews including earlier studies, see Hussian, 1984; Burgio and Burgio, 1986; and Karuza and Katz, 1991; for specific intervention protocols, see Lundervold and Lewin, 1992). Studies were identified in the following two general areas: functional issues (exercise/ambulation, incontinence, bathing, eating) and psychiatric disorders (dementia, depression). The primary interventions identified were behavioral, with the few cognitive applications occurring for depression. Each clinical area is reviewed below, followed by a section on special issues in implementing these techniques.

Functional Issues

Exercise/Ambulation

Physical activity and physical fitness have been related to reduced mortality for the population in general (Blair et al., 1989) and for older adults specifically (Rakowski and Mor, 1992). Exercise may exert its protective effect through its impact on coronary artery disease, blood pressure, glucose metabolism and insulin resistance, bone density, and other factors. Further, exercise can improve muscle strength and function, which is particularly relevant for older populations who are at risk for falls, fractures, and reduction in activities of daily living (ADLs) related to muscle dysfunction (Fiatarone and Evans, 1993). Finally, exercise has been shown to enhance psychological function in both younger (Doyne et al., 1987; Ossip-Klein et al., 1989) and older (Powell, 1974) adults.

Behavioral interventions to increase exercise among nursing home patients have typically targeted ambulation, muscle strength, and flexibility/endurance. Interventions with community-dwelling elderly have also included aerobic or aerobic-type exercise programs (e.g., Stevenson and Topp, 1990).

Ambulation. Ambulation studies have demonstrated that walking can be increased through simple behavioral procedures. An early study by MacDonald and Butler (1974), using a single-subject design, showed that verbal prompts to walk, and interaction with staff contingent on walking, increased ambulation in two nursing home residents who had been previously transported by wheelchair. Burgio et al. (1986) extended these procedures to eight nursing home residents who were physically capable of walking but were transported to meals by wheelchair. Nursing home staff were trained to prompt subjects to walk from the entrance to the dining area to the table, and to verbally reinforce any walking. Significant increases in walking occurred and were maintained through the 4-month follow-up. Further, as the study progressed, seven of the subjects did not require staff assistance for most sessions. Although these results suggest that resident ambulation can be increased through behavioral intervention, Baltes et al. (1983) reported that staff are more likely to reinforce dependent behaviors, such as requests for assistance, and less likely to reinforce independent behaviors, such as walking. Thus, programs targeting staff as well as patients may be critical to affecting ambulation.

Muscle Strength. The recent position statement of the American College of Sports Medicine (1990) now includes recommendations for both muscle-strengthening as well as endurance exercises for adults of all ages. Several studies have demonstrated that high-intensity resistance training produces dramatic increases in muscle strength in older individuals, including frail elderly up to 100 years of age

(Fiatarone and Evans, 1993). Using an 8-week weight lifting protocol based on standard rehabilitation principles of progressive-resistance training, Fiatarone et al. (1990) showed significant increases in muscle strength, size, and functional mobility among 10 frail nursing home residents averaging 90 years of age. Subjects exercised three times per week, with three sets of eight repetitions per leg at each session. The load was adjusted to provide 50% of a one-repetition maximum at week 1, and 80% at subsequent weeks. Such high-intensity protocols may be necessary, as little or no increase in muscle strength has been shown with low- to moderate-resistance training in older adults. While not specifically a behavioral therapy treatment, effective implementation of exercise programs can be enhanced by incorporation of behavioral and cognitive approaches to motivate and reinforce patients' initiating and maintaining weight lifting. Such techniques include provider education and encouragement of patients, using patient-determined daily weight-lifting goals (within provider-set guidelines), and the provision of feedback on patient progress.

A novel approach to muscle strength maintenance has been reported by Bruemmer and colleagues (1993), who are conducting bedside exercise in hospitalized older adults in an attempt to prevent muscle atrophy associated with reduced mobility.

Flexibility/Endurance. A behavioral procedure to enhance stationary bicycle riding was reported by Perkins et al. (1986). Subjects were eight male residents in a nursing home care unit at the Jackson Mississippi VA Medical Center who ranged from 46 to 78 years of age. Treatment involved prompting bicycle riding through posting distance goals and providing immediate feedback and gold stars to subjects on whether these goals were met, providing colored buttons for met goals during the first 3 weeks, providing T-shirts for four consecutive weeks of met goals, and announcing successful exercisers in an in-house newsletter distributed to staff and residents. Prompts and rewards were gradually eliminated over time to examine maintenance of exercise. Results showed significant increases in bicycle riding during the course of treatment, which was consistently maintained in six of eight subjects. While health outcomes were not assessed, this study supported the effectiveness of behavioral strategies in promoting exercise in nursing home residents. Improved grip strength, spinal flexion, chair-to-stand time, ADLs, and self-rating of depression was reported for 20 nursing home residents following a 7-month program of twice-weekly 45-minute exercise sessions (McMurdo and Rennie, 1993). Exercise involved repetitive upper- and lower-limb range of motion and muscle strengthening in a seated position. Notable in this study was the 64 to 100% attendance rate (averaging 91%) at sessions and the 75% completion rate for exercise participants at 7 months.

Overall, exercise interventions appear to be both physiologically sound and feasible for even frail nursing home residents. Sample sizes in most studies reviewed were small, and further research is needed to identify strategies to enhance maintenance of exercise in older (as well as younger) populations. Nevertheless, a number of behavioral approaches to implementing programs to enhance activity are currently available for incorporation in nursing home settings.

Incontinence

One of the most serious problems in nursing home residents is incontinence, with prevalence rates pegged at 50% (Mohide, 1986). The economic cost of managing incontinence has been estimated at $2 billion a year (Ouslander and Kane, 1984; Hu, 1990). Typically, the problem is assumed to be an inevitable and irreversible consequence of aging and treated by use of long-term indwelling catheters or diapers. With attendant risks of infection and skin ulceration, neither of these approaches is ideal. Behavioral-based approaches offer the promise of being effective management alternatives for at least some residents.

At the outset, it is important to distinguish among the common types of incontinence, since the relevance and effectiveness of behavioral techniques will vary with the type of incontinence. Of the four basic types of persistent urinary incontinence—overflow, stress, urge, and functional incontinence—behavioral interventions are seen as potentially relevant for all but overflow incontinence, which typically requires surgical intervention or catheterization (Ouslander, 1991).

A number of behavioral techniques have been developed that vary in the involvement of the patient and staff members. These have been described extensively elsewhere (e.g., Burgio and Burgio, 1986; National Institutes of Health Consensus Development Conference, 1990; Ouslander, 1991) and include pelvic muscle exercises, biofeedback, bladder training, bladder retraining, and prompted voiding.

Pelvic Muscle Exercises. This approach provides exercises that strengthen the pelvic floor muscles; it results in greater closing force on the urethra. The efficacy of this treatment has ranged from 30 to 90% in reported studies (Wells, 1990).

Biofeedback Techniques. Biofeedback has been used to teach patients to exert greater control over urine storage. Patients are given muscle exercises and are provided with immediate feedback on how well they are controlling sphincter, detrusor, and abdominal muscles. Patients with stress or urge incontinence benefit from these techniques, with complete control achieved by 20% of the patients and improvement in urinary control found in an additional 30% (National Institutes of Health Consensus Development Conference, 1990).

Bladder Training. This approach teaches patients to void at regular times during the day. The logic is to "catch the patient" before the incontinence occurs. This is especially relevant to those patients who suffer from urge and functional incontinence. Cure rates of 10 to 15% have been found using these techniques (National Institutes of Health Consensus Development Conference, 1990).

Bladder Retraining. This method attempts to restore the normal pattern of urination by teaching the patient to gradually expand the intervals between voiding by techniques such as learning to resist the sensation of urgency or developing a voiding schedule by the clock (Burgio and Burgio, 1986). To be successful, bladder retraining interventions call for a patient who is cooperative and motivated and who has sufficient mental function to participate in the training program. Overall, studies of bladder training efficacy report high cure rates, ranging from 44 to 90%. The outcomes, however, do vary with initial bladder capacity (Burgio and Burgio, 1986). While this approach is more demanding on the patient, it has the advantage of less direct staff involvement.

Prompted Voiding. In this approach, staff develop a frequent voiding schedule for residents, periodically check the residents' dryness, prompt the resident to void, and reinforce the resident for voiding. Although the typical schedule for prompted voiding is 1 to 2 hours, a recent study suggested that a less intensive 3-hour schedule may be effective for some residents (Burgio et al., 1994).

Prompted voiding has been shown to be most relevant for incontinence that is due to the poor functional level of patients. Up to 75% of all nursing home patients show significant reductions in incontinence with this procedure (Schnelle et al., 1983; Schnelle, 1990).

While behavioral techniques have been found to have the greatest potential for success, several caveats should be noted. Most of the studies on the efficacy of behavioral techniques have been tested on younger, community-based, more functional adults (Burgio and Burgio, 1986). The rates of efficacy with nursing home residents is less clear. The cost-effectiveness of behavioral techniques compared to other approaches, such as use of diapers, is also a consideration (Schnelle et al., 1993). A major barrier to the success of behavioral techniques is the cognitive impairment and low level of functioning of residents (Ouslander, 1990, 1991). An important consideration in maximizing the effectiveness of behavioral approaches to the management of incontinence in nursing homes is the appropriate selection of patients who can benefit from behavioral techniques and the development of an effective staff organization to monitor and implement the intervention. Guidelines for the selection process and specific intervention procedures are available (e.g., Schnelle et al., 1993).

Bathing

Downs and colleagues tested two modeling interventions to reduce avoidance of whirlpool baths among nursing home residents (Downs et al., 1988). Residents, who had previously demonstrated apprehension and resistance toward the lifting and lowering of their chairs (needed to enter and exit the whirlpool bath), were randomized to one of two modeling conditions, participant modeling or filmed modeling, or to no treatment. Participant modeling involved breaking the bath time into small, incremental steps that the therapist demonstrated and the residents then practiced with verbal reinforcement and assistance as needed. Participant modeling was conducted in both group and individual formats. Filmed modeling involved presenting the same information as in participant modeling but using a film of peers demonstrating these procedures. Consistent with empirical guidelines, filmed models first displayed apprehensiveness about the bath but then modeled coping skills that enabled them to complete the bathing routine successfully. Both modeling approaches have been shown to be effective for a range of fears and avoidance behaviors (Bandura, 1986). Results showed the greatest improvements with participant modeling, followed by filmed modeling, and no significant change for the no-treatment group. Participant modeling appeared most effective when administered in individual format, as single residents who remained fearful were shown to disrupt the progress of other group members. Further, some family members objected to the group bathing format, even though groups consisted of same-sex residents and residents remained clothed throughout the procedure. The authors suggest means of reducing barriers to group participant modeling, including screening or pretraining the most disruptive residents, and preceding participant modeling with filmed modeling of both individual and group approaches.

Eating

There is some evidence that eating dependency among nursing home residents can be successfully addressed by employing behavioral interventions (Baltes and Zerbe, 1976; Lewin et al., 1989). For example, in a recent series of single-case-design studies by Lewin et al. (1989), behavioral techniques were successful in reducing food dependence in two of three severely cognitively impaired female nursing home residents. A behavioral strategy of prompting coupled with social reinforcement was used with two women who were largely dependent on staff for feeding. The intervention was successful with one woman, who increased her rate of independent feeding behaviors at meals from 25 to 50% during baseline to 75 to 100% following the intervention. The third woman, who fed herself independently but had low food intake at meals, was found to significantly increase her food consumption after an intervention that consisted of serving her preferred foods in small containers and giving her verbal praise for eating.

These case studies show the promise of behavioral interventions as ways to increase the feeding independence of nursing home residents. The pattern of results also highlights the difficulty of implementing behavioral strategies with residents who are severely impaired cognitively. The paucity of recent studies examining behavioral approaches to facilitate feeding independence among nursing home residents is puzzling, given the prevalence of feeding dependence and its associated costs. Further work is clearly needed to develop and evaluate new behavioral techniques.

Psychiatric Disorders

Dementia

Behavioral interventions have targeted several behavioral and cognitive difficulties associated with dementia, including conversational skills, wandering/inappropriate behaviors, and disruptive/assaultive behaviors.

Conversational Skills. Memory aids have been one approach used to improve patterns of conversation with demented patients. For example, using a single-subject design, Bourgeois (1993) reported that a ''memory book'' consisting of simple statements and photographs of familiar people and events resulted in improved quality of conversations between pairs of demented patients. Similarly, providing a card with a listing of relevant names or daily routines, combined with prompting to use the card, increased conversation among residents (Bourgeois, 1990).

Wandering/Inappropriate Behaviors. Hussian (1988) used environmental cues and verbal prompts with five demented male patients in an attempt to reduce inappropriate voiding, climbing into the beds of other patients, entering the nursing station, and attempting to leave a protective environment; these techniques were also used to increase ability to locate relevant ward items (e.g., patient's own bed). Cues included a bright yellow sign on the door of the rest room, a bright sign with the patient's name over his bed, tape on the floor in front of the exit door, and colored signs near other relevant ward items. During the first phase of study, staff prompted the patients to attend to the cues; in a subsequent phase, cues alone were provided. All patients showed at least an 86% improvement in problem behaviors relative to periods when no interventions were provided; these improvements persisted even when cues alone (without prompts) were provided. Similarly, Hussian and Brown (1987) demonstrated that placing an eight-strip grid of clearly visible, horizontal masking tape stripes 57.2 cm from exit doors significantly reduced exiting from the ward by demented patients. The investigators attribute this effect to the observation that demented patients often see two-dimensional patterns as three-dimensional and thus pause or stop at flat grid patterns that non-demented patients would cross over.

These interventions are relatively straightforward and logical. In settings in which hallways and rooms look alike, the environment is handicapping, particularly to cognitively impaired patients. Patients can easily become confused about which is the correct room to enter or exit. Changing the environment by providing clear signs identifying key areas, combined with staff reinforcement of the patients' attending to these signs or, in some cases, providing clear floor grids, produces clear changes in patient behavior. Whether these changes will be maintained over long periods of time using the above protocols or whether additional maintenance efforts are needed remains to be studied.

Disruptive/Assaultive Behaviors. Behavioral models and approaches for decreasing disruptive and assaultive behaviors among nursing home patients have been described. For example, Cariaga et al. (1991) identified specific impairments among disruptive vocalizers as well as staff-reported utilization and perceived effectiveness of various existing interventions. Using a behavior-analytic perspective and drawing from literature with other populations, the authors suggested behavioral interventions that could be tested for dealing with this clinically meaningful problem. In addition, Lundervold and Lewin (1992) provide specific examples of behavioral programs for decreasing such inappropriate behaviors.

Empirical data on the effectiveness of these procedures were reported by Lundervold and Jackson (1992), who conducted an applied behavioral analysis of a nursing home resident with Huntington's disease and depression. The resident had frequent episodes of hitting, kicking, and biting and had been placed in restraints for approximately 8 hours after each episode. Pharmacological intervention had been unsuccessful. An applied behavioral analysis revealed that staff demands (e.g., to take a bath) and staff responses to his requests reliably precipitated aggressive acts. Aggression appeared to be maintained by avoidance of the undesired task and by staff attention. Intervention involved the following components: (1) staff were trained to change their response to the resident's requests by explaining why they could not immediately respond, telling him they would return to assist him, and verbally praising him for being patient; (2) a reinforcement schedule was developed to reinforce behaviors incompatible with aggression and enhance cooperation with instructions (cigarette smoking was used to reinforce cooperative behavior and the lack of aggression); (3) since nursing staff would not agree to elimination of restraints, each aggressive episode was followed by 5 minutes of soft wrist and chest restraints in bed and a loss of the opportunity to smoke. The intervention resulted in a significant decrease in aggressive episodes, to less than 4 per month (average of 1.16), with the resident remaining restraint-free about 99% of the time. Thus, this intervention appeared effective in reducing behaviors that were time-consuming and dangerous to staff, and it meaningfully improved quality of life for the patient. It should be noted, however, that the choice of a more healthful alternative to cigarette smoking as a reinforcer would be desirable.

Examples of behavioral treatment of aggressive behaviors in elderly patients in settings other than nursing homes are available. For example, Vaccaro (1988) developed a behavioral treatment program targeting six elderly aggressive/assaultive men in a state-operated developmental center. During the treatment phases, the patients were observed in group activities. At 10-minute intervals, patients were rewarded with fruit, cookies, or juice (individualized to each patient's preferences) for the absence of aggressive behavior during this period. Any aggressive behavior was immediately followed by a verbal reprimand and removal from the group activity (i.e., sitting alone at one end of the room) for a period of 10 minutes. Results showed a 76 to 78% improvement in aggressive behavior, with number of aggressive incidents dropping from 399 to 407 during baseline periods to 89 to 97 during treatment periods. In addition, improvements in aggressive behavior generalized to the patients' wards even as active treatment for aggression was phased out.

Reducing aggression during bathing was described by Lundervold and Lewin (1992). The resident was an elderly woman with Alzheimer's disease in a foster care setting who would bite, hit, and/or pinch her caregiver during the morning routine of bathing and dressing. These behaviors would occur while she was sitting, with caregivers leaning in front of her to undress, toilet, sponge-bathe, and dress her. To change this routine, the resident was instructed to stand facing away from the caregiver and hold onto the towel bar to prevent herself from falling. If she let go of the bar, the caregiver lowered her to the floor so she would not injure herself and instructed her to stand and grab the bar again. For bathing, the resident was placed in the bath, again facing away from the caregiver and holding onto the bar, and instructed to wash herself with her other hand. This new routine had several features: by having the resident face away from the caregiver, it removed a stimulus for hitting (i.e., having the caregiver bend down in front of the resident), and having the resident hold onto the bar and bathe herself did not leave her hands free to harm the caregiver.

Depression

The effectiveness of behavioral and cognitive-behavioral therapies for depression has been clearly demonstrated for the population in general (e.g., Elkin et al., 1989; Sotsky et al., 1991) as well as for the elderly (e.g., Gallagher and Thompson, 1982, 1983; Thompson et al., 1987). For example, Gallagher and Thompson (1982) randomly assigned older adult outpatients with a major depressive disorder to cognitive therapy, behavioral therapy (Lewinsohn, 1974), or brief insight psychotherapy in order to compare various psychotherapies in the absence of antidepressant medications. The therapy took place over a 12-week period and consisted of 16 one-on-one sessions. Pre-post comparisons indicated that a significant decrease in depression was found for patients enrolled in each of the three treatments, with no difference in depression among the three treatments at termination. However, long-term follow-up, 1 year later, indicated that cognitive and behavioral therapy patients maintained their gains more than the brief insight group. Further, two-thirds of the patients in the cognitive and behavioral therapy groups reported using the specific skills they learned in therapy to deal with depressive situations. In a follow-up controlled study, Thompson et al. (1987) assigned older adult patients, who met criteria of a major depressive disorder, to behavioral, cognitive, brief psychotherapy, and wait-list control. Therapy lasted between 16 to 20 individual sessions. The findings paralleled the original study. After completing therapy, subjects in the treatment groups improved and the wait-list controls did not. The gains were held 1 year after therapy.

Further, in the general population, these therapies have been at least as effective or superior to pharmacotherapies in treating mild, moderate, and, in some studies, even severe nonpsychotic depressions. For example, Beutler et al. (1987) compared group cognitive therapy with supportive intervention and a pharmacological treatment using alprazolam, a minor tranquilizer. Improvement in depression was found under all treatments, with the greatest improvement found in the cognitive therapy group.

Finally, cognitive therapies may reduce relapse rates relative to pharmacotherapies, and both cognitive and behavioral therapies may improve functional work capacity (Munoz et al., 1994).

Behavioral Approaches to Depression. Behavioral approaches typically view depression as resulting from a loss of previous reinforcers (Lewinsohn, 1974), a process that often accompanies aging, particularly for frail, institutionalized patients. Treatment focuses on helping patients increase the availability of pleasant activities. Goddard and Carstensen (1986) applied this approach to the treatment of an 86-year-old depressed nursing home resident who was confined to a wheelchair and had recently broken her wrist. An applied behavior analysis indicated significant loss of reinforcers, particularly during morning and evening hours. Treatment involved increasing the patient's access to self-initiated pleasant activities (identified by the patient), with special focus on the morning and evening, and verbally reinforcing her positive self-statements and actions. Improvements were found in daily mood ratings, which persisted through a 6-week follow-up. Anecdotally, staff and visitors commented about the positive changes in the patient. It should be noted, however, that her score on the Geriatric Depression Scale (Brink et al., 1982), though improved, was still in the mildly depressed range.

Cognitive Therapy for Depression. The basic premise of cognitive therapy with depressed patients is that depression is a result of a systematic mindset that misinterprets events to make them consistent with patients' negative beliefs about themselves as failures, the world as joyless, and the future as hopeless. Consequently, the main components of cognitive therapy are to teach patients to identify their automatic thought patterns, challenge their negative and illogical thoughts, and interpret events more rationally. Developing a friendly and mutually respectful therapeutic relationship is important, so that the interrelations among the patients' thought, feelings, and actions can be explored and changed (Thompson et al., 1986).

Prior to treatment (Newman and Beck, 1990), a comprehensive diagnostic evaluation is recommended to make sure that the depression is not secondary to another psychological disorder or that there is not an underlying organic disorder, such as hypothyroidism. The severity of the depression, especially if it is associated with suicidal tendency, should be determined. In more severe cases, medication may be indicated.

Cognitive therapy is short-term, lasting an average of 12 to 16 sessions (e.g., Beck and Young, 1985). The first session typically focuses on developing the therapeutic rapport, defining the problem and setting the goals of the treatment, and educating the patient about the relationship between thoughts, moods, and behaviors. Early on, patients are taught self-observational skills to help identify automatic thinking. Often patients are given "homework," where they track frequent negative thoughts or record their thoughts in depressive situations in a "daily thought record." Imagery techniques, where patients imagine solving current problems or dealing with threatening situations, can be helpful in altering negative beliefs. Behavioral techniques, especially at the start of therapy, are often used. Schedules for activities, assertiveness practice, and teaching of problem-solving techniques are used to engage the patient in changing his or her behavior and to overcome the lethargy and inactivity that result from feelings of hopelessness.

Fears of relapse are not uncommon. Thompson et al. (1986) recommend several ways to deal with relapse, including reinterpreting a mild depressive episode as a chance to practice the skills learned in therapy or scheduling a few "booster" sessions a month apart before the termination of therapy.

Cognitive Therapy in the Nursing Home. Patient age (Jarrett et al., 1991; Sotsky et al., 1991), and intelligence (Haaga et al., 1991) have been found to be unrelated to cognitive therapy outcome, although these conclusions are best treated as preliminary (Whisman, 1993). The track record would suggest that cognitive therapy could be an effective treatment modality with nursing home residents. The irony is that, given the prevalence of depression among nursing home residents, there has been a paucity of controlled studies of cognitive interventions in this setting.

One recent report (Abraham et al., 1992) examined group-based psychotherapeutic interventions in nursing homes. This controlled study tested the effectiveness of nurse led 24-week cognitive, focused imagery, and discussion group interventions with depressed patients. Subjects were enrolled if they had a score of 11 or higher on the Geriatric Depression Scale (or a score of 10 with clinical evidence of depressive symptomalogy); sufficient hearing, verbal, and comprehension skills to participate in group sessions; absence of major cognitive impairment; absence of antidepressant medication, and no history of endogenous depression. While no significant changes were found in depression, hopelessness, or life satisfaction scores for the patients enrolled in the three treatment groups, there were significant increases in cognitive scores after treatment in the cognitive therapy and focused visual imagery groups. The results suggest that an added secondary gain (i.e., improved cognition) may result from cognitive therapy. Cognitive therapy, by virtue of its limited duration, can be potentially cost-effective in the nursing home context. Especially if patients are screened, the therapy can be done in a group setting.

Cognitive and Behavioral Therapy for Depression: Summary. Studies with outpatient geriatric populations have generally supported the effectiveness of both behavioral and cognitive-behavioral therapies for clinically depressed patients, with effects of these therapies most notable at follow-up (e.g., Gallagher and Thompson, 1982). In addition, psychotherapies, and particularly cognitive therapy, have been shown to be at least as effective as pharmocotherapy for depression in the general population (Munoz et al., 1994). The few studies in nursing homes have suggested the utility of these approaches with this group, although consistent effects on depression measures have not been demonstrated. For the above studies, this may be due to the insensitivity of the depression measures (e.g., the Geriatric Depression Scale) to change (particularly since the patients may not have met standard criteria for clinical/major depression), the small sample sizes, insufficient follow-up, or shortcomings of the treatments themselves. Despite these potential flaws, positive changes in some areas were demonstrated. Clearly, more controlled studies that compare behavioral and cognitive therapies to pharmacological interventions (Chapters 3 and 6), as well as to other psychotherapeutic approaches (Chapter 14) in older populations are called for. Nevertheless, the broader positive results with these therapies for depressed patients in general, and the positive changes noted with nursing home groups, make behavioral and cognitive-behavioral therapies potentially usable as treatment options for depression in nursing home patients.

The recent clinical practice guidelines for the detection and treatment of depression in primary care, developed by the Agency for Health Care Policy Research (Depression Guideline Panel, 1993a,b,c,d), have been praised for their potential to enhance the identification and pharmacological treatment of depression by primary care physicians. However, these guidelines have also been criticized on a number of grounds, including insufficient information on drug dosages for elderly patients and the emphasis on pharmacotherapy as the first line of treatment, with a lack of emphasis on psychotherapies as viable alternatives or complements (Munoz et al., 1994). The range of medical conditions, medications, difficult life situations, and psychosocial issues that are particularly prevalent in nursing home residents underscores the importance of incorporating cognitive and behavioral therapies rather than relying on pharmacological management alone. A major advantage of both behavioral and cognitive therapies for nursing home residents is that they provide an alternative to pharmacological treatment, with its attendant dangers of polypharmacy. (The reader is referred to Chapter 6 for a more complete discussion of depression, and to Chapter 3 for psychopharmacological considerations.)

Special Issues in the Implementation of Behavioral and Cognitive Interventions

Staff Training

One question that arises in using both cognitive and behavior therapy in the nursing home is who will be doing the therapy. Studies have used different therapists, ranging from psychologists to nurses, nursing assistants, and other health care providers. As the list of eligible providers of mental health services in long-term-care settings expands, a question can be raised regarding whether the outcomes are equivalent with different professional providers. In a therapeutic approach, such as cognitive therapy, a special set of skills is necessary to assess patients appropriately and to conduct the therapeutic sessions. How much training and at which level best prepares therapists and produces the best patient outcomes is an important question for future research.

Implementation of behavioral and cognitive interventions may be done individually in the context of typical therapy sessions, in group settings, or through more general implementation by nursing home staff under the supervision of a behavioral/cognitive specialist (e.g., psychologist). Programs to train staff in these interventions have been reported. Ray and colleagues (Ray et al., 1993) conducted a controlled trial of a program to reduce antipsychotic drug use in nursing homes. Direct-care staff (physicians, nurses, nursing assistants, and others) were trained in medication withdrawal/monitoring and concurrent behavioral management approaches. Results showed decreases in antipsychotic medication use and physical restraint and no increase in behavior problem frequency. Mixed results have been reported for nursing assistant training. Cohn et al. (1990) found that a five-session program in behavioral management resulted in increases in both knowledge and self-reported use of these skills among nursing assistants. However, Smyer et al. (1991) reported that this program produced improvements in knowledge but did not improve performance. This last study provides an important caveat that reflects a common behavioral principle that information alone is often insufficient to change behavior. Producing meaningful changes in the behavior of health care providers may be best accomplished by combining training with appropriate and ongoing prompts and reinforcers to staff for using the new skills.

The Patient's Role

Another consideration in developing both cognitive and behavioral therapeutic approaches is the tendency for older adults to think that psychotherapy is a "medical treatment," to shift responsibility for the cure of the problem onto the health professional (Karuza et al., 1992), and to take a respectful but passive role. This tendency, if anything, can be expected to be more pronounced in a nursing home, with its "medical" overtones, and the tendency of staff to reinforce dependent behaviors (Baltes et al., 1983). Given the dynamics of cognitive and behavioral therapy, such a passive stance by older adults may make it difficult to develop collaborative therapeutic relationships between therapists and patients. Setting up the ground rules, assumptions, and expectations of these therapies at the outset becomes very important.

Perspectives: Keep It Simple (KIS) Is Often Best

A range of physical, mental health, and adjustment problems are responsive to formal interventions, which include behavioral and cognitive as well as more traditional medical and psychiatric/psychological therapies. However, it is important to note that "just because a hammer is available, not every problem is necessarily a nail." These points have been made by several authors in poignant ways. The late B. F. Skinner, a father of behavioral approaches, provided a series of behavioral insights on his own aging (e.g., Skinner, 1983; Skinner and Vaughan, 1983), in which he described a number of minor and practical environmental adjustments to compensate for changing capacities associated with aging. Similarly, Oneal (1986) presented a series of case studies illustrating the sometimes easily overlooked simple solutions. For example, she described a nursing home resident who refused to remain in bed at night. Instead, this resident continuously jumped up, ripped off her nightgown, and walked around the room nude and mumbling. The author ultimately determined that the resident hated the nightgown, which had been a gift from a sister whom she also hated. The social worker asked the patient to pick out a new nightgown from a catalogue and then purchased it for the resident; thereafter, the resident's nighttime problems disappeared. Although a behavioral intervention could have been developed to reinforce staying in bed, this social worker's simple solution was correct, sensitive to the patient's needs, and effective. Finally, Dallam (1987) gave examples of disruptive behaviors that were calmed by the nurse's touch or kind words or by the presence of another resident. In the efforts to provide clinically and cost-effective interventions for complex problems, these examples underscore the need to allow for the possibility that simple, humane solutions sometimes exist. It is when these solutions cannot be found that behavioral, cognitive, and traditional psychotherapy and medical interventions become necessary.

References

Abraham IL, Neundorfer MM, Currie LJ. Effects of group interventions on cognition and depression in nursing home residents. *Nurs Res* 41:196–202, 1992.

American College of Sports Medicine. The recommended quantity and quality of exercise for developing and maintaining cardiorespiratory and muscular fitness in healthy adults. *Med Sci Sports Ex* 22:265–274, 1990.

APA. *Reform of the Mental Health Delivery System: Essential to Health Care Reform.* Washington, DC: Government Relations Practice Directorate, 1993.

Baltes MM, Honn S, Barton EM, et al. On the social ecology of dependence and independence in elderly nursing home residents: A replication and extension. *J Gerontol* 38:556–564, 1983.

Baltes MM, Zerbe MB. Independence training in nursing home residents. *Gerontologist* 16:428–432, 1976.

Bandura A. *Social Learning Theory.* Englewood Cliffs, NJ: Prentice-Hall, 1977.

Bandura A. *Social Foundations of Thought and Action: A Social Cognitive Theory.* Englewood Cliffs, NJ: Prentice-Hall, 1986.

Beck AT. *Depression: Clinical, Experimental, and Theoretical Aspects.* New York: Harper & Row, 1967.

Beck AT, Young JE. Cognitive therapy of depression. In: Barlow D, ed. *Clinical Handbook of Psychological Disorders: A Step by Step Treatment Manual.* New York: Guilford, 1985:206–224.

Beutler LE, Scogin F, Kirkish P, et al. Group cognitive therapy and alprazolam in the treatment of depression in older adults. *J Consult Clin Psychol* 55:550–556, 1987.

Blair SN, Kohl HW III, Paffenbarger RS Jr, et al. Physical fitness and all-cause mortality: A prospective study of health men and women. *JAMA* 262:2395–2401, 1989.

Bourgeois MS. Enhancing conversation skills in patients with Alzheimer's disease using a prosthetic memory aid. *J Appl Behav Anal* 23:29–42, 1990.

Bourgeois MS. Effects of memory aids on the dyadic conversations of individuals with dementia. *J Appl Behav Anal* 26:77–87, 1993.

Brink TL, Yeasavage JA, Lum O, et al. Screening tests for geriatric depression. *Clin Gerontol* 1:37–43, 1982.

Bruemmer V. The impact of exercise on physical frailty in the nursing home setting. In: Innovations in Long-Term Care. Symposium presented at the State Society of Aging of New York 21st Annual Conference, Albany, NY, 1993.

Burgio LD, Burgio KL. Behavioral gerontology: Application of behavioral methods to the problems of older adults. *J Appl Behav Anal* 19:321–328, 1986.

Burgio LD, Burgio KL, Engel BT, Tice LM. Increasing distance and independence of ambulation in elderly nursing home residents. *J Appl Behav Anal* 19:357–366, 1986.

Burgio LD, McCormick KA, Scheve AS, et al. The effects of changing prompted voiding schedules in the treatment of incontinence in nursing home residents. *J Am Geriatr Soc* 42:315–320, 1994.

Burgio LD, Sinnott J. Behavioral treatments and pharmacotherapy: Acceptability ratings by elderly individuals in residential settings. *Gerontologist* 30:811–816, 1990.

Cariaga J, Burgio L, Flynn W, Martin D. A controlled study of disruptive vocalizations among geriatric residents in nursing homes. *J Am Geriatr Soc* 39:501–507, 1991.

Cohn MD, Horgas AL, Marsiske M. Behavior management training for nurse aides: Is it effective? *J Gerontol Nurs* 16:21–25, 1990.

Dallam LL. Touching you, touching me. *Am J Nurs* 87:140, 1987.

Depression Guideline Panel. *Depression in Primary Care.* Vol 1. *Diagnosis and Detection* (Clinical Practice Guideline No. 5, AHCPR Publication No. 93-0550). Rockville, MD: Department of Health and Human Services, Public Health Service, Agency for Healthcare Policy and Research, 1993a.

Depression Guideline Panel. *Depression in Primary Care.* Vol 2. *Treatment of Major Depression* (Clinical Practice Guideline No. 5, AHCPR Publication No. 93-0551). Rockville, MD: Department of Health and Human Services, Public Health Service, Agency for Health Care Policy and Research, 1993b.

Depression Guideline Panel. *Depression in Primary Care. Detection, Diagnosis and Treatment: Quick Reference Guide for Clinicians* (Clinical Practice Guideline No. 5, AHCPR Publication No. 93-0552). Rockville, MD: Department of Health and Human Services, Public Health Service, Agency for Health Care Policy and Research, 1993c.

Depression Guideline Panel. *Depression Is a Treatable Illness. A Patient's Guide* (AHCPR Publication No. 93-0553). Rockville, MD: Department of Health and Human Services, Public Health Service, Agency for Health Care Policy and Research, 1993d.

Downs AFD, Rosenthal TL, Lichstein KL. Modeling therapies reduce avoidance on bathtime by the institutionalized elderly. *Behav Ther* 19:359–368, 1988.

Doyne EJ, Ossip-Klein DJ, Bowman ED, et al. Running vs. weight lifting in the treatment of depression. *J Consult Clin Psychol* 55:748–754, 1987.

Elkin I, Shea MT, Watkins JT, et al. NIMH treatment of depression collaborative research program: General effectiveness of treatments. *Arch Gen Psychiatry* 46:971–982, 1989.

Ellis A. *Reason and Emotion in Psychotherapy.* New York: Lyle Stuart, 1962.

Fiatarone MA, Evans WJ. The etiology and reversibility of muscle dysfunction in the aged. *J Gerontol* 48(special issue):77–83, 1993.

Fiatarone MA, Marks EC, Ryan ND, et al. High-intensity strength training in nonagenarians—Effects on skeletal muscle. *JAMA* 263:3029–3034, 1990.

Gallagher D, Thompson L. Treatment of major depressive disorder in older adult outpatients with brief psychotherapies. *Psychother Theory Res Pract* 19:482–490, 1982.

Gallagher DE, Thompson LW. Effectiveness of psychotherapy for both endogenous and nonendogenous depression in older adult outpatients. *J Gerontol* 38:707–712, 1983.

Goddard P, Carstensen LL. Behavioral treatment of chronic depression in an elderly nursing home resident. *Clin Gerontol* 4:13–20, 1986.

Guy DW, Morice HO. A comparative analysis of behavior management in the nursing home. *Clin Gerontol* 4:11–17, 1985.

Haaga DAF, DeRubeis RJ, Stewart BL, Beck AT. Relationship of intelligence with cognitive therapy outcome. *Behav Res Ther* 29:277–281, 1991.

Hu T. Impact of urinary incontinence on health care costs. *J Am Geriatr Soc* 38:292–295, 1990.

Hussian RA. Behavioral geriatrics. *Progr Behav Modif* 16:159–183, 1984.

Hussian RA. Modification of behaviors in dementia via stimulus manipulation. *Clin Gerontol* 8:37–43, 1988.

Hussian RA, Brown DC. Use of two-dimensional grid patterns to limit hazardous ambulation in demented patients. *J Gerontol* 42:558–560, 1987.

Jarrett RB, Eaves GG, Grannemann BD, et al. Clinical, cognitive and demographic predictors of response to cognitive therapy for depression: A preliminary report. *Psychiatry Res* 37:245–260, 1991.

Karuza J, Zevon MA, Gleason T, et al. Models of helping and coping, responsibility attributions and well being in community elderly and their helpers. *Psychol Aging* 5:194–208, 1992.

Karuza J, Katz PR. Psychosocial interventions in long-term care: A critical overview. In: Katz PR, Kane RL, Mezey MD, eds. *Advances in Long-Term Care* Vol 1. New York: Springer, 1991.

Krasner L. Behavior therapy. *Annu Rev Psychol* 22:483–582, 1971.

Labouvie-Vief G, Gonda J. Cognitive strategies, training, and intellectual performance in the elderly. *J Gerontol* 31:327–332, 1976.

Lewin LM, Lundervold D, Saslow M, Thompson S. Reducing eating dependency in nursing home patients: The effects of prompting, reinforcement, food preference and environmental design. *J Clin Exp Gerontol* 11:47–63, 1989.

Lewinsohn PM. Clinical and theoretical aspects of depression. In: Calhoun KS, Adams HE, Mitchell K, eds. *Innovative Treatment Methods in Psychopathology.* New York: Wiley, 1974.

Lundervold DA, Jackson T. Use of applied behavior analysis in treating nursing home residents. *Hosp Commun Psychiatry* 43:171–173, 1992.

Lundervold DA, Lewin LM. *Behavior Analysis and Therapy in Nursing Homes.* Springfield, IL: Charles C Thomas, 1992.

MacDonald ML, Butler AK. Reversal of helplessness: Producing walking behavior in nursing home wheelchair residents using behavior modification procedures. *J Gerontol* 29:97–101, 1974.

Mahoney MJ. *Cognition and Behavior Modification. Cambridge, MA: Ballinger, 1974.*

McMurdo MET, Rennie L. A controlled trial of exercise by residents of old people's homes. *Age Ageing* 22:11–15, 1993.

Meichenbaum D. *Cognitive Behavioral Modification.* Morristown, NJ: General Learning Press, 1975.

Mohide EA. The prevalence and scope of urinary incontinence. *Clin Geriatr Med* 2:639–655, 1986.

Munoz RF, Hollon SD, McGrath E, et al. On the AHCPR Depression in Primary Care Guidelines—Further considerations for practitioners. *Am Psychol* 49:42–61, 1994.

National Institutes of Health Consensus Development Conference. *J Am Geriatr Soc* 38:265–272, 1990.

Newman CF, Beck AT. Cognitive therapy of affective disorders. In: Wolman B, Stricker G, eds. *Depressive Disorders*. New York: Wiley, 1990:343–367.

Oneal E. A simple way to modify behavior. *Geriatr Nurs* 7:45, 1986.

Ossip-Kelin DJ, Doyne EJ, Bowman ED, et al. Effects of running or weight lifting on self-concept in clinically depressed women. *J Consult Clin Psychol* 57:158–161, 1989.

Ouslander JG. Urinary incontinence in nursing homes. *J Am Geriatr Soc* 38:289–291, 1990.

Ouslander JG. New approaches to the diagnosis and treatment of incontinence in the nursing home. In: Katz PR, Kane RL, Mezey MD, eds. *Advances in Long-Term Care*. Vol 1. New York: Springer, 1991:61–80.

Ouslander JG, Kane RL. The costs of urinary incontinence in nursing homes. *Med Care* 22:69–77, 1984.

Pavlov IP. *Conditioned Reflexes* (Aurep GV, trans). London: Oxford, 1927.

Perkins KA, Rapp SR, Carlson CR, Wallace CE. A behavioral intervention to increase exercise among nursing home residents. *Gerontologist* 26:479–481, 1986.

Phan TT, Reifler BV. Psychiatric disorders among nursing home residents—Depression, anxiety, and paranoia. *Clin Geriatr Med* 4:601–611, 1988.

Powell RR. Psychological effects of exercise therapy upon institutionalized geriatric mental patients. *J Gerontol* 29:157–161, 1974.

Rakowski W, Mor V. The association of physical activity with mortality among older adults in the Longitudinal Study of Aging. *J Gerontol Med Sci* 47:M122–M129, 1992.

Ray WA, Taylor JA, Meador KG, et al. Reducing antipsychotic drug use in nursing homes—A controlled trial of provider education. *Arch Intern Med* 153:713–721, 1993.

Schnelle JF. Treatment of urinary incontinence in nursing home patients by prompted voiding. *J Am Geriatr Soc* 38:356–360, 1990.

Schnelle JF, Ouslander JG, Osterweil D, Blumenthal S. Total quality management: Administrative and clinical applications in nursing homes. *J Am Geriatr Soc* 41:1259–1266, 1993.

Schnelle JF, Traughber B, Morgan DB, et al. Management of geriatric incontinence in nursing homes. *J Appl Behav Anal* 16:235–241, 1983.

Skinner BF. *About Behaviorism*. New York: Knopf, 1974.

Skinner BF. Intellectual self-management in old age. *Am Psychol* 38:239–244, 1983.

Skinner BF, Vaughan M. *Enjoy Old Age: A Program of Self-Management*. New York: Norton, 1983.

Smyer M, Brannon D, Cohn M. Improving nursing home care through training and job redesign. *Gerontologist* 32:327–333, 1991.

Sotsky SM, Glass DR, Shea MR, et al. Patient predictors of response to psychotherapy and pharmacotherapy: Findings in the NIMH Treatment of Depression Collaborative Research Program. *Am J Psychiatry* 148:997–1008, 1991.

Stevenson JS, Topp R. Effects of moderate and low intensity long-term exercise by older adults. *Res Nurs Health* 13:209–218, 1990.

Thompson LW, Davies R, Gallagher D, Krantz SE. Cognitive therapy with older adults. *Clin Gerontol* 5:245–279, 1986.

Thompson LW, Gallagher D, Breckenridge JS. Comparative effectiveness of psychotherapies for depressed elders. *J Consult Clin Psychol* 55:385–390, 1987.

Vaccaro FJ. Application of operant procedures in a group of institutionalized aggressive geriatric patients. *Psychol Aging* 3:22–28, 1988.

Watson JB. *Behaviorism.* New York: Norton, 1925.

Wells T. Pelvic (floor) muscle exercise. *J Am Geriatr Soc* 38:333–337, 1990.

Whisman M. Mediators and moderators of change in cognitive therapy of depression. *Psychol Bull* 114:248–265, 1993.

Zimmer JG, Watson N, Treat A. Behavioral problems among patients in skilled nursing facilities. *Am J Public Health* 74:1118–1121, 1984.

15

Working with Families

Marion Zucker Goldstein

The need for psychiatric services in nursing homes is well established (Rovner et al., 1986; Borson et al., 1987; Chandler and Chandler, 1988; Parmelee et al., 1989; Curlik, et al. 1991). This need and its relative absence of appropriate psychiatric care in nursing homes in the United States has also been addressed legislatively in the Nursing Home Reform Act of the Omnibus Budget Reconciliation Act (OBRA) of 1987 and the 1989 Health Care Financing Administration (HCFA) regulations. These limit access to nursing homes for nondemented patients with mental health problems unless appropriate psychiatric services are available. More psychiatrists need to be trained in geriatric psychiatry to service the ever increasing mental health needs of the elderly and their families.

Psychiatric literature on assessment, education, support, participation, therapy and other family interventions for residents of nursing homes is available (Goldstein 1989; Goldstein et al., 1993) but not widely used. Though much research on depressive symptoms in family caregivers has been done (Deimling and Bass, 1986; Deimling et al., 1989; Fitting et al., 1986; George and Gwyther, 1986; Zarit et al., 1986; Gallagher et al., 1989; Pruchno and Resch, 1989; Stommel, 1990; Rosenthal et al., 1993), ongoing therapeutic interventions are still the exception rather than the rule. The opportunity to work with families of elderly residents in the nursing home ranges from admission through death. Mental health needs should be addressed with knowledge, sensitivity, and empathy, to enhance the quality of life of nursing home residents, as well as their families.

This chapter addresses the needs of families with elderly relatives residing in nursing homes. Through a series of case vignettes, various assessment and intervention strategies are discussed.

Family needs in the nursing home vary considerably and depend on the following:

1. The current mental, physical, legal, financial, and social status of the elderly person and the family
2. The current residence from which the recommendation for nursing home placement is made—e.g., own home, relative's home, retirement home, acute care hospital, other nursing home
3. The family demographics, past and present relationships
4. Acceptance and understanding of the condition of the elderly relative by various family members
5. Patient and family's resources, stresses, and responsibilities
6. Knowledge of nursing home facilities, staff training and patterns, physical plant, locations, cost
7. Duration of nursing home resident's declining condition

These issues are to be considered when an elderly patient is first admitted to a nursing home and remain important throughout the entire stay.

Entering the Nursing Home: A Difficult Adjustment

> Name me no names for my disease
> With uninforming breath.
> I tell you I am none of these,
> But homesick unto death.
> *Witter Bynner*

It is difficult for most adults, regardless of age, to give up the privacy and autonomy they have in the familiar surroundings of home and neighborhood. Caring for a home contributes to a feeling of mastery and self-esteem for most. Opportunities to engage in homemaking activities are lost with relocation to a nursing home.

It is very important for families and nursing home staff to understand the nature of attachment to the residence from which an older person is being relocated. The painful, repetitive litany of "I want to go home, I want to go home," or "take me home, take me home," so often expressed by nursing home residents, especially during the first 6 months following admission, is all too familiar to those visiting or working in nursing homes. Attention to remaining capacity to engage in previously valued activities and opportunities to keep in touch with familiar objects and remaining friends can facilitate adaptation to a new environment for young and old, fit and disabled alike.

Living arrangements before admission to nursing homes of residents, aged 65 and over with next of kin are illustrated in Figures 15.1, 15.2, and 15.3. These figures show the distribution by private or semiprivate living arrangements, by other health-related facilities, and by whether the elderly lived alone or with others, as reported from the 1985 National Nursing Home Survey (Hing, 1989).

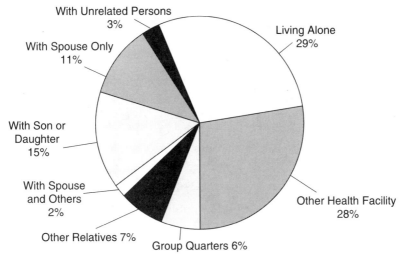

FIGURE 15.1. Living arrangement before admission to nursing home of residents age 65 and over (living alone or with others, *N* = 1,306,800). (From Hing et al., 1989.)

It is of particular interest to note that more than one-half of nursing home residents who have family came from their own homes or apartments and almost one-third from a relative's home. Far more than one-half of those who already were in a health-related facility came from other nursing homes and considerably fewer from hospitals.

Who initiates these moves from one nursing home to another? How do families deal with these moves? What stresses does this relieve or create? Are these partially a reflection of the need for different levels of care? Though statistics

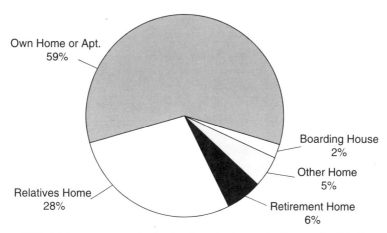

FIGURE 15.2. Living arrangement prior to admission to nursing home of residents age 65 and over with next of kin (private or semiprivate living quarters, (*N* = 948,100). (From Hing et al., 1989.)

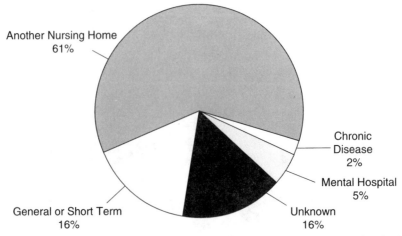

Another Nursing Home
61%

Chronic
Disease
2%

Mental Hospital
5%

General or Short Term
16%

Unknown
16%

FIGURE 15.3. Living arrangements prior to admission to nursing home (other health facilities, N = 358,700). (From Hing et al., 1989.)

do not give us the answers to such questions, they stimulate a need for further efforts to facilitate adaptation to relocations in late life. Figure 15.1 shows that about one-third of residents of nursing homes lived alone prior to admission; when the next of kin of another third were asked where their elderly relatives had resided prior to admission, they said that they did not know. Of those who lived with next of kin prior to nursing home admission, most had lived with a daughter or son than a spouse.

Table 15.1 reveals that more women than men and more Caucasians than others lived alone, more men than women lived with a spouse, as did more Caucasians than others, more women lived with a son or daughter, more African Americans and others lived with relatives other than offspring, than did Caucasians.

TABLE 15.1. Type of Living Arrangement Prior to Admission to Nursing Home by Gender and Race (N = 1,306,800)

Living arrangement	% Male	% Female	% White	% Black/Other
Alone	18.3	29.7	27.0	21.0
With spouse	17.0	7.9	10.8	6.1
Spouse and other relatives	3.6	1.1	1.7	
Son/daughter	6.9	16.2	13.7	13.0
Other relatives	9.4	8.1	7.8	15.8
Unrelated persons	2.9	3.2	2.9	6.0
Group quarters	5.0	6.1	5.9	
Another health facility or unknown	36.9	27.7	30.2	31.0
	100.0	100.0	100.0	100.0

Source: Hing et al. (1989).

Vignettes

Vignette 1: The Guilt-Ridden Family

K. L., an 81-year-old white widowed woman who had had several falls, has occasionally left the stove turned on and allowed food to rot in the refrigerator. She complains of loneliness and does not like to eat alone but refuses to socialize with a neighbor. She has lost weight. She is on several medications: one for arthritis, one for anxiety, and eyedrops for her glaucoma. Her married daughter has her over for dinner several times a week. Her single daughter brings her food, monitors her medications, and takes her to doctors when necessary. Her son oversees her finances and occasionally, when he has time, helps with home maintenance. A home health aide comes twice a week for 5 hours but does not drive. K. L. sees her grandchildren on occasion and is taken to family celebrations. Lately, she has felt more fatigued, has become more hard of hearing, and has asked to be brought home early.

K. L. complains frequently that she does not see enough of her children, since they all work and have their own busy lives to lead, making her feel that she is not very important to them and might as well be dead. She is the youngest and only survivor of seven siblings. She is quite attached to her home and her belongings but dreads the many lonely hours and has let her children convince her that it is time to give up the family home and move to a nursing home. The primary care physician agrees and has recommended a nursing home where he is on the staff.

Soon after the move, she has terrible regrets that she has agreed to go, has crying spells, insomnia, lack of appetite, and diminished interest. She feels that no one understands her. The social worker recommends that the family bring family pictures and familiar objects. The nursing staff states they have difficulty bathing her in the high-tech bathroom and that she seems to be afraid. The family members feel very guilty that they have admitted her to the nursing home and start blaming each other for the decision. This is especially evident when one of the daughters notices that her mother is wearing a dress that belongs to one of the other residents, that her dentures are missing, and that her nails are not cut.

The primary care physician has meanwhile requested a consultation from a geriatric psychiatrist upon the request of one of the daughters. After a thorough mental status assessment of K. L. with the help of an amplifier (Goldstein, 1990; Silver and Hermann, 1991), the psychiatrist met with the patient's children and with the nursing home staff. K. L. was treated with antidepressants and milieu therapy. In conjunction with the intake social worker, the family history was reviewed with highlighting of developmental milestones in the patient's life as well in the lives of the adult children. The three adult children with available spouses and older grandchildren were seen by themselves as well as with their mother. Over time, the hopeless and helpless feelings to which this family interaction had contributed was alleviated and a sense of empowerment instilled in K. L. and her adult children.

Methods used were those of *psychoeducation* and *task orientation with follow-up*. The patient's condition was explained in terms of the series of losses she had sustained, including those of physical health, those of autonomy by each activity involved, and those of relationships and familiar surroundings. The tasks were assigned with attention to K. L.'s interests, motivation, level of stress, and ability to experience satisfaction from a successful outcome.

It was recommended that one adult child (R. T.) obtain durable power of attorney for K. L. by consensus. K. L. needed help with advanced directives, including her will and health proxy. The adult children decided, with the help of the nursing home social worker and with K. L.'s participation, who would assume responsibility for these tasks. Another adult child (S. P.) took responsibility to take K. L. to an audiologist to obtain a hearing aid so staff could help her adjust to it on a day-to-day basis with family participation. Physical therapy was ordered to maintain range of motion and ambulation. New dentures were made with K. L.'s name imprinted on them. The dietitian came to discuss K. L.'s favorite foods with her and the family. The recreational therapist discussed K. L.'s past and present interests with her and the family.

The clothing and bathroom situations needed to be addressed. The family was encouraged to discuss this directly with the nursing staff. The availability of an Ombudsman (Netting et al., 1992) assigned to the nursing home was also brought to their attention, so that they could turn to this resource if there was no improvement in the situation. This situation was most likely not unique to their mother but possibly represented a repetitive problem, endured by others as well. Subsequently the adult children and grandchildren were given an opportunity to schedule the frequency and length of their visits with K. L. They decided whether they would visit as individuals or as a group, so it would optimize the patient's pleasure and satisfaction. In this way, the visits could be predicted by K. L. and were less likely to be perceived as "never enough." A calendar was obtained to mark down important family events and the next scheduled visit. A follow-up visit was arranged by the consulting psychiatrist with the family after 6 weeks, followed by another in 2 months. Subsequently, the family was referred to an open monthly family group that the social worker had started under the supervision of the psychiatrist.

A geriatric psychiatry fellow from a neighboring medical school sat in on the family group once a month to help identify and discuss behavioral and other mental health concerns the families were experiencing with their relatives in the nursing home; family members who lived locally as well as those living out of town were included in this group.

Points of Relevance: Vignette 1

The doctor-patient relationship has been held supreme since time immemorial. Laudatory as it may be, this attitude needs modification as soon as frailty and any level of dependence is detected in the elderly patient, while joint decision making with patient and family can take place. Optimally, work with family must start prior to the patient's admission to the nursing home, so all options can be explored and all concerned can be comfortable with the decisions made.

The majority of elderly want to stay in their own homes and are often willing to take greater risks than the family will allow or is able to tolerate. The home health care industry (Mor, 1987) is rapidly expanding but generally lags behind in attention to mental health care, as do many nursing homes. Early detection of depression with appropriate intervention, as in this example, could conceivably have prevented what may well have been premature institutionalization.

Vignette 2: The Overstressed Family

M. N. is a 78-year-old white woman with a progressive dementia who lived with her married daughter, recently unemployed son-in-law, and their four children.

The family depended on M. N.'s savings to pay their expenses. She used to help with the children while their parents went to work until she became progressively more forgetful, untidy, unable to cook and find her way, and required supervision herself. The primary care physician said it was "senility and they should put her away."

They had not been asked about financial circumstances and were embarrassed to reveal their current problems. The daughter had given up a responsible position to look after her children and her mother, while her husband was still employed. They now decided to use the remaining family savings to get the mother into a nursing home near their house where they could assure her of frequent visits. The daughter went back to work to support the family and advance her career, which required her to be out of town a great deal of the time.

The nursing home made space available to one of the family support groups of the local Alzheimer Association, which met every other week (Fenchak, 1989). The patients's family was asked to participate and was eager to learn about the stages of a progressive dementia of the Alzheimer type or related disorders and to get answers to their concerns about the hereditary nature of the disease and the availability of memory-enhancing drugs. The grandchildren learned how to communicate with their grandmother and remained affectionate without feeling rejected when she failed to remember their names or recognize their faces. The son-in-law had an opportunity to talk about his shame over having lost his temper with his frail mother-in-law and having verbally abused her in sheer frustration over his own situation while having to listen to her repeat herself over and over while she was living with them.

On admission, the intake social worker had taken an extensive history of the patient from the daughter and filed it in the admissions office. Many of the nurses and aides on the unit knew little about the person that the patient had once been.

Points of Relevance: Vignette 2

The family and the nursing home staff have a great deal to offer each other on an ongoing basis. In this instance, attention was paid to family stresses and little was asked of them in terms of involvement in the care of the patient. However, the family was offered a great deal of education and support by the Alzheimer Association's family support group in the nursing home setting. The son-in-law was able to reveal his shame over verbally abusing a frail elderly woman. The family were able to rebuild their own relationships while remaining advocates for quality of care and quality of life for the nursing home resident. The grandchildren maintained contact with the person who had helped raise them. The problem posed by the fact that those caring for the demented resident did not know the person she had once been was not addressed or resolved.

Vignette 3: The Family at Odds with One Another

O. P. was an 85-year-old white widowed mother of two married sons who had fallen in her own home, fractured her hip, and required an emergency hip replacement. Following her husband's death 3 years earlier, her mental status had declined rapidly. She frequently hallucinated her deceased husband's presence and would talk to him as though he were still living. She would call other family members who visited by his name. One of her daughters-in-law did all her shopping for her and, during recent months had had to prepare O. P.'s meals in order for her to eat. O. P. would go once a week to the hairdresser down the street and religiously attend church on Sundays, but her attendance at social functions had become more and more sporadic. Her conversation had become limited and repetitive and she expressed concerns that money was being stolen from her.

Immediately following her hip replacement, O. P.'s speech was described as incoherent and rambling, she was very restless, misinterpreted what went on around her, and saw people who were not there.

The family and primary care physician, who came to see the patient postoperatively, decided that the patient required long-term institutionalization. The patient was put on haloperidol 2 mg once a day and discharged with this medication.

The son, who had power of attorney, sold the patient's antiques and put her house on the market while she was recovering from surgery in the hospital. The hospital social worker recommended a nursing home where physical therapy would be available for the patient and where the patient could be accepted after the necessary paperwork was complete. For the time being, only a double room was available at the nursing home, but since O. P. had no reported post-operative complications, her hospital days were used up. The patient was under the impression that she would return home following her hospitalization and was quite distraught to find herself with a roommate in a nursing home. She had fearful recollections of the immediate postoperative period and was relieved to "have her mind back." She refused to take haloperidol while in the nursing home because it made her feel stiff, and she was written up as "non-compliant" by the nursing staff. She was angry at her son and daughter-in-law and felt that they had robbed her.

Her two sons were 15 years apart in age and had little in common. One of the sons was rather intellectual and the other an outdoor type with little formal education. He was eager for the mother's house and resources for his own four children, one of whom was learning-disabled and would never be self-sufficient.

While this scenario evolved, the nursing home was in a quandary as to who would pay the bill. Their notary had apparently witnessed a paper that withdrew power of attorney from one son and gave it to the other, thus alienating the family who had cared for O. P. for many years while she was living in her own home. Neither the issue of O. P.'s competency nor that of her level of cognitive functioning had been formally addressed.

She was delighted with the renewed interest of her oldest son, who brought his wife and children to visit her. Her grandchildren were a delight to her, and the slightest token of affection from them made her day. She had soon forgotten her other daughter-in-law's years of dedicated care.

It was only after the youngest son hired a lawyer that a geriatric psychiatrist was asked to assess the patient's mental status to assist the court in deciding whether O. P. was competent to make decisions on her own behalf and, if not, who would be a suitable guardian.

Points of Relevance: Vignette 3

What went wrong here and why? It appears that the knowledge base of aging, dementia, delirium and depression, of normal aging and the psychopathology of late life, of the professionals this family encountered was as limited as that of the family themselves. The primary care physician who had been the family doctor for 30 years did not address the patient's mental health issues or family concerns. The orthopedic surgeon, the hospital discharge social worker, and the admitting social worker of the nursing home all "did their job." Each in his or her own way had overlooked essentials. The patient's youngest son was left feeling that he had not taken good care of his mother. O. P. was left with much resentment for not being included in the decision-making processes on her own behalf. Harm was done by oversight and much is to be learned from hindsight. This is a case in which the family was not worked with and needed to be, at many steps on the way to nursing home placement from an acute care hospital and during the relative's nursing home residence. It should also be noted that the patient no longer needed haloperidol after the postoperative delirium subsided, and that it should have been discontinued.

This particular scenario exemplifies the legitimate fear and aversion that the elderly and their families have about getting involved in the "formal care-giving system."

Vignette 4: Spousal Devotion, Decline, and Discord

S. T., age 90, was admitted to a geriatric psychiatry unit from the emergency room of a general hospital because she had hit her now wheelchair-bound husband, to whom she had been married for 67 years.

The couple lived in their own home and were able to manage with the help of home health care aides around the clock. S. T.'s husband had had a stroke several years earlier and she insisted that the help was necessary only for him— that she was just fine. As a matter of fact, she perceived the aides as being in her way, running her household, and wanting to get rid of her. The couple were quite devoted to each other and she made light of her physically uncontrolled behavior toward him as a playful gesture. Other than a severe scoliosis and a moderately severe dementia, S. T. was in good health. She had a good appetite and slept well. She was socially pleasant and gracious but extremely forgetful. The couple would speak to each other on the telephone and she would alternate between being affectionate, verbally abusive, and tearful. After a visit from her husband, she remained tearful and heartbroken as she described her feelings and requested discharge to go home, wanting to be with him. There were no other relatives. During the course of a complete dementia workup, magnetic resonance imaging (MRI), extensive neuropsychological testing, kitchen skills assessment, and survival skills testing, arrangements were made, at the husband's request, to find three nursing homes from which he could choose and where the couple could reside together. Every time the topic of a move to a nursing home was raised with her by her husband, she insisted that he had never discussed it with her but had told her he would when the time had come. She recalled neither the ambulance ride for her MRI, her resistance to having it done, nor the conversation with her husband about going together to a nursing home. Moving her to a nursing home would require guardianship because it would have to occur over her objections. However, she would be willing to go if it meant joining her husband. Though bewildered at the prospect, it appeared that she could be transferred willingly. The legal help invoked by the husband consisted of a retired judge and a semiretired lawyer, both family friends but not familiar with the procedures required by current state guardianship laws. Because of transportation problems in getting the couple together to work these problems through and prevent undue and prolonged depression, the task of assisting the adaptation to nursing home life for this couple (while also preventing abusive behaviors) had to be left up to the nursing home staff. The husband was advised to choose the one of three nursing homes he was considering that had a medical director who was a geriatrician and a geriatric psychiatrist as a consultant on a weekly basis. Because of the husband's handicap and S. T.'s tendency to abuse him physically, it was recommended that they room near but not with each other. The discharge summary was sent to the administrator, intake social worker, medical director, and geriatric psychiatrist. The husband was given time to arrange his affairs, so he could be at the nursing home upon the patient's arrival and the patient would not have to be taken over her objections, having to wait for guardianship in an acute care geriatric psychiatry unit.

Over the years, the couple has been a challenge to the nursing home staff. The husband was liked for his rational, gentle, and accepting manner, the wife for her ability to sustain social graces for short periods of time. As long as possible, they were given regular brief private time together, as they wished. A bell was placed in proximity to the husband in case his wife's behavior became abusive. Adjusting to the loss of a familiar environment and activities and adapting to the nursing home environment, staff, and other residents required new learning. This took almost a year and was accomplished by establishing structured and predictable daily routines with minimal changes of staff and explicit communications between staff and between shifts.

Points of Relevance: Vignette 4

The wishes of a couple who have been married for 67 years had to be respected within the context of prudence and safety. Though help from elderly trusted friends and professionals is understandably sought and must be accepted as much as is feasible and practical, assistance from younger professionals to their seniors should be readily available.

It must also be recognized that the younger generation must allow sufficient time for the elderly to express their feelings, resentments, and wishes while allowing as much preservation of autonomy as is realistic, safe, practical, and legal.

In situations like this, where one spouse goes to a nursing home and the other remains in the community, yet the couple remain intensely attached to one another regardless of failing mental status, the nursing home staff must facilitate the couple's socialization if that is what they choose to do "till death do us part." Value systems of the younger generation, with emphasis of "making a new life" may not be acceptable during the lifetime of the partner, no matter how incapacitated.

The consistency of a simplified life-style and minimization of unexpected events stabilized this couple's relationship in their decline.

Vignette 5: The Aggressive Patient for Whom the Nursing Staff Has Decided They Are Unable to Care

A. B. was moved from a health-related facility to a skilled nursing facility because of the onset of fecal and urinary incontinence. He was taken out of a familiar environment with familiar staff and other residents to an unfamiliar environment with staff who were unfamiliar with him. He was 78 years of age, had been a widower for 5 years, had four married children and eight grandchildren. He had once been a teacher and musician. Until recently, he would sing children's songs on occasion, enjoyed musicals, and would respond to staff who sang to him. Singing to him while assisting him with toileting, bathing, dressing, and grooming would alleviate some of the humiliation he still experienced when he was assisted with these activities. Fiercely independent and proud in his younger years, he disliked being touched by strangers but had gotten used to one of the aides in the health-related facility. He trusted this aide and would usually cooperate.

The staff in the skilled nursing facility had just had several discharges, both "living and dead"; most worked 12-hour shifts and looked forward to their breaks more than to their work. After a month on the floor of the nursing home, A. B. got the reputation of being "hard to handle." He would hit staff when they were providing physical care and grunt at them.

The staff complained to the nursing supervisor, who brought the matter to the attention of the administration. A. B.'s daughter, who visited frequently, was asked to come to an "administrative" meeting. Here, she was told that the family would have to look for another nursing home, since the father was injuring staff members. Fortuitously, she had started psychotherapy several years ago for depression and had gained a great deal of insight into her relationship with her father. She described him as historically having an authoritarian manner. She now had the fortitude and wit to turn this administrative meeting around and had those present listening spellbound to stories describing her father the way he once was. She gained their interest in helping staff to find effective ways to deal with A. B. They decided to assign one or two staff to him who were able to get along with him and seemed to like him.

Points of Relevance: Vignette 5

The outcome of a scenario like this is not always a happy one and causes inordinate stress to most families. Few families are prepared to deal with threats from a nursing home to discharge their relative because of "misbehavior," for which the relative is inappropriately held responsible. Most often in these situations, nursing home staff can learn from the family, who have known the patient considerably longer and in a great variety of situations. The nursing home must turn the situation into one of collaboration with the family, where learning must take place among all who have the capacity.

Vignette 6: The Distant, Resistive Family

R. S. is an 82-year-old white widowed woman whose progressive Parkinson's disease has led to neurological features of subcortical dementia. R. S.'s gait had become progressively more unsteady, her posture had become stooped. She had hypophonia, lost her usual drive and initiative, and suffered from psychomotor retardation. She had lived in a nursing home for the preceding 2 years. She spoke highly of the general environment and the food but complained bitterly about the infrequency and brevity of her adult children's visits. She complained repetitively of her weak voice, stating that other residents could not hear her or just didn't answer. Meals were no longer a social time, and she avoided other communal activities. She sat and stared a considerable part of the day or took short walks with her walker. She grieved over her home, her antiques, her ability to get in her car and go places. She enjoyed one old-time friend, who was a resident in the same nursing home and who, occasionally, came over spontaneously to give her a hug and tell her she loved her. Her children dutifully took her from physician to physician for various complaints. She was found to have 40 to 60% occlusion of her carotid arteries. She was on meclizine for dizziness and digoxin and furosemide for cardiac problems. She was on sertraline (zoloft) for possible depression. She complained about her slow gait, which made it difficult for her to get to the bathroom on time, especially at night. Above all, she complained about her children not letting her "just be 82 years old" but constantly being "on her case." They reprimanded her for not speaking up more forcibly, for not being more sociable, and, overall, for not trying hard enough. She was smart and witty enough to understand that they were giving her the "stand up straight" routine that she may have given them when they were teenagers. Staff at the nursing home did not perceive R. S.'s disabilities as personal failures and helped her function within the realm of her limitations. Nursing home staff supplied R. S. with a commode near her bed at night and a walker with wheels. Also, quiet one-on-one time with a volunteer was arranged for her on a daily basis. The children reported staff members for infantilizing their mother and not making her try hard enough. These family members were unable to accept the irreversible limitations of their mother's decline. They wanted their mother the way they had known her in the past, lively and engaging, giving and caring for them and others. Their concern and request was always for yet another pill to bring that situation about. Their own personal development had not reached that stage during which parent care can be carried out in a reality-oriented manner, with acceptance and responsiveness to parental dependency needs. Their mother needed their respect and tenderness, neither of which they were able to supply. They were unable to accept nursing staff expertise or physicians' explanations of R. S.'s conditions.

Points of Relevance: Vignette 6

This family created an adversarial situation with nursing home staff because of their own emotional needs. They did not have the fortitude to deal with their mother's decline. They feared their own grief and denied the reality of her condition, thus making themselves emotionally unavailable to her and the nursing home staff while getting on with their own busy and rewarding lives. Each adult child would have to be willing to have one-on-one or brief group psychotherapy to overcome this resistance. Psychoeducation does not suffice here. They would have to admit possible misperceptions and be motivated to grieve over the loss of the person their mother once was.

Hospice, Death, and Bereavement

Attending to terminally ill patients and their families and dealing with death and bereavement is a frequent occurrence in nursing homes. Most families of patients with a progressive dementia have already undergone partial bereavement during the various phases of decline. It is not unknown for families to receive correspondence from the nursing home, following the relative's death, that the resident has been "discharged." Frequently the relative's room has been emptied before family gets a chance to do so, and belongings placed in plastic bags, in order to make room for the next resident.

It has been recognized for some time now that the increased role of nursing homes as permanent places of residence, with death as the inevitable outcome for the majority of patients admitted, require effective educational programs and supports for residents as well as for families, staff, and administrators if they are to provide sensitive and appropriate care at the time of terminal illness and death (Brody et al., 1984). In reality, in many nursing homes, neither residents nor family members are routinely given choices between aggressive treatment approaches to maintain life regardless of quality and a hospice approach with emphasis on comfort and quality of life during its terminal phase. Both treatment modalities have Medicare coverage with certain restrictions and Joint Commission on Accreditation of Healthcare (JCAH) criteria (Mor, 1987). A routine question asked of family members on admission of a relative to a nursing home is what funeral arrangements will be made in the event of death. This question is asked right along with the question about DNR (do not resuscitate) wishes in case of cardiac arrest, availability of health proxy documentation, and who will be responsible for the nursing home bill.

Each nursing home must institute special training programs to support staff in their own bereavement when patients they have cared for pass away. Only if staff are sufficiently supported can they be sensitive and supportive of the needs of dying patients and their families and to respond attentively to each situation they may encounter.

Summary

In this chapter several situations have been discussed to highlight both the flawed and successful ways in which nursing homes deal with or support the families of their residents. Since all nursing home residents must have a primary care physician, it is this physician who can seek the necessary consultation for the nursing home and help guide staff in assuring a humane and sensitive environment in the nursing home for both residents and their families. When available, it is the multidisciplinary professional team that ensures that everyone is treated sensitively and who maintains emotional support and education for the residents and their families.

The requisite administrative initiative and infrastructure, to enable nursing home staff to collaborate with and support families of residents on an ongoing basis, is essential.

Acknowledgment

I wish to thank Marsha Clark for her skillful application of Harvard Graphics and for manuscript preparation.

References

Borson S, Liptzin B, Nininger J, et al. Psychiatry and the nursing home. *Am J Psychiatry* 144:1412–1418, 1987.

Borson S, Liptzin B, Nininger J, et al. *Report of the Task force on Nursing Homes and the Mentally Ill Elderly.* Washington DC: American Psychiatric Association, 1989.

Brody EM, Lawton MP, Lebowitz B. Senile dementia—Public policy and adequate institutional care. *Am J Public Health* 74:1381–1383, 1984.

Chandler JD, Chandler JE. The prevalence of neuropsychiatric disorders in the nursing home population. *J Geriatr Psychiatry Neurol* 1:71–76, 1988.

Curlik SM, Frazier D, Katz IR. Psychiatric aspects in long-term care. In: Sadavoy J, Lazarus LW, Jarvik LF, eds. *Comprehensive Review of Geriatric Psychiatry.* Washington DC: American Psychiatric Press, 1991:547–564.

Deimling G, Bass D. Symptoms of mental impairment among elderly adults and their effects on family caregivers. *J Gerontol* 41:778–784, 1986.

Deimling G, Bass D, Townsend A, Noelker L. Care-related stress: A comparison of spouse and adult-child caregivers in shared and separate households. *J Aging Health* 1:67–82, 1989.

Fenchak B. M. Mutual support groups for families of Alzheimer's disease patients. In: Goldstein MZ ed. *Family Involvement in the Treatment of the Frail Elderly.* Washington DC: American Psychiatric Press, 1989:109–156.

Fitting M, Rabins P, Lucas MJ, Eastham J. Caregivers for dementia patients: A comparison of husbands and wives. *Gerontologist* 26:253–259, 1986.

Gallagher D, Rose J, Rivera P, et al. Prevalence of depression in family caregivers. *Gerontologist* 29:449–456, 1989.

George L, Gwyther L. Caregiver well-being: A multidimensional examination of family caregivers of demented adults. *Gerontologist* 26:253–259, 1989.

Goldstein MZ, Colenda CC, Kennedy GJ, et al. *Select Models of Practice in Geriatric Psychiatry: A Report of the American Psychiatric Association Task Force on Models of Practice in Geriatric Psychiatry.* Washington, DC: American Psychiatric Press, 1993.

Goldstein MZ. Evaluation of the elderly patient. In: Bienenfeld D, ed. *Verwoerdt's Clinical Geropsychiatry,* 3rd ed. Baltimore: Williams & Wilkins, 1990:47–58.

Goldstein MZ, ed. *Family Involvement in the Treatment of the Frail Elderly.* Washington DC: American Psychiatric Press, 1989.

Hing E, Sekshenski E, Strahan J. National Center for Health Statistics. *The National Nursing Home Survey: 1985 Summary for the United States. Vital and Health Statistics.* Series 13, No.97 DHHS Pub. No. (PHS)89-1758. Public Health Service. Washington, DC: U.S. Government Printing Office, 1989.

Mor V. Hospice: The older person as patient and caregiver. *Generations* Spring: 19–21, 1987.

Netting FE, Paton RN, Huber R. The long-term care ombudsman programs: What does the complaint reporting system tell us? *Gerontologist* 32:843–848, 1992.

Parmelee PA, Katz IR, Lawton MP. Depression among institutionalized aged: Assessment and prevalence estimation. *J Gerontol* 44:M22–M29, 1989.

Pruchno R, Resch N. Husbands and wives as caregivers: Antecedents of depression and burden. *Gerontologist* 29:159–165, 1989.

Rosenthal CJ, Sulman J, Marshall VW. Depressive symptoms in family caregivers of long-stay patients. *Gerontologist* 33:249–247, 1993.

Rovner BW, Kafonek S, Filipp L, et al. Prevalence of mental illness in a community nursing home. *Am J Psychiatry* 143:1446–1449, 1986.

Silver IL, Hermann N. History and mental status examination. In: Sadavoy J, Lazarus LW, Jarvik LF, eds. *Comprehensive Review of Geriatric Psychiatry.* Washington, DC: American Psychiatric Press, 1991:149–169.

Stommel M, Given C, Given B. Depression as an overriding variable explaining caregiver burdens. *J Aging Health* 2:81–102, 1990.

Zarit S, Todd P, Zarit J. Subjective burden of husbands and wives as caregivers: A longitudinal study. *Gerontologist* 26:260–266, 1986.

16

Psychiatric Consultation and Liaison

Hilary T. Hanchuk

In the nursing home geriatric psychiatry is often practiced as a consultative service. The need for such a consultative service is supported by surveys that have demonstrated the prevalence of psychiatry disorders within this setting to be nearly 80% (Rovner et al., 1992). Despite the apparent need, expert and readily available psychiatric consultation and liaison are not available in most nursing homes. This chapter illustrates the roles of the psychiatrist within the nursing home setting. Particular attention is devoted to consultative and liaison functions as they relate to the identification and treatment of mental disorders of nursing home residents.

Consultation-Liaison Psychiatry

Consultation-liaison psychiatry is defined in *The American Psychiatric Association's Psychiatric Glossary* (1984) as an area of special interest that addresses the interpersonal, psychological, and psychosocial aspects of all medical care, particularly in a general hospital setting. The liaison psychiatrist works closely with other physicians and nonphysician staff to enhance the diagnosis, treatment, and management of the patient with illness considered primarily nonpsychiatric. Consultation may be to any part of the health care system that affects the patient and the family. It typically consists of short-term intervention by a "liaison team" with a biopsychosocial approach to illness.

Lipowski (1986) summarized consultation-liaison psychiatry as encompassing four major models: (1) a patient-oriented consultation in which the referred patient is the focus of the consultant's inquiry, (2) a crisis-oriented therapeutic consultation—one involving a rapid assessment of the patient's problem and coping style as well as active therapeutic intervention, (3) consultation focused on the consultee's problem, and (4) a situation-oriented consultation. Unfortunately, one specialized setting not discussed in Lipowski's comprehensive review was consultation-liaison psychiatry within the nursing home setting.

Within a nursing home, a consulting psychiatrist will function as a consulting mental disorder diagnostician, as a consulting psychopharmacologist, and as a psychotherapist. The role of the geriatric psychiatrist is also to be an integral and active participant of an evaluating and treating team of health care providers. His role is to assess cognition and mental status, to diagnose the various dementias, to rule out delirium, and to diagnose various other psychiatric conditions—disorders such as mood disorders, anxiety disorders, psychotic disorders, and personality disorders. Once a diagnosis or workable differential diagnosis is achieved, treatment is decided upon. This treatment will often include education of the staff and family, therapy recommendations for the patient and caregivers, behavioral modifications to be carried out, and pharmacological interventions.

Although often essential, the liaison functions of the consulting psychiatrist are frequently forgotten. Liaison is defined as teaching nonpsychiatric caregivers what they need to know about psychiatric management of the patient. However, Hackett and Cassem (1987) have argued that the term ''liaison'' is confusing and unnecessary, as no other medical consultative service employs this term for its activities. The essence of liaison—that is, teaching nonpsychiatrists psychiatric and interpersonal skills—should be done as a matter of course during routine consultation (Hackett and Cassem, 1987). In this chapter the concept of liaison in the nursing home emphasizes the psychiatrist's relationship to and support of long-term-care nonpsychiatric staff. Liaison to the nursing home facility's staff includes educating nurses, nursing aides, social workers, and others with regard to psychiatric disorders. Staff are also supported in their roles as primary care providers burdened by the stress of the milieu and their difficult patients. Liaison activities also involve attempts to resolve, with education and support, the frequent conflicts that arise between families and nursing home staff.

Consulting psychiatrists must carefully integrate multiple roles and relationships. Patients, relatives, nurses, social workers, internists, and administrators may have very different agendas for care and different notions about psychiatry as a discipline. As a result, much of the consultant's work requires sustained interaction with pertinent individuals. Unfortunately, geriatric psychiatric consultation is poorly reimbursed by third-party payers in comparison with the psychiatric interventions targeted to younger patients. As a result, economic pressures for the service to be provided in an efficient fashion are often, unfortunately, at the expense of thorough understanding and complete patient care.

The Need for Consultative Psychiatry

Psychiatric disorders are so common within nursing homes that analogies to psychiatric hospitals have been proposed. (See Chapter 1 on the role of the nursing home as a psychiatric hospital.) From a psychiatrist's perspective, nursing homes share many characteristics with a geriatric psychiatry inpatient facility. Due to factors such as the closing of state psychiatric facilities and society's difficulties in managing community-residing mentally ill, elderly patients with psychiatric disorders are often placed in nursing homes. Studies examining who receives placement conclude that after matching for cognitive abilities, patients with higher scores on standardized psychiatric rating scales are more likely to receive placement in an institution (Steele et al., 1990; Pruchno et al., 1980; Knopman et al., 1988; Morriss et al., 1990). However, the contemporary long-term-care facility and acute geriatric psychiatric inpatient unit differ in several key dimensions. Acute care is usually only 1 to 6 weeks in duration. Additionally, inpatient units have more generous staffing patterns than nursing homes, with better ratios of health care providers to patients. The model of medical management by physicians in the inpatient setting includes near immediate availability and daily visits. In the nursing home, in contrast, it is most often occasional consultative care, perhaps with rounds occurring once per month. Given this structure, the psychiatrist rarely provides direct patient care in most long-term care facilities but instead offers diagnostic impressions and treatment recommendations to be carried out by others.

Consulting the Psychiatrist

A consultation is requested due to a perceived problem. Unfortunately, when a consultation request is initially generated, the problem is rarely clearly delineated. Often, consultation is not requested until the symptoms are quite severe. Psychiatric diagnosis within nursing homes is often associated with the use of restraints and neuroleptics to assist in managing severe behavioral disorders. The patients are often labeled problematic and uncooperative. Rovner and colleagues (1992) reported that residents referred to as uncooperative frequently had many psychiatric disorders, particularly dementia syndromes complicated by delusions, depression, or delirium. Few patients were truly uncooperative, indicating that such a diagnostic category—of being "uncooperative" alone—does not sufficiently describe the behavior to be treated.

Though psychiatric disorders in the long-term-care setting are common, very few individuals receive initial psychiatric evaluations for screening or treatment purposes. The most common reasons stated are a set of very difficult behaviors identified by nursing staff. Each difficult behavior deserves a differential diagnosis. Some of these behaviors involve comorbid behavioral sequelae to the patient's defensive mechanisms that accompany lifelong personality traits—axis II in the *Diagnostic and Statistical Manual of Mental Disorders*, 4th ed. (APA, 1994), behaviors common to the respective dementia and its stage, or non-dementia–related axis I diagnoses.

From a nursing perspective, Hogstel (1990) described the reason for consultation as often being due to bizarre or troublesome behavior and overt signs of psychiatric disorders. She subdivided these troublesome behaviors into (1) withdrawal and depressive, (2) aggressive and combative, (3) paranoid and delusional, (4) confusion, and (5) altered sleep. Loebel and colleagues (1991) described their experience examining 197 patients at six nursing homes and found the following reasons generating a consultation: (1) behavioral problems, (2) mood-related problems, (3) request by involuntary treatment services, (4) psychotic features, (5) physical signs, and (6) impaired activities of daily living. In addition, they concluded that requests for referral were weak predictors of diagnosis.

In one of several published nursing home psychiatric consultation experiences, Goldman and Klugman (1990) reviewed their first 60 psychiatric consultations provided to a university-affiliated teaching nursing home. As is often the case in such reports, all patients seen had a clear, diagnosable mental disorder. The frequency of depression was significant, with over 40% of cases suffering from major affective illness. Consultation to the nursing home resulted in a critical change in diagnosis and management in more than one-third of the patients seen.

As a result, the primary task for the psychiatrist is to define the problem. The next is to examine the patient, review records, and interview informants. Once this is accomplished, the consultant attempts to explain the behavior and educate staff while defusing potential conflicts. Finally, therapeutic recommendations are advised.

Who Consults the Psychiatrist?

The nursing home consultation request to a geriatric psychiatrist may arrive from one of several routes. In may originate from the patient's family, the primary physician, the nursing staff, the social worker, or even the administration. Several points regarding the origin of consultation deserve emphasis. The consult is usually generated by an individual who has knowledge of the geriatric psychiatrist's work or of the field. Other health care providers are often surprised that such evaluation and treatment are indeed possible. This, of course, argues for the importance for those who provide any type of care to this patient population of having knowledge of the various psychiatric manifestations likely to emerge in the nursing home and the diagnostic and treatment approaches that are potentially useful.

Timing and Availability of Consultation

The number, frequency, and extent of psychiatric problems within a nursing home are commonly a function of the size and culture of the institution. Some facilities will perceive that they do not need psychiatric consultation, while other facilities appear to require several full-time psychiatrists. Nearly all nursing homes will have occasional psychiatric emergencies that necessitate expedient attention. As automatic and immediate availability to a facility would be optimal, such availability from a psychiatrist in private practice is frequently impossible. Scheduled rounds, conducted by the consultant for a half day every 2 weeks are often attainable. The frequency with which the consultant visits the facility and the length of time spent there depend on the acuity of the patients, the number of patients, and the personal practice style of the psychiatrist. Nonetheless, scheduling a predictable frequency of consultation at the nursing home alleviates many of the nursing staff's concerns. This also clarifies the psychiatrist's commitment to the nursing home while resolving office scheduling difficulties.

Consultation Regarding the Cognitively Impaired Resident

The psychiatric care provided in the long-term-care setting is often the diagnosis and treatment of individuals with cognitive impairment. Before suggesting a course of treatment for a disturbing behavior, one must attempt to understand the patient better. Such an understanding is a multidimensional undertaking. This model has been referred to as the biopsychosocial model. Many recent advances in psychiatry have concentrated on the biological aspects of behavioral disorders, but the psychosocial aspects of behavior continue to be an essential part of the evaluation. A psychosocial evaluation will attempt to derive an understanding of the patient's premorbid personality characteristics. Often, behavior that is not understandable in the face of dementia can be better understood if one knew the patient prior to the onset of cognitive impairment. An inquiry into familial temperamental traits is often left out of an evaluation but yet may offer important information. As a patient with dementia often seems to dwell in the past, an understanding of the patient's childhood, young adulthood, and prior psychological traumas is helpful. As the long-term-care setting is a setting of communal living, information about the character of the patient's interpersonal relationships and the way in which emotional crises are handled can be of great help. Simple features, such as the examination of a patient's likes, hobbies, hates, and things guaranteed to upset him or her should be noted. The consultant's evaluation of the resident's mental status at a single point in time may be limited in the amount of perspective it offers. Thus, to approach an understanding of a patient's cognitive "baseline," his or her educational and employment history should be reviewed. Another crucial aspect of a patient's history is, of course, the psychiatric history of evaluation and treatment. When Pietrukowicz and Johnson (1991) studied the effect on nursing home staff of having a resident's life history to refer to, they found that those that reviewed such a history rated the resident as more instrumental, autonomous, and personally acceptable.

Treatment Rules of Thumb

Sakauye and Camp (1992), in their experience of conducting a consultation-liaison psychiatry program in a teaching-nursing home, emphasized the following guiding principles in such a clinical practice. The first is the importance of making the patient human to the staff. Second, always assume that no behavior is random. Constantly look for depression or psychosis as a source of problems, as these entities are invariably responsive to intervention. Due to the neurophysiological sensitivities of the aged, reduce the number of medications and their dosages whenever possible. Never underestimate the importance of creating a more home-like environment. Finally, look for and use conditions in which learning still occurs, even in dementia.

The American Association of Geriatric Psychiatry Board of Directors and others (AAGP et al., 1992) propose five positions to define appropriate treatment of geriatric patients in nursing homes. Position 1 notes that to optimize the use of psychotherapeutic medications requires additional support for clinical training and research. Position 2 notes the importance of appropriate use of psychotherapeutic medications for the treatment of patients with diagnosed psychiatric disorders. Position 3 states that the principles underlying the treatment of psychiatric disorders and behavioral problems in nursing homes are identical to those for the treatment of geriatric patients in other settings. Position 4 notes that residents with Alzheimer's disease or other dementias should be evaluated to determine whether they are experiencing affective, psychotic, and behavioral symptoms and then be treated accordingly. Position 5 states that functional psychiatric disorders are common in residents of nursing homes and require treatment that makes long-term care necessary.

Consultations and Pharmacological Treatment Recommendations

Many patients within nursing homes are given psychotropic medications. In a review of psychotropic medication use, Lantz and coworkers (1990) reported that 50% of patients had been placed on some psychotropic within a 5-year span, with approximately 25% taking such agents continuously. In a 1-month survey of 850 residents in intermediate-care facilities in Massachusetts, each patient was prescribed an average of 8.1 medications; more than 50% were taking psychotropics, 26% were on antipsychotics, 28% on sedative/hypnotics, 26% on diphenhydramine, plus a typical benzodiazepine equivalent to 7.3 mg of diazepam per patient per day. In addition, the most common antidepressant prescribed was amitriptyline (Beers et al., 1988). In another study of 55 rest homes, Avorn and colleagues (1989) found that 55% of the residents were taking at least one psychoactive drug, 39% were taking an antipsychotic, and 18% were taking two or more. The authors questioned the continued use of the medications, as 6% of these patients had moderate or severe tardive dyskinesia and 50% had no evidence of physician participation in decisions of mental health treatment. In addition, staff had a poor understanding of the purpose and side effects of the medications. As psychotropic medication use will continue to be common, given the prevalence of mental disorders within nursing homes, the consulting psychiatrist has an essential role in advising on the appropriate use and monitoring of psychotropic medications.

Consultations and Nonpharmacological Treatment Recommendations

Psychiatrists should offer long-term-care settings their expertise in psychopharmacological interventions while also championing nonpharmacological treatments for mental illness. Katz (1976) elegantly demonstrated a program of multimodal group interactive therapy that was started in an extended-care facility. They found that 44% of the participating patients were judged improved. They argued that their results warrant a redefinition of the psychotherapeutic approach to include factors other than the severity and chronicity of disease in determining the prognosis for behavioral change in geriatric institutionalized residents. Avorn and colleagues (1992) described an educational program targeted to physicians, nurses, and aides that reduced the use of psychoactive drugs in nursing homes without adversely affecting the overall behavior and level of functioning of the residents.

Therapeutic trials of well documented nonbiological interventions (change of room, selection of dining companions, visitation schedules, talking therapies, recreational therapies, and so on) should be undertaken with suggested lengths of trial and documentation of observable benefit. Often, the problem that initiated the psychiatric consultation is quite severe by the time it is recognized as warranting intervention. Therefore the choice is usually not "psychosocial" instead of "biological" treatment but rather needing to offer and initiate several plans and modes of intervention simultaneously. The need for the psychiatric consultant to develop and oversee the implementation of these integrated approaches cannot be overemphasized. As multiple interventions are initiated, several liaison relationships between the psychiatrist and the other parties in the health care team must also be initiated and fostered.

The "L" (Liaison) of "C-L" (Consultation Liaison) Psychiatry

The consultant's liaison relationship to the nursing home is essentially a series of ties to numerous staff who represent different aspects of the long-term-care system. Essential aspects of the patient's care include the consultant's establishment of relationships to the facility's nurses, aides, social workers, psychologists, recreational therapists, administration, and other physicians. To optimize the essential input of all those whose activities contribute to the well-being of the resident, it is desirable to build a team, with each individual representing a specific aspect of the resident's care.

To work as a team necessitates a level of skill and knowledge of psychiatric aspects of the patients by all the team members, with clear communication between nursing home staff, the resident's family, and all treating physicians. Such an approach works best when the psychiatrist meets the patients at a known time (constant intervals) and place (an interview room), with representatives of the various members of the caregiving team present or easily available. Identification of troublesome behaviors requires observations by the social worker, head nurse, nurses from the various shifts, and resident's family. Members of the team should compare answers to the following questions: When does the behavior occur? What are the triggers? How long does the behavior last and what makes it better? To receive all this information and decide on a course of action can be done only with an organized team approach.

The Consultant's Liaison Relationship to Other Physicians

That psychiatric consultation is available within the home should be common knowledge to all the physicians on staff. A recent trend in psychopharmacology is the proliferation of medications with such low side-effects profiles that their use by primary care physicians has increased dramatically. In facilities where consultation psychiatry is an available resource, all individuals treated with psychotropic medications should be initially examined by a psychiatrist to evaluate and document the treatment rationale underlying such an intervention. This initial baseline assessment may prove to be very useful in the case of treatment failure or when it is necessary to consider the rationale for future continuation or discontinuation of treatment. It is exclusively the consultant psychiatrist who can provide a comprehensive assessment of present behavioral symptoms and thorough documentation of the resident's prior psychiatric history, familial psychiatric risk factors, and psychosocial history. The psychiatrist can then develop and oversee the implementation of a treatment plan that addresses the resident's biological, psychological, and social mental health needs.

The relationship between the consultant and other physicians calls for special care. The psychiatrist's office support staff may occasionally have to interrupt patient sessions for physician calls in order to expedite requested consultations. Such an accommodation fosters a closer working alliance between physicians. Frequent contact between medical providers consolidates and expedites treatment. Many believe that all residents should have their medical orders funneled through one physician, who then is in the position to manage the overall picture. In this context, the psychiatrist must pass his or her recommendations through the primary care physician, who then writes the appropriate orders. When only one physician writes orders (except for emergencies), confusion for the nursing staff is minimized. At times, residents may be seen more frequently by the psychiatrist than by the primary care physician because their problems are mostly in the behavioral realm. This being true, the primary care physician may become upset at serving as a mere clerk to the psychiatrist. It may also contribute to anxiety among primary practitioners as treatments are being signed for that the primary physician does not fully understand. In such circumstances, the matter of which physician is the consultant and which is the primary order-writing physician of record must be clarified among the facility's staff. On the other hand, the primary care physician sometimes disregards the consulting psychiatrist's recommendations without feedback or documentation. The consulting psychiatrist, who feels that his or her consultations are ignored in the facility, may ultimately cease consulting to the home. These issues no doubt produce interpersonal conflicts between the physicians. In such difficult situations, physician roles must be reorganized, with clear boundaries as to responsibilities and privileges. Invariably the solutions to such problems lie in the ability of all parties to communicate in the spirit of patient care as collaborating members of the health care team.

The Consultant's Relationship to Administration

Frequently consulting psychiatrists find it difficult to provide psychiatric consultation to nursing homes due to relatively poor levels of reimbursement by Medicare and Medicaid. Hence, many psychiatrists are requesting that their time be additionally compensated by the nursing home administration for their consistent availability and the liaison and educational activities they provide within the facility. Though mental health care is often included or bundled into nursing home rates, such care may not be implemented. With consistently available psychiatric services, mental health care is expedited, prevention of psychiatric hospitalization becomes a reality, and quality of individual care is improved. Agitated patients who are not successfully treated—through their screaming, kicking, biting, and hitting of other residents and staff—have a way of negatively influencing the environment. Such behavior is often contagious among residents and has a deleterious effect on staff and visitors. No doubt such problems lead to lower morale, higher staff turnover, and a drain on available staff resources. Visiting families, especially privately paying families, are not eager to place their loved ones in facilities with very agitated, psychotic, or depressed residents. Such disturbances may also influence state reviewers negatively. Such compelling arguments for added compensation for the consultant psychiatrist often escape the attention of nursing home administrators. These administrators may value (like many administrators) a decrease in the number of problems rather than a proliferation of problems. They may not like to hear about poor mental health care within the facility, but they may appreciate having a consistent psychiatric resource to deal with these issues.

The Consultant's Relationship to the Nurses

Smith and colleagues (1990) emphasized that, from a nursing perspective, the treatment of mental health problems is a growing concern in long-term-care facilities. Up to 80% of nursing home residents suffer form some type of mental illness, but most receive no active treatment. They also note that nursing home staff do not receive sufficient training on mental health issues, the aging process, and the assessment and management of psychiatric symptoms in the elderly.

In addition, issues of staff burnout deserve more consideration. Working in a team approach has much to offer in fostering empathic nursing care. In one of the few publications regarding nursing burnout, Astrom and associates (1990) reported that registered nurses had a significantly lower degree of burnout compared to the nurses' aides and licensed practical nurses. Of all respondents in their investigation, 27.4% were assessed to be at risk for burnout. The authors found a weak negative correlation between staff burnout and their empathy with the residents' difficulties.

The following structure is one model of nursing's potential relationship to the consultation-liaison psychiatrist, which may improve the delivery of mental health services. One nurse is identified as the psychiatric nurse. This is often one of the most clinically skilled nurses in the facility, someone who may have had some psychiatric inpatient experience. Such a nurse is crucial to the flow and monitoring of mental health care. The functions of this identified nurse included (1) determining the residents to be seen; (2) preparing the residents for the psychiatrist's evaluation; (3) collecting the medication record; (4) reporting on the efficacy of the medications used; (5) reporting communications from the other nurses, aides, and therapists to the consultant; (6) translating the recommendations to the other nurses and aides; (7) encouraging relevant nurses and aides to attend the consultant's rounds and to share data; (8) and communicating to the psychiatrist's office the resident's status. Through this role, the nursing home's psychiatric nurse may accumulate prestige among the nursing house staff. Thus the nurse's knowledge base and importance to the facility grows. As the nurse's experience with psychiatric treatments and evaluations improves, so does the level of care within the facility.

The Consultant's Relationship to the Nursing Home Psychologist

A few nursing homes will have the luxury of a psychologist who works or consults at the facility. Referrals for individual supportive therapies, behavioral treatment plans, and group therapy are often possible. Consulting psychologists will also refer patients back to the psychiatrist for pharmacological consultation. This may occur when the "talk therapies" fail to bring about sufficient improvement in the resident. If the psychologist has the ability to conduct structured neuropsychological evaluations, such data can be used when deciding the appropriate level of functioning that the facility may expect for a given resident.

The Consultant's Relationship to the Social Worker

The initial social work assessment on the patient's record is frequently the most thorough and useful information regarding the resident in the chart. Even more informative than the written record is the social worker's intimate knowledge of the family and the operating dynamics within the family. Quite often the social worker will have evaluated the family and resident on the phone and in person during the lengthy nursing home admission process. The social worker is often aware of visitations by the resident's family and is frequently the recipient of any complaints that are forthcoming. Evaluation of the appropriateness of prospective nursing home applicants or the prior assessment and treatment of especially difficult patients or families have proliferated in geriatric psychiatrist's offices. The social worker frequently functions as the facility's essential intermediary between health care providers and the resident's family.

The Consultant's Relationship to the Families

The consultant's availability to families also requires a clear structure. Some psychiatrists prefer to be available only through the facility's social worker. Clearly, many families need to be contacted concerning patient behavior, past history, and medication use. Asking the social worker to request that family members call the office is frequently the best course. The consultant must be prepared to educate the relatives of a nursing home resident about a chosen course of treatment or to address their concerns about their loved one's care. For very distraught families, scheduling an office visit is best. Family members have often been in the caregiver's role for an extended period of time. The care of a senior is never trivial and almost always very stressful. It is not uncommon for caregivers to develop major depressions. The consulting psychiatrist must be willing to assess such relatives and offer treatment when indicated.

The Consultant's Relationship to the Resident

To the extent possible, the consultation should be a pleasant experience for the resident. A sense of caring and interest should be conveyed. One must introduce oneself and conduct the interview in a cordial fashion, with profuse thanks and best wishes at the end of the evaluation. Due to the patients' cognitive impairment and accompanying mistrust of strangers, such exaggeration of the norms of the affective components of normal human interaction is frequently necessary. Though patients with dementia may have severe memory deficits and gaps in other areas of cognitive functioning, they will frequently maintain a memory for the affective quality of the interaction. If the patient feels insulted, demeaned, belittled, or threatened, they will often carry that emotional tone for quite a while and may remember the consultant with that first impression. This must be avoided, as the patient's cooperation during a thorough mental status evaluation is essential. In addition, the sense of listening, interest, and caring in the healing arts can never be overly encouraged. It is important for the consultants to keep an eye on their own cordiality and to assess patients' complaints and level of insight early. It is also helpful to attempt to obtain a mental status examination with the permission of the patient (i.e., "You have felt that there is nothing wrong with you or your memory. I routinely check the memory of all patients. Would you mind if I asked some questions to help me better understand your memory ... ?''). If the patient is uncooperative, assessment of mental status may be obtained in a less direct and formal process. The flow of the interview is also important. Once into the mental status exam, it is best to continue at a good pace before the patient refuses to go on because of difficulties that are being encountered. The patient may be encouraged with quick, polite statements such as "Please try ... trying is more important than no answer ... I know you can do it ... very good [even with wrong answers]. ... I'm sorry that it strikes you that it's a stupid question, but questions such as this one [serial sevens, spelling words backwards, digit span, etc.] help me understand your ability to sustain attention [or whatever the task is eliciting].''

Conclusion

In this chapter, several of the roles of the consultation-liaison psychiatrist in the nursing home are reviewed. Importantly, the psychiatrist serves to provide expert mental health assessment. He or she develops comprehensive treatment plans that address the resident's biological, psychological, and social needs. Finally in no small measure, he or she educates nursing staff and resident's families regarding the contemporary approaches to identifying and treating mental disorders in the elderly.

References

AAGP, AGS, APA. Psychotherapeutic medications in the nursing home. *J Am Geriatr Soc* 40:946–949, 1992.

The American Psychiatric Association's Psychiatric Glossary. Washington, DC: American Psychiatric Press, 1984.

APA. *Diagnostic and Statistical Manual of Mental Disorders,* 4th ed. Washington, DC: American Psychiatric Association, 1994.

Astrom S, Nilsson M, Norberg A, Winblad B. Empathy, experience of burnout and attitudes towards demented patients among nursing staff in geriatric care. *J Adv Nurs* 15:1236–1244, 1990.

Avorn J, Dreyer P, Connelly K, Soumerai SB. Use of psychoactive medication and the quality of care in rest homes. *N Engl J Med* 320:227–232, 1989.

Avorn J, Soumerai SB, Everitt DE, et al. A randomized trial of a program to reduce the use of psychoactive drugs in nursing homes. *N Engl J Med* 327:168–173, 1992.

Beers M, Avorn J, Soumerai SB, et al. Psychoactive medication use in intermediate-care facility residents. *JAMA* 260:3016–3020, 1988.

Bienenfeld D, Wheeler BG. Psychiatric services to nursing homes: A liaison model. *Hosp Commun Psychiatry* 40:793–794, 1989.

Goldman LS, Klugman A. Psychiatric consultation in a teaching nursing home. *Psychosomatics* 31:277–281, 1990.

Hackett TP, Cassem NH. *Massachusetts General Hospital Handbook of General Hospital Psychiatry,* 2nd ed., St. Louis: Mosby, 1987.

Hogstel M. *Geopsychiatric Nursing.* St. Louis: Mosby, 1990.

Katz MM. Behavioral change in the chronicity pattern of dementia in the institutional geriatric resident. *J Am Geriatr Soc* 24:522–528, 1976.

Knopman DS, Kitto J, Deinard S, Heirig J. Longitudinal study of death and institutionalization in patients with primary degenerative dementia. *J Am Geriatr Soc* 36:108–112, 1988.

Lantz MS, Louis A, Lowenstein G, Kennedy GJ. A longitudinal study of psychotropic prescriptions in a teaching nursing home. *Am J Psychiatry* 147:1637–1639, 1990.

Lipowski ZJ. Consultation-liaison psychiatry: The first half century. *Gen Hosp Psychiatry* 8:305–315, 1986.

Loebel JP, Borson S, Hyde T, et al. Relationships between requests for psychiatric consultations and psychiatric diagnoses in long-term-care facilities. *Am J Psychiatry* 148:898–903, 1991.

Pietrukowicz ME, Johnson MM. Using life histories to individualize nursing home staff attitudes toward residents. *Gerontologist* 31:102–106, 1991.

Pruchno R, Michaels JA, Potashnik SL. Predictors of institutionalization among Alzheimer's disease victims with caregiving spouses. *J Gerontol* 45:259–266, 1990.

Rovner BW, Steele CD, German PS, Clark R. Psychiatric diagnosis and uncooperative behavior in nursing homes. *J Geriatr Psychiatry Neurol* 5:102–105, 1992.

Sakauye KM, Camp CJ. Introducing psychiatric care into nursing homes. *Gerontologist* 32:849–852, 1992.

Smith M, Buckwalter KC, Albanese M. Geropsychiatric education programs providing skills and understanding. *J Psychosoc Nurs Ment Health Serv* 28:8–12, 1990.

Steele C, Rovner B, Chase GA, Folstein M. Psychiatric symptoms and nursing home placement of patients with Alzheimer's disease. *Am J Psychiatry* 147:1049–1051, 1990.

17

Ethical Issues

Teresa M. Schaer

As our population ages and as more elderly spend the last years of their lives in nursing homes, physicians and physician extenders will become increasingly involved in crucial and sensitive medical/ethical decision making in the long-term-care setting. At present, the literature on medical ethics concentrates on ethical dilemmas in the hospital setting, leaving those working in nursing homes to draw on this information, though much of it does not readily extrapolate to the nursing home. As stated in the 1991 *Hastings Center Report on Nursing Home Ethics,* "It is important to explore how notions based on acute care . . . can be modified so that they resonate more fully with the predicaments of nursing home residents, caregivers, and family members" (Collopy et al., 1991).

We begin this chapter with a discussion of basic ethical principles and how they apply in the long-term-care setting. The concepts of competence versus decision-making capacity and of proxy decision maker and substituted judgment are defined and explained. The remaining sections deal with the practical issues of advance directives, do-not-resuscitate orders, do-not-hospitalize orders, nutrition and hydration, and ethics committees; they provide suggestions for dealing with ethical dilemmas encountered in daily practice in the nursing home. (The reader is referred to Chapter 18 for a thorough discussion of the legal underpinnings of decision making in nursing homes.)

Application of Ethical Principles in the Nursing Home

Among the basic ethical principles that guide medical decision making in all patient-care settings, autonomy and beneficence remain paramount. Although the application of these two principles in nursing homes is ideally the same as in hospitals, the characteristics of individuals who reside in nursing homes, as well as their goals of management, further complicate the decision-making process (Uhlmann et al., 1987).

The principle of *autonomy* refers, in essence, to the right of self-determination—i.e., the right to make decisions for oneself. This right is threatened for the elderly who reside in nursing homes for a number of reasons. Some 40 to 80% of nursing home residents have a type of cognitive dysfunction (Glasser et al., 1988; Miller and Cugliari, 1990; Rifkin et al., 1992). Those elderly who are not demented when admitted are at high risk for developing confusional states due to their underlying frailty. Furthermore, patients in this setting often are not allowed to make decisions for themselves simply because they are thought to be "too old and frail" and thus incapable of participating in the decision-making process (Uhlmann et al., 1987; Kloezen et al., 1988; Kapp, 1990).

The second principle, that of *beneficence,* refers to promotion of the patient's well-being. In the nursing home, deciding what constitutes "well-being" or what is "good" for the individual can be a difficult process, as becomes apparent below. Unfortunately, the nursing home resident is often unable to verbalize wishes and values due to confusion, impaired speech, or sensory impairments. In addition, family or friends (who are often looked upon as surrogate decision makers) are often not available—a reflection of the social isolation that affects substantial numbers of nursing home residents. In situations such as these, applying the principle of *proportionality,* wherein one weighs the benefits and burdens of a given intervention, becomes problematic.

Competence/Decision-Making Capacity

Among the most misunderstood but important concepts in medicine is that of *patient competence.* "Competence" is a legal rather than a medical term, which refers to a pronouncement by the courts that an individual lacks the capacity for independent decision making. "Decision-making capacity," on the other hand, refers to a patient's ability to understand the nature and consequences of a given course of action. Decision-making capacity (DMC) is issue- or event-specific and does not have the global connotations of a judge's pronouncement of "incompetence." In medicine it is determined at the bedside by an individual's primary care provider and does not necessarily require a specialist's (i.e., psychiatrist's) intervention.

The evaluation of DMC has become increasingly important in this era of autonomy. In fact, the evaluation to determine capacity has been described as "the foundation for every other ethical issue in geriatrics" and "for exercising many of the resident rights" under the nursing home regulations legislated by the Omnibus Budget Reconciliation Act (OBRA) of 1987 (Levenson, 1990).

Unfortunately, there are few generally accepted guidelines describing how the clinician is to perform this evaluation (Kloezen et al., 1988; Mahler and Perry, 1988; Searight, 1992).

Any practitioner who has been asked to determine an individual's DMC will readily say that identifying individuals at either end of the spectrum—that is, clearly capable of making decisions for themselves or clearly incapable of making such decisions—is, in general, not a difficult task. Little formal testing is needed to ascertain their DMC. It is the individual in the middle or "gray zone" who is difficult to identify. These individuals may retain some degree of DMC or may fluctuate in this respect (Rifkin et al., 1992; Marson et al., 1993). Kloezen and coworkers (1988) call this group "marginally competent" and states that these individuals are at risk for being considered incompetent and losing all of their rights to self-determination. On the other hand, they may be called competent inappropriately and be deprived of the protection they need from a proxy decision maker.

In evaluating DMC, one must be aware that capacity to make decisions can fluctuate over time (Kloezen et al., 1988; Mahler and Perry, 1988; Farnsworth, 1989). It is well known that a person with dementia has good days and bad days. Even in the course of one day, an individual may have more lucid moments in the morning as opposed to the evening hours. Discussions aimed at discovering a person's preferences regarding specific medical treatment can be broached during these more lucid times. In some cases, multiple examinations may be necessary because of these problems (Farnsworth, 1989). The goal is to at least obtain some idea of what that individual would want if he or she were fully competent.

Finally, an otherwise fully capable individual may temporarily lack DMC due to a reversible underlying condition such as delirium caused by an acute illness (Mahler and Perry, 1988). Resolution of the acute problem can render that individual capable of again making decisions. Depression, which is pervasive among nursing home residents, can also affect an individual's DMC and must be carefully considered.

There is agreement in the literature that some sort of mental status examination, such as the Folstein screening Mini-Mental State (Folstein et al., 1975), should be included during the evaluation for determining capacity (Farnsworth, 1989; Levenson, 1990; Marson et al., 1990; Rifkin et al., 1992). There is also agreement that testing cognitive abilities is not enough (Fitten et al., 1990; Searight, 1992). One study showed that "patients who score low on a Folstein may still retain some level of DMC as demonstrated by other assessment tools of cognitive function" and "a normal score on a Folstein may not be synonymous with full DMC" (Rifkin et al., 1992). There is also some consensus that the evaluation should include a multidisciplinary approach with input from other members of the health care team. In a nursing home, it is important to obtain, from nurses and nurses' aides, information about resident function and behavior (Levenson, 1990).

Some tests of competency include a psychiatric battery of questions that test the ability to abstract (describe similarities and differences, explain proverbs) and demonstrate appropriate insight and good judgment. Although these questions give some clue to the mental capabilities of an individual, they do not relate directly to the question at hand: Is this person capable of making decisions regarding a specific medical treatment whether in the present or in the future, as in the case of the advance directive?

Roth and colleagues (1977) first described five "tests for competency" in 1977. These categories were used and modified into four "levels of decision-making capacity" by Levenson in (1990). They include the following:

1. *Evidencing a choice.* At this level, an individual can be described as meeting at least the minimum criterion for capacity. Such a person must exhibit a preference for or against a treatment and thus be demonstrating a positive interest in making a decision.

2. *Factual appreciation of the issues.* In this level, the individual is capable not only of demonstrating a preference but also shows an awareness of the medical situation and its implications.

3. *Rational manipulation of information.* The individual manifests this level of capacity if he or she not only meets the criteria set forth above but also exhibits a set of values/opinions in addition to logical reasoning that takes into account these values. The individual must also be relatively free of coercion or excessive dependence on another person.

4. *Appreciation of the consequences of the decision.* At this level the individual must demonstrate the above and comprehend the consequences of the decision to consent or refuse a medical treatment. He or she must also recognize the need for additional information and employ it in the decision-making process (Levenson, 1990).

Levels 2 through 4 are described throughout the psychiatric and legal literature (Farnsworth, 1989). Levenson added level 1, and this level can be very important for the geriatric population.

It has been stated that, in general, the more serious and irreversible the anticipated consequences of a decision may be, the higher the level of capability required (Levenson, 1990). For example, an individual may be competent enough to decide what to wear but be unable to decide upon a medical treatment. Although this may be true in most circumstances, this notion should not be applied rigidly to questions regarding life-sustaining treatments. A nursing home resident may, for instance, express a strong opinion about respirators or tube-feeding due to a long held point of view but at the same time may no longer understand the implications of his or her words due to a dementing process. For example:

An 85-year-old male with mild to moderate dementia of the Alzheimer type states that he would never want to be kept alive on "one of those breathing machines." When asked if he understands that refusal of such life support under certain circumstances would lead to his death, he demonstrates poor understanding of the issues and just states he doesn't want to talk about it anymore.

This man is at level 1 described above; i.e., he is evidencing a choice without factual appreciation of the issues and outcome of the choice. His preferences should not be ignored but rather appreciated in the context of working with a surrogate decision maker. This should include discussions of how consistent this opinion has been over time and how it fits with the individual's lifelong pattern of conduct.

Just as a decision made by a person who is judged to be incapacitated by being at level 1 does not validly authorize a physician to perform a medical treatment, likewise a physician cannot force treatment upon the same person who refuses a treatment unless reasonable action is taken to obtain valid consent from a proxy decision maker (Roth et al., 1977). Even then, the individual's preference should be given adequate weight, taking into account the consistency of that preference based on historical information known about that individual.

Although the levels described above can be helpful and provide some guidelines as to *what* to evaluate during an evaluation of DMC, more is needed regarding *how* to determine the level at which an individual is appropriately placed. Several studies have been published describing methods of evaluating competency using essays and vignettes (Kloezen et al., 1988; Fitten et al., 1990; Janofsky et al., 1992; Searight, 1992; Marson et al., 1993), but each has its limitations and none has become widely accepted.

To complicate the situation further, an article by Silberfeld and colleagues (1993) makes a distinction between capacity to consent to a treatment being offered in the present and the capacity to complete an advance directive involving treatments in the future. They argue that the two activities are different and that an individual may not be able to decide upon a specific decision at hand but may still be capable of filling out an advance directive.

Unfortunately there is no standard method for the evaluation of DMC. Whatever the method, clinical experience and judgment must play an important role. More studies are needed, as are recommendations by noted organizations such as the American Geriatric Society and the American Psychiatry Association.

Proxy Decision Makers and Substituted Judgment

For the nursing home resident who either completely lacks DMC or exhibits a low level of DMC, a surrogate decision maker is needed. The resident who retains a higher degree of DMC should make his or her own decisions. Many, however, either request or may benefit from some assistance from loved ones (Kapp, 1991).

Under the *Guidelines on the Termination of Life-Sustaining Treatment and the Care of the Dying* (Hastings Center, 1987), after the first step of assessing DMC, the health care provider must identify one of the following as the surrogate decision maker:

1. A person designated by the patient in an advance directive or in another written or oral statement
2. A court appointed surrogate if one has been so appointed with the appropriate authority granted
3. If neither of the above exists, a family member or concerned friend

In the process of selecting a family member to act as the surrogate decision maker, the health care provider will have to refer to individual state laws to see if a priority order is legislated. In general, those listed include the spouse, daughter or son, a parent (invariably not applicable for an elderly nursing home resident), a sibling, or a niece or nephew. The relation of the person is not as important as is the involvement of that person in the life of the resident. In a nursing home, there is often the mistaken impression that the individual chosen to be the surrogate decision maker is the "responsible party" listed at the front of the chart. This is not always the case (Kapp, 1990). The role of surrogate decision maker optimally should be filled by an individual who is knowledgeable about the resident's values and preferences and who can theoretically make "the decision that the incompetent patient would make if he or she were comepetent" (*In re Jobes*, 1987). In legal terminology, this is called substituted judgment.

Although the concept of surrogate decision making has been historically endorsed, most strongly by Justice O'Connor in the Cruzan decision (*In re Cruzan*, 1990), there are objections to this concept in the literature (Emanuel and Emanuel, 1992). Some accumulated data reveal that family members who attempt to make decisions regarding life-sustaining measures for their elderly loved ones often disagree and choose incorrectly what that individual would want. In one study, agreement on specific preferences ranged from 59 to 88% (Seckler et al., 1991). In another study, spouses were found to have overestimated subjects' preferences in the area of resuscitation, with disagreement ranging from 10 to 47% of the time (Uhlmann et al., 1988). These studies also revealed that few elderly had discussed preferences with their families. Although it has not been proven, it is likely that prior discussions with family would improve concordance rates.

In the meantime, the large majority of nursing home residents require that the health care provider work with a proxy decision maker. In doing so, it is very important that the health care provider avoid using certain phrases or questions. For example, one should try not to say, "What should we do?" Instead, one might phrase it, "Has the resident ever told you about what he or she would want in a situation such as this one?" This helps to take the burden of total responsibility off of the proxy and leads that person to decide what the resident would want (Sachs and Siegler, 1991).

The conversation should focus on what is known about the resident's prior wishes. Written statements in the form of advance directives are the best evidence of individual preferences; unfortunately, however, few residents in nursing homes have such documents. In lieu of something written, the proxy should be asked about (1) spoken directives made to any family member, friend, or health care provider that could serve as evidence; (2) voiced reactions about others being kept alive on ventilators or with tube-feeding; (3) deductions that can be made about the individual based on a knowledge of the person's spiritual or personal beliefs or based on a lifelong pattern of conduct.

If the proxy is unable to make a decision based on the "substituted judgment" standard, then a decision must be made based on the "best interest" standard. This means that the decision must be what the proxy believes to be the best for the resident. Since most decisions in a nursing home revolve around the withholding and withdrawal of life-sustaining treatments, it would be important for the physician to guide the decision maker to see the resident as a whole; to realize that decisions favoring prolongation of life may or may not be in the resident's best interest; and to understand that palliative/comfort care is available and can be actively provided by the health care team.

During such discussions, another phrase that should be avoided is, ''Do you want us to do everything possible?'' This leads the proxy to believe that the alternative is to ''do nothing,'' which is often interpreted as abandonment (Sachs and Siegler, 1991). The choice is actually between specific treatment options that should be outlined for the proxy and should necessarily include aggressive interventions, conservative treatment modalities, and palliative care, each with its possible and probable consequences. It is important to mention that in the ''palliative care'' alternative, the providers will ''do everything possible'' to keep the resident comfortable and pain-free (Sachs and Siegler, 1991).

Situations may arise in which there is dispute over who should act as a proxy decision maker, as when there are several family members. The potential for significant conflict then arises. Most conflicts are due to poor communication, misunderstandings, and misperceptions (Sachs and Siegler, 1991). These should be recognized as being amenable to intervention, and this can best be done with a team approach, bringing the disputing parties together and talking openly about the conflict. When this fails, the ethics committee should be called together to evaluate the case and problem at hand. The role of the ethics committee in such a situation is discussed below.

Advance Directives in the Nursing Home

The Patient Self-Determination Act (PSDA) went into effect on December 1, 1991; since that time, all health care institutions, including nursing homes, have been required to ask about the presence of an advance directive when an individual is admitted. The PSDA was a much-needed and welcome development for long-term-care facilities because the issues of end-of-life decisions had been avoided for many years (Weiss, 1991). In addition, the law has made it necessary for nursing homes to develop institutional policies on advance directives, resuscitation, and the withholding and withdrawal of life-sustaining treatments. (See Chapter 18 for additional information on these legal mandates.)

There are three types of advance directives:

1. The instruction directive, also known as a living will, provides written instructions regarding what an individual would want in terms of life-sustaining measures in the event that person becomes incapable of making decisions.

2. The proxy directive, also known as a durable power of attorney, allows for the appointment of a health care representative or a proxy decision maker for health care decisions in the event that one becomes incapable of making decisions for oneself.

3. The combined directive provides for written instructions as well as the appointment of a proxy decision maker.

The requirements of the federal PSDA do not extend to the physician, but there is at least one state advance directive statute (New Jersey's) that also makes it incumbent upon the physician to discuss advance directives at the time of admission. In most states, this is not the case, and it is therefore up to personnel at the nursing home to first ask if an advance directive has been filled out and also to make a copy of the advance directive available to the doctor. Although the physician may not be the first professional to broach the issue of advance directives, this in no way detracts from the primary care provider's pivotal role in this process.

It has been argued that the time of admission to a nursing home is very traumatic for the potential resident and family, making it a sensitive time to raise the topic of advance directives. To make this discussion easier, the resident and family should be contacted as much in advance of the admission as possible to explain the new law and how the facility supports the resident's right to participate in healthcare decisions (Weiss, 1991). Unfortunately, advance discussions are difficult for the admission that takes place straight from a hospital to the nursing home (Batchelor et al., 1992). In such cases, there is short notice, with little lead time to contact the resident and/or family about these issues.

The essential fact remains that the PSDA mandates that these issues be addressed. The initial question of whether an advance directive has been filled out or not should be asked immediately upon admission. Any follow-up discussion can take place at a later date if it appears that the issue is too sensitive to discuss at the time of admission. If an advance directive has been filled out, a copy should be reviewed and placed on the chart. This is usually done by a social worker or nurse during the admissions interview process.

When the form is being reviewed, it is important to note the type of directive, the date it was completed, and whether the document conforms to state law. The type and style of document is important because there are many varieties of forms available, including some that are vague and easily misinterpreted. If this is the case and the prospective resident is cognitively intact (i.e., DMC is not questioned), the resident should be encouraged to update the advance directive on a document recommended by the state or institution. If the individual carries a diagnosis of moderate to severe dementia and/or there is a question regarding DMC, the form, whether it is vague or specific, cannot be changed but must rather be accepted as is. A follow-up discussion with the family by the physician is then necessary to discuss the meaning or intentions of that individual at the time the form was filled out.

The PSDA applies only to new admissions to a hospital or other institution. For a nursing home, this means that the residents already in the facility are excluded from the law. Since many cognitively intact residents live for several years in a nursing home, these individuals should be helped to complete an advance directive if this has not already been done. It is also important that these same residents be given an opportunity, on a yearly basis, to change their treatment wishes. If a change is made, the physician and family should be notified of these changes (Weiss, 1991).

For those individuals who lack DMC and do not have an advance directive, there is no formal mechanism for arriving at guidelines for future decision making. The time of admission is probably the best time to address these issues—i.e., the very time that the surrogate is being asked whether the incoming resident has an advance directive.

In response to this problem, an investigational form was tested by Janns and Schaer (1993) to help formalize discussion with families. The form has the appearance of an advance directive but is entitled Guidelines Regarding Life-Sustaining Measures for the Resident with Impaired Decision-Making Capacity. On this form, surrogates were asked to fill in what they believed to be the wishes of the resident regarding resuscitation, ventilation, feeding tubes, and other life-sustaining treatments and then to fill in how they arrived at their conclusion (i.e., did they base the decision on a spoken directive, verbal reaction, religious beliefs, or lifelong pattern of conduct). Results of the study showed that the form was readily accepted by surrogate decision makers, who were grateful for the opportunity to discuss those end-of-life issues that are usually not raised until it is too late. This type of form, although not strictly an advance directive written by the resident, performs a similar function. It is not, however, binding or strictly ''legal.'' Its purpose is to serve as a guide for the clinician in times of crisis and to be used in conjunction with further discussion with the proxy (Janns and Schaer, 1993).

A common misconception about advance directives is that if an individual has one placed in the chart, it automatically means that the resident is a ''no

Guidelines Regarding Life-Sustaining Measures for the Resident with Impaired Decision-Making Capacity

I, _____, _____,
    Name of person filling out form   Relationship to resident

am aware that _____
              Name of resident

is unable to make decisions for herself or himself at this point in her or his life. Based on the information that I know about this resident, I believe that she or he would want the following with regard to life-sustaining measures:

Initial *one* of the following two statements.

1. _____   All medical measures should be provided to sustain her or his life, regardless of her or his physical or mental condition.

OR

2. _____   At this point in the life of _____, life-sustaining measures should not be initiated. If they have been, they should be withdrawn, recognizing that this may hasten her or his death.

(continued)

If #2 is chosen, initial any or all of the following that apply:

a. _____ No CPR (cardiopulmonary resuscitation, which can only be initiated by emergency medical services and is not done at the nursing home). This involves chest thrusts, drugs, or electric shock to get the heart to start beating again.

b. _____ No artificial breathing (also known as breathing by ventilator, which involves placing a tube within the lungs)[a]

c. _____ Avoid hospitalization

d. _____ No feeding tubes, either through the nose or directly into the stomach

e. _____ No dialysis or chemotherapy[a]

f. _____ Artificial breathing[a] and feeding tubes may be used only on a temporary basis for what appears to be an acute condition (e.g., pneumonia)

[a]These procedures can only be implemented in a hospital and cannot be done at the nursing home.

Additional Instructions: _____

_____

The above statements were completed based on the following information.

Initial and describe any of the following that may apply:

1. _____ A living will/advance directive
2. _____ A spoken directive to family, friend, or health provider

An example of a statement heard: _____

_____

_____

3. _____ A voiced reaction to knowledge about someone being kept alive by artificial means. An example of a statement heard:

_____

4. _____ Deductions from the resident's personal and spiritual beliefs
5. _____ Lifelong pattern of conduct
6. _____ Other

THE DIRECTIVES ABOVE CAN ACT ONLY AS A GUIDELINE IN THE CARE OF THE ABOVE-NAMED RESIDENT. IT IS NOT A TRUE "LIVING WILL" OR "ADVANCE DIRECTIVE" BECAUSE IT IS NOT WRITTEN BY THE RESIDENT AND IT IS NOT LEGALLY BINDING.

Guidelines Regarding Life-Sustaining Measures for the Resident with
Impaired Decision-Making Capacity (*continued*)

This form may be revised or updated at any time by the person completing this form.

_____   _____

Date   Signature

                                                 _____

                                                 Relationship to resident

Additional signatures of concerned others if applicable:

_____   _____

Date   Signature

                                                 _____

                                                 Relationship to resident

_____   _____

Date   Signature

                                                 _____

                                                 Relationship to resident

_____   _____

Date   Witness

code''—i.e., that a do-not-resuscitate (DNR) order should be written (Schaer et al., 1992). This is not always true. The two must be addressed separately, either with the cognitively intact resident or with the proxy decision maker. When an individual fills out an advance directive, that person is expressing directions for care in the event that he or she becomes unable to make decisions. For the mentally intact individual, it is a directive regarding treatments in the *future*. Furthermore, most advance directives request that life-sustaining treatments be withheld only if the person is permanently unconscious, terminally ill, or diagnosed as having an irreversible, incurable condition (which can include severe mental deterioration). In comparison, a DNR order withholds resuscitation in the *present*. If a nursing home resident is no longer able to make decisions *and* has an advance directive, the surrogate and physician must then interpret the instructions in that advance directive to determine if indeed a DNR order should be written.

Do-Not-Resuscitate Orders in the Nursing Home

In the early 1980s the do-not-resuscitate (DNR) order was a controversial issue in acute care hospitals. More recently, the issue has become controversial in the nursing home (Levinson et al., 1987). Despite this, there seems to be some agreement in the literature regarding specific aspects of the order. (In this chapter, the initials "DNR" mean do not resuscitate after *cardiopulmonary* arrest, not after respiratory arrest, which may result from choking or respiratory distress.)

Many studies have demonstrated a low survival rate for elderly undergoing cardiopulmonary resuscitation (CPR) in the hospital. The futility of initiating CPR on an elderly nursing resident has also been demonstrated in several studies. Applebaum and associates (1990) conducted a retrospective study on 117 nursing home residents for whom CPR was attempted over a 1-year period in Baltimore County. Only two (1.2%) survived, and they had extremely poor outcomes despite their survival. The authors concluded that "The benefit of CPR initiated in nursing homes is extremely limited." In Washington, D.C., Awoke and associates (1992) found that of 45 subjects who suffered cardiac arrest and received CPR, none survived.

A subsequent study by Tresch and associates (1993), done in 68 Milwaukee nursing homes, demonstrated more optimistic statistics. Of 196 nursing home residents who received CPR, 37 (19%) were successfully resuscitated. When this group was broken down into two groups—witnessed and unwitnessed arrests—the breakdown revealed that 27% of the residents who had a witnessed arrest survived while only 2.3% of those who had an unwitnessed arrest survived (Tresch et al., 1993). At face value, the 27% statistic for witnessed arrests seems encouraging; however, upon closer scrutiny, this may not extrapolate to nursing homes throughout the country. In the study, 68% of the witnessed arrests were observed by nursing home personnel and *basic* CPR was started by a nurse (Tresch, 1993). Few if any long-term-care facilities throughout the country have the ability to provide *advanced* life support (Miller and Cugliari, 1990). Furthermore, many nursing homes do not require that nursing personnel be certified in *basic* CPR. Often, nursing homes have the policy (written or unwritten) that the emergency medical service (EMS) be called and CPR initiated when they arrive. This would, in most cases, cause an unacceptable delay between the arrest and CPR.

Applebaum and Awoke conclude from their findings, described above, that CPR should not be offered in nursing homes (Awoke et al., 1992). Justification for a unilateral decision by the physician to write DNR orders on all nursing home residents is based on the low survival rates cited and the fact that several ethics articles now advocate that physicians should not be required to provide futile therapy (Murphy, 1988). Miles (1990) argues that the prediction of futility should rest more "on personal frailty than on institutional residence."

Most health care providers will agree on the futility of CPR in the resident of advanced age and/or frailty, but it is very unlikely that this will become standardized in the near future. The current legal environment and fear of malpractice that encourages physicians to "do everything," regardless of what an individual's quality of life may be, discourages the adoption of standards to limit emergency interventions. However it remains to be seen whether society will mandate guidelines in this era of cost containment.

Despite the findings described previously, it has been shown that CPR is rarely initiated in nursing home residents who die (Finucane et al., 1991; Finucane and Denman, 1989). In many nursing homes, it is recognized that the frail, chronically ill elderly who reside there are close to death and the burden of "overtreatment with violent, generally ineffective interventions" such as CPR, is unwarranted (Finucane, 1993).

It is unfortunate but perhaps not surprising to learn that many DNR orders are written without resident or surrogate participation in the decision (Finucane and Denman, 1989; Meyers et al., 1990). As with all decisions regarding medical treatment, the individual who retains DMC should play a role in the decision-making process. Those residents who are capable of making decisions are often more informed than we want to admit. Many have already thought about their impending death and welcome the opportunity to discuss it—often expressing wishes to "let nature take its course" and "leave me alone when the time comes."

For the majority of nursing home residents—i.e., those who lack DMC—surrogates are relied on to make the decision about a DNR order. In practice, although studies show that surrogates often do not know what their elderly loved one would want (Uhlmann et al., 1988; Seckler et al., 1991), they generally welcome the chance to discuss the issues of dying and death, which are often paramount in their minds (Janns and Schaer, 1993). Consumers are becoming much more versed in these issues than ever before and decisions are often made even before explanations are given and discussions are held.

In practice, the much larger problem lies in getting physicians to even address the issue with residents and their families, and not necessarily in getting residents and families to understand. Although physicians may be aware that the DNR order is an important option to discuss with residents and surrogates, it is not placed high on their list of priorities, or they blame lack of time for not discussing it. They also may avoid the issue for fear of an ombudsman (see below) or other regulatory agencies. The first step toward getting physicians to address the issue of DNR is for the nursing home to have a policy in place.

One study showed that implementation of a DNR policy "can shorten time to physician documentation of a DNR order" (Batchelor et al., 1992). The medical director and director of nursing are responsible for making the physician staff aware of this policy and encouraging them to address the issue with every resident. Unfortunately, studies reveal that it is not standard for long-term-care facilities to have DNR policies (Levinson et al., 1987; Lipsky et al., 1988; Brunetti et al., 1990; Miller and Evans, 1991), but they are fast becoming a necessity.

Do-Not-Hospitalize Orders in the Nursing Home

Few empirical studies have focused on do-not-hospitalize (DNH) orders. Lipsky and associates (1990) proposed that the order offers a tremendous benefit for those residents of nursing homes who do not wish to be hospitalized or for those "carefully selected" residents who would gain little therapeutically if they were hospitalized. It is stated that a DNH order preserves patient autonomy and, in addition, is a way to limit health care costs (Lipsky et al., 1990). At face value, this makes sense; however, "great caution is needed here," as stated in an accompanying editorial (Nolan, 1990). Rejection of the hospital as a site for treatment can be misinterpreted as a rejection of all forms of treatment. More importantly, each situation must be viewed individually, even those where it seems clear that hospitalization would be ineffective. The following two case histories are illustrative of this fact.

> An 84-year-old woman, with severe dementia residing in a nursing home, and still ambulating, is found lying on the floor in the hallway. Her right leg is foreshortened and externally rotated, causing the patient extreme pain when it is moved. She has a DNH order on her chart and the nurses are confused as to how to proceed.

> An 87-year-old man who is chair- or bed-bound and has moderate dementia is visited daily in a nursing home by his wife, who obtains great joy from each visit. He develops a urinary tract infection and is treated with an antibiotic. During this period, his oral intake of fluids declines temporarily and he becomes dehydrated. He continues to deteriorate and then stops eating. He has a DNH order on his chart.

In each case, identifying the general goal of medical management is the "critical initial step" (Nolan, 1990). The context of each situation is extremely important in the decision-making process in order to determine whether hospitalization will or will not further the management goals identified. Based on these arguments, Nolan (1990) has suggested that instead of a global DNH order, a "hospital query" order would be a better way to ensure that each case is individualized. An order such as this, however, may be too general. It does little to guide a covering physician when a primary attending is not available. A better wording might be "avoid hospitalization"—a phrase which clearly indicates that hospitalization is not a desired alternative for a particular nursing home resident but that each situation should be analyzed carefully, considering the resident's and surrogate's goals. Another problem with the DNH order is the possible misinterpretation of the letters DNH to say DNR. Although this is a theoretical problem, it is hard to imagine a case where a DNR order would not accompany a DNH order.

Currently, many nursing homes do not use or are unfamiliar with the order DNH. They do, however, have the "practical equivalent" (Lipsky et al., 1990). The practice of keeping an individual at a nursing home and not transferring him or her to a hospital without a specific order is very commonplace, and it is assumed that this is done in an individualized fashion after discussion with family. Health care providers in nursing homes must work against the common tendency to transfer residents to hospitals without any question as to whether treatment at that site would benefit the person overall or whether the resident or surrogate would even want the transfer (Nolan, 1990).

Nutrition and Hydration in the Nursing Home

Artificial nutrition and hydration are the most controversial of life-sustaining treatments. Currently in our society, it is not only legal but also ethical for health care providers to respect the right of patients to refuse artificial nutrition and hydration (Lynn and Childress, 1983; Campbell-Taylor and Fisher, 1987, U.S. Congress, 1987; Scofield, 1991).

One of the major reasons for the intense controversy within and among nursing homes regarding feeding tubes is the fact that many individuals who live or work in these facilities harbor many misconceptions about this life-sustaining measure. A study by Kayser-Jones (1990) revealed that 70% of the nursing home nurses interviewed thought that if a resident was unable to eat, a tube should be placed. Their reasons included the belief that tube feeding is a necessary comfort measure. Importantly, this study also revealed that tubes were placed more out of fear of receiving a citation from inspectors or investigation by an ombudsman than any other factors. The most glaring misconception was that death from dehydration and malnutrition was a horrible way to die. There are reports suggesting that hospice nurses have a more positive perception of dehydration in the terminal patient and that terminally ill patients with end-stage dehydration actually experience less discomfort than patients receiving hydration (McCann et al., 1994; Andrews and Levine, 1989; Printz, 1988).

Important recommendations emerged from the Kayser-Jones (1990) survey; they include the following:

1. Residents in nursing homes who have eating problems should receive a thorough evaluation.
2. Residents and their families should be given an opportunity to express their wishes.
3. Information on artificial nutrition and hydration should be presented to residents and families in an "unbiased, understandable manner at an appropriate time."
4. Nursing homes should develop "in-service programs that focus on eating problems and artificial nutrition" for the nurses and nurse's aides.
5. "Decisions regarding artificial nutrition should be made collaboratively, with patients, their families, the physician, and the nursing home staff participating.

A sixth recommendation can be added: that the decision maker should attempt to discover what the individual would want—either from written advance directives, verbal statements, or knowledge from religious belief and past behavior. It is also important that health care providers help residents of nursing homes as well as their families to realize that the true cause of death is the primary disease process, not the withholding of artificial nutrition and hydration (Printz, 1988).

In situations where a conflict exists or where health care providers are uncomfortable about withholding treatment, the physician and staff need not feel alone in the decision-making process. Either the expertise of a geriatric team can be called in for guidance (Watts and Cassel, 1984) or an institutional ethics committee may be asked to review the case (Printz, 1988).

Ethics Committees in Long-Term-Care Facilities

In the 1960s and 1970s, very few hospitals throughout the country could boast of the existence of ethics committees within their walls (Doudera, 1986). During the 1980s, more and more hospitals developed such committees in the aftermath of the Quinlan case in New Jersey, in which ethics/prognosis committees were recommended and "delegated immunity-granting authority" (Annas, 1991). Such committees were practically unheard of in long-term-care facilities, and only in the 1990s has the need become apparent. A national survey of nursing homes, published in 1988, revealed that only 2% of the sample had established ethics committees (Glasser et al., 1988).

The structure and function of ethics committees within hospitals has been the subject of much debate over the past decade. The setting of long-term-care facilities, so different from hospitals, provides an even bigger challenge because of the relatively low level of physician participation in resident care, stronger nursing involvement, and fewer administrators with more concentrated authority (Miller and Cugliari, 1990).

The challenges presented within this setting first include the question of who should serve on such a committee. Most long-term-care facilities already have several mandatory committees, and it seems that three individuals form the core of each committee: the administrator, the director of nursing and the medical director. These three individuals would likely also form the core of the ethics committee. Unfortunately, it does not naturally follow that these three individuals have sufficient (or any) training in ethics or understanding of ethical issues qualifying them to serve on such an important committee. It is for this reason that some nursing homes are turning to nearby or affiliated hospitals. An agreement is reached such that the hospital ethics committee serves the needed functions of writing and sharing ethics policies, reviewing controversial and difficult ethical cases, and educating staff and community. Other nursing homes are utilizing ethics departments within local universities or seminaries.

For those long-term-care facilities that are not affiliated with or close enough to a hospital or university which could serve in such a role, regional ethics committees are being created. It is unknown how many of these are being formed throughout the country, and the few that have been created are still in their infancies. Such a committee is usually formed by a group of local nursing homes, each sending representatives. The membership of the committee should be multidisciplinary. Commitment and desire should not be enough for membership. Members must develop a knowledge base in the area of medical ethics. The presence of an ethicist and enlightened attorney on the committee is key to this educational process. Appointment of nurse's aides and a nursing home resident representative is also important.

The functions of the ethics committee have already been alluded to. They include but are certainly not limited to policy and guideline development; education of committee members, staff, and community; and case review and consultation, both retrospective and prospective (Doudera, 1986; Glasser et al., 1988; Miller, 1990). These functions are often delegated to subcommittees for the extensive work needed to put together policies. The role of the larger committee is to review, make changes, and improve on the work of the subcommittes. Case review can be a function of the full committee or an ad hoc subcommittee that is called together as needed.

When specific cases are reviewed, the role of the ethics committee is not to provide a solution or make the final decision but rather to serve as a forum for discussion, opening up communication where communication has been poor or has failed, educate those involved with the case about the legal and ethical issues surrounding each decision, and assist in weighing the benefits and burdens of treatment. There is also an unwritten "therapeutic" role that helps the health care team handle the stress of dealing with these cases (Fost, 1987). The final role of the committee is to provide guidelines with recommendations for a decision.

As an adjunct to the education of committee members, nursing home staff, residents, and family, it has been suggested that an ethics manual be developed and distributed. Such a manual might define important terms, discuss ethical rights and individual responsibilities, and give examples of case studies and analyses (Zweibel et al., 1987).

As an alternative to the ethics committee, The Jewish Home for the Aged in New York City utilizes an approach that involves an ethics consult team and case review via "ethics rounds." The rounds include multidisciplinary participation, a resident/family interview, and team discussion. They conclude with a formal presentation or overview by an ethicist (Libow et al., 1991; Olson et al., 1993).

Ethics consultation is another service that can be found in some hospitals throughout the country (LaPuma and Schiedermayer, 1991), but it is very rare in the long-term-care facility. One individual ethicist performing such a service for several nursing homes could be viewed as an alternative to those having difficulty forming an ethics committee or as a needed adjunct to such a committee (Siegler and Singer, 1988).

The Ombudsman

The Office of the Ombudsman for the Institutionalized Elderly is a state agency, created to protect the rights and welfare of elderly residents in long-term-care facilities. In some states, most notably New Jersey, the rights of residents with regard to life-sustaining treatments are also overseen by this agency. It behooves anyone working in a nursing home to become aware of the rules and regulations regarding ethical issues in one's state and through one's ombudsman.

Conclusion

Decision making in nursing homes remains an extremely complex endeavor. Attention to but a few basic overriding ethical principles in the context of a working partnership between patient, family, and health care team will go a long way toward optimizing each resident's overall quality of life.

References

Andrews MR, Levine AM. Dehydration in the terminal patient: Perception of hospice nurses. *Am J Hosp Care* 31–34, January/February 1989.

Annas G. Ethics committees: From ethical comfort to ethical cover. *Hastings Cent Rep* 21:18–21, 1991.

Applebaum GE, King JE, Finucane TE. The outcome of CPR initiated in nursing homes. *J Am Geriatr Soc* 38:197–200, 1990.

Awoke S, Mouton C, Parrott M. Outcomes of skilled cardiopulmonary resuscitation in a long-term care facility: Futile therapy? *J Am Geriatr Soc* 40:593–595, 1992.

Batchelor AJ, Winsemius D, O'Connor PJ, Wetle T. Predictors of advance directive restrictiveness and compliance with institutional policy in a long-term-care facility. *J Am Geriatr Soc* 40:679–684, 1992.

Brunetti LL, Weiss MJ, Studenski SA, Clipp EC. Cardiopulmonary resuscitation policies and practices: A statewide nursing home study. *Arch Intern Med* 150:121–126, 1990.

Campbell-Taylor I, Fisher RH. The clinical case against tube feeding in palliative care of the elderly. *J Am Geriatr Soc* 35:1100–1104, 1987.

Collopy B, Boyle P, Jennings B. New directions in nursing home ethics. *Hastings Cent Rep* 21:1–15, 1991.

In re Cruzan v. *Director,* Missouri Department of Health, 110, S CT 2841, 1990.

Doudera AE. Developing issues in medical decision making: The durable power of attorney and institutional ethics committees. *Prim Care* 13:315–326, 1986.

Emanuel EJ, Emanuel LL. Proxy decision making for incompetent patients, an ethical and empirical analysis. *JAMA* 267:2067–2071, 1992.

Farnsworth MG. Evaluation of mental competency. *Am Fam Physician* 39:182–190, 1989.

Finucane TE. Attempted cardiopulmonary resuscitation in nursing homes. *Am J Med* 95:121–122, 1993.

Finucane TE, Boyer JT, Bulmash J, et al. The incidence of attempted CPR in nursing homes. *J Am Geriatr Soc* 39:624–626, 1991.

Finucane TE, Denman SJ. Deciding about resuscitation in a nursing home: Theory and practice. *J Am Geriatr Soc* 37:684–688, 1989.

Fitten LJ, Lusky R, Hamann C. Assessing treatment decision-making capacity in elderly nursing home residents. *J Am Geriatr Soc* 38:1097–1104, 1990.

Folstein MF, Folstein SE, McHugh PR. "Mini-Mental State": A practical method for grading the cognitive state of patients for the clinician. *J Psychiatr Res* 12:189–198, 1975.

Fost N. Life and death decisions: Part 2. *Hosp Phys* 37–38, August 1987.

Glasser G, Zweibel NR, Cassel CK. The ethics committee in the nursing home: Results of a national survey. *J Am Geriatr Soc* 36:150–156, 1988.

Hastings Center. In: Smith DH, Veatch RM, eds. *Guidelines on the Termination of Life-Sustaining Treatment and the Care of the Dying*. Bloomington, IN: Indiana University Press, 1987.

Janofsky JS, McCarthy RJ, Folstein MF. The Hopkins Competency Assessment Test: A brief method for evaluating patients' capacity to give informed consent. *Hosp Commun Psychiatry* 43:132–136, 1992.

Janns C, Schaer T. Evaluating surrogate decision-making for the cognitively impaired nursing home resident. *J Am Geriatr Soc* 41:SA52, 1993.

In re Jobes, 108 New Jersey 394, 1987.

Kapp MB. Health care decision making by the elderly: I get by with a little help from my family. *Gerontologist* 31:619–623, 1991.

Kapp MB. Liability issues and assessment of decision-making capability in nursing home patients. *Am J Med* 89:639–642, 1990.

Kayser-Jones J. The use of nasogastric feeding tubes in nursing homes: Patient, family and health care provider perspectives. *Gerontologist* 30:469–479, 1990.

Kloezen S, Fitten LJ, Steinberg A. Assessment of treatment decision-making capacity in a medically ill patient. *J Am Geriatr Soc* 36:1055–1058, 1988.

LaPuma J, Schiedermayer DL. Ethics consultation: Skills, roles, and training. *Ann Intern Med* 114:155–160, 1991.

Levenson SA. Evaluating competence and decision-making capacity in impaired older patients. *Older Patient* 11–15, Winter 1990.

Levinson W, Shepard MA, Dunn PM, Parker DF. Cardiopulmonary resuscitation in long-term care facilities: A survey of do-not-resuscitate orders in nursing homes. *J Am Geriatr Soc* 35:1059–1062, 1987.

Libow LS, Olson E, Neufeld RR, et al. Ethics rounds at the nursing home: An alternative to an ethics committee. *J Am Geriatr Soc* 40:95–97, 1992.

Lipsky MS, Hickey DP, Browning G. Treatment limitations in nursing homes in northwest Ohio. *Arch Intern Med* 148:1539–1541, 1988.

Lipsky MS, Hickey DP, Browning G, Taylor C. The use of do-not-hospitalize orders by family physicians in Ohio. *J Fam Pract* 30:61–64, 1990.

Lynn J, Childress JF. Must patients always be given food and water? *Hastings Cent Rep* 10:17–21, 1983.

Mahler J, Perry S. Assessing competency in the physically ill: Guidelines for psychiatric consultants. *Hosp Commun Psychiatry* 39:856–861, 1988.

Marson D, Ingram BS, Duke L, Harrell L. Consistency of physician competency decisions in Alzheimer's-type dementia. *J Am Geriatr Soc* 41:SA55, 1993.

McCann RM, Hall WJ, Groth-Juncker A. Comfort care for terminally ill patients: The appropriate use of nutrition and hydration. *JAMA* 272:1263–1266, 1994.

Meyers RM, Lurie N, Breitenbucher RB, Waring CJ. Do-not-resuscitate orders in an extended-care study group. *J Am Geriatr Soc* 38:1011–1015, 1990.

Miles SH. Resuscitating the nursing home resident: Futility and pseudofutility. *J Am Geriatr Soc* 38:1037–1038, 1990.

Miller J, Evans T. Some reflections on ethical dilemmas in nursing home research. *West J Nurs Res* 13:375–381, 1991.

Miller T, Cugliari AM. Withdrawing and withholding treatment: Policies in long-term-care facilities. *Gerontologist* 30:462–468, 1990.

Murphy DJ. Do-not-resuscitate orders: Time for reappraisal in long-term-care institutions. *JAMA* 260:2098–2101, 1988.

Nolan K. Do-not-hospitalize orders: Whose goals? What purpose? *J Fam Pract* 30:31–32, 1990.

Olson E, Chichin ER, Libow LS, et al. A center on ethics in long-term care. *Gerontologist* 33:269–274, 1993.

Printz LA. Is withholding hydration a valid comfort measure in the terminally ill? *Geriatrics* 43:84–88, 1988.

Rifkin J, Naughton T, Schaer T. The evaluation of decision making capacity in a nursing home population. *J Am Geriatr Soc* 40:SA79, 1992.

Roth LH, Meisel A, Lidz CW. Tests of competency to consent to treatment. *Am J Psychiatry* 134:279–284, 1977.

Sachs GA, Siegler M. Guidelines for decision making when the patient is incompetent. *J Crit Illness* 6:348–359, 1991.

Schaer T, Armstrong P, Lynn J. Misconceptions and problems regarding the use of advance directives. *Gerontologist* 32(spec issue II):301, 1992.

Scofield GR. Artificial feeding: The least restrictive alternative? *J Am Geriatr Soc* 39:1217–1220, 1991.

Searight, HR. Assessing patient competence for medical decision making. *Am Fam Physician* 45:751–759, 1992.

Seckler AB, Meier DE, Mulvihill M, Cammer-Paris BE. Substituted judgment: How accurate are proxy predictions? *Ann Intern Med* 115:92–98, 1991.

Siegler M, Singer PA. Clinical ethics consultation: Godsend or "God squad?" *Am J Med* 85:759–765, 1988.

Silberfeld M, Nash C, Singer P. Capacity to complete an advance directive. *J Am Geriatr Soc* 41:1141–1143, 1993.

Tresch CC. Personal communication, 1993.

Tresch CC, Neahring JM, Duthie EH, et al. Outcomes of cardiopulmonary resuscitation in nursing homes: Can we predict who will benefit? *Am J Med* 95:123–130, 1993.

Uhlmann RF, Clark H, Pearlman RA, et al. Medical management decisions in nursing home patients. *Ann Intern Med* 106:879–885, 1987.

Uhlmann RF, Pearlman RA, Cain KC. Physician's and spouses' predictions of elderly patients' resuscitation preferences. *J Gerontol* 43:M115–M121, 1988.

U.S. Congress, Office of Technology Assessment Project Staff. *Life-Sustaining Technologies and the Elderly*, OTA-BA-306. Washington, DC: U.S. Government Printing Office, July 1987.

Watts DT, Cassel CK. Extraordinary nutritional support: A case study and ethical analysis. *J Am Geriatr Soc* 32:237–242, 1984.

Weiss SM. The PSDA: A long-term-care view. *J Clin Ethics* 2:196–199, 1991.

Zweibel NR, Cassel CK, Glasser G. Mechanisms for responding to ethical issues in nursing homes. *Long-Term-Care Currents* 10:7–9, 1987.

18

Medicolegal Issues

Marshall B. Kapp

Mental Health Needs of the Nursing Home Population: Assessment and Treatment Requirements

A substantial proportion of current nursing home residents in the United States need mental health services (Burns et al., 1993). The large cognitively and emotionally impaired population of older persons in long-term-care institutions today derives from two main sources (Mental Health Law Project, 1991): (1) individuals who have developed mental health problems relatively late in life as a result of specific illnesses associated with the aging process and (2) individuals with a long history of mental health problems who, during the past three decades, have been transinstitutionalized (Kanter, 1991–92) from large state psychiatric hospitals to places within the present nursing home industry. While many factors have contributed to the transinstitutionalization phenomenon, legal developments have played a major role in at least two respects: (1) judicial decisions and legislative enactments tightening up on the authority of states to involuntarily commit persons to, and keep persons within, public psychiatric hospitals and (2) cases and statutes intended to improve conditions within state psychiatric facilities but which, in fact, set quality standards that would be so expensive to comply with that states have chosen to reduce their institutional censuses instead (Grob, 1991).

In recognition of the widespread mental health needs of nursing home residents, Congress included special provisions addressing this problem as part of its massive overhaul of nursing home regulation found in the Omnibus Budget Reconciliation Act (OBRA) of 1987 (Public Law No. 100-203). Relevant amendments were added in OBRA 1990 (Public Law No. 101-964).

Assessment Requirements

Specifically, OBRA 1987 contains a requirement (codified at 42 U.S.C. §1396[a]–[h]) for the states to conduct preadmission screening and annual resident reviews of all nursing home applicants and residents suspected of having serious mental illness (but excluding dementia), mental retardation, or a related disorder. This process, which became legally mandatory in 1989, is known as PASARR and is intended to prevent inappropriate placement of persons with mental disabilities in Medicaid (Title 19)–certified nursing facilities. PASARR entails two determinations for individuals found to have a mental disorder. The state mental health or retardation authority must determine first whether the person requires nursing home services and, second, whether specialized services are needed to address the disability.

An applicant who is found not to need nursing facility services—that is, health-related services above the level of room and board that can only be provided in an institutional setting—may not be admitted to a Medicaid certified nursing home under any conditions. Applicants needing nursing facility services who additionally need specialized services may be admitted, but the state must then ensure that the specialized services are provided.

If a person has resided in a nursing facility for less than 30 months before the date of the initial review determination and that person is found to need specialized services but not nursing facility services, the state must work with the resident's family or legal representative for safe and orderly discharge from the facility, prepare and orient the resident for discharge, and provide or arrange for the provision of specialized services. Such discharge need not be immediate. States have alternative disposition plans (ADP), approved by the federal Health Care Financing Administration (HCFA), in which appropriate community residences are identified. States, however, cannot delay providing specialized services to an individual awaiting discharge to a more appropriate setting because the better alternatives are not yet available.

People who have resided in a particular nursing facility for more than 30 months prior to a PASARR finding that they need specialized, but not nursing facility, services are given more leeway. The state must (1) inform them of the institutional and noninstitutional alternatives covered under the state plan, (2) offer the choice of remaining in the facility or of receiving covered services in an alternative setting, (3) clarify the impact of leaving the facility on the resident's eligibility for services (including implications for readmission to the facility), and (4) provide or arrange for indicated specialized services, whether inside or outside of the nursing facility. States may not delay informing residents of alternatives because the alternatives are not yet ready for use.

Several studies have speculated about the impact of PASARR requirements on the potential displacement of present and future nursing facility residents (Freiman et al., 1990; Eichmann et al., 1992). Most of this speculation was predicated on the very expansive definition of mental illness incorporated in the Proposed Rule promulgated by the Department of Health and Human Services in 1990 (55 *Federal Register* 10951, March 23, 1990) to implement OBRA 1987,

TABLE 18.1.   Criteria for Serious Mental Illness Under 57 Fed. Reg. 56450
(November 30, 1992)

A major mental disorder diagnosable under DSM-III-R of schizophrenic, mood, paranoid, panic, or other severe anxiety disorder; somatoform disorder; personality disorder; other psychotic disorder; or other mental disorder that may lead to a chronic disability.

Such diagnosable mental disorder does *not* include a primary diagnosis of dementia, including Alzheimer's disease or a related disorder, and does *not* include a non-primary diagnosis of dementia unless the primary diagnosis is a major mental disorder.

The disorder results in functional limitations in major life activities within the past 3 to 6 months and the individual typically has problems in at least one of the following areas on a continuing or intermittent basis: (a) interpersonal functioning, (b) concentration, persistence, and pace, or (c) adaptation to change.

The treatment history indicates that the individual has experienced at least one of the following: (a) psychiatric treatment more intensive than outpatient care more than once in the past 2 years, or (b) within the last 2 years, due to the mental disorder, experienced an episode of significant disruption to the normal living situation, for which supportive services were required.

namely "a primary or secondary diagnosis of a mental disorder as defined in the Diagnostic and Statistical Manual, 3rd Edition [DSM-IIIR]." In the Final Rule, 57 *Federal Register* 56450 (November 30, 1992), the definition of mental illness was narrowed considerably to mean a "serious mental illness [as defined by the Secretary of DHHS in consultation with the National Institute of Mental Health]." The criteria for considering a person to have a serious mental illness under this latter definition are set forth in Table 18.1.

The PASARR process is distinct from OBRA's requirement for an initial and annual "comprehensive, accurate, standardized, reproducible assessment of each resident's functional capacity" by the nursing facility, 42 U.S.C. §1396r(b)(3)(C)(i). This latter assessment describes the resident's capacity to perform daily life functions, notes significant impairments in functional abilities, and identifies medical problems. The facility must use the assessment "in developing, reviewing, and revising the resident's plan of care," 42 U.S.C. §1396r(b)(3)(D). Proposed regulations implementing this assessment stress that it should be coordinated with the PASARR process, 57 *Federal Register* 61614, 61620 (December 28, 1992). The Proposed Rule includes, among others, Resident Assessment Protocols (RAPs) for psychotropic drug use (p. 61718), physical restraints (p. 61728), mood state (p. 61681), delirium (p. 61650), and cognitive loss/dementia (p. 61654).

Treatment Requirements

Compliance with the mental disorder assessment requirements imposed by PASARR is the state's responsibility, as is providing any specialized services needed by admitted and retained residents. "Specialized services" are defined in the PASARR regulations as intensive interventions meant to treat individuals experiencing an acute episode of severe mental illness. The state may directly provide or arrange for the delivery of these services anywhere within or outside of the nursing facility, in another institution, or in a community setting.

In contrast to what the state must provide, the nursing facility itself is required to provide "mental health" services to the many residents (Eichmann et al., 1992) who need them, regardless of the diagnosis. These services are less intensive and frequent than those which the state must provide—a difference of degree, not kind, between "specialized" and "mental health" services. Mental health services may include nontechnical interventions such as group or individual counseling, family therapy, and regular companionship.

Informed Consent and Compromised Capacity

Federal and state resident rights statutes and regulations, as well as common-law decisions and professional organization principles statements, encourage nursing home residents to participate in decisions concerning their own lives, including choices about medical care. These choices may involve specific treatments to be provided within the nursing facility as well as questions concerning discharge from the facility or transfer to another treatment setting. For many residents, though, compromised cognitive or emotional capacity makes it difficult, if not impossible, for them to provide legally effective and ethically valid informed consent to or refusal of particular medical interventions or placements. This situation presents challenges for clinicians who endeavor to manage the care of those individuals (Ouslander et al., 1991).

As a practical matter, the attending physician functions as a gatekeeper for the resident's autonomy (Post, 1992). Although only a court may legally find a person decisionally incompetent and appoint a substitute decision maker with official authority (i.e., a guardian or conservator), ordinarily the clinician's working assessment regarding the resident's decisional incapacity will trigger reliance on the surrogate for acceptance or refusal of medical intervention (see discussion of advance directives, below). Such reliance, in turn, triggers questions concerning confidentiality and the sharing of information with others absent the resident's express permission (Post, 1992).

In most situations, a working assessment of a resident's decisional capacity may be performed adequately by a primary care physician—i.e., a nonpsychiatrist. Indeed, the resident's attending physician ordinarily knows the resident much better than would a consultant psychiatrist meeting the resident for the first time. Nonetheless, following initial assessments by the primary care physician, a separate psychiatric consultation is often requested (although this is almost always limited to situations where the resident has disagreed with the physician's treatment recommendations) (Knight, 1991). The consultation request is sometimes motivated by the physician's free-floating anxiety about potential legal liability and the desire for a documented second opinion by someone whose expertise a court is likely to respect (Searight, 1992). Utilizing a psychiatric consultation may be especially advisable for residents who have been determined by the PASARR process (see above) to suffer from some mental disorder but who appear at least marginally capable of making and expressing their own opinions about medical care. (See Chapter 16 for a thorough discussion of the role of the consultant psychiatrist.)

Practice guidelines for the clinical assessment of decisional capacity abound in the medical and legal literature (e.g., Freedman et al., 1991; Galen, 1993; Smyer, 1993). (A thorough exposition of this topic is offered in Chapter 17.)

Nursing facilities should consult with their medical staffs and nursing and social service departments, as well as institutional legal counsel, to utilize the professional literature and any relevant case law or statutes in the particular jurisdiction to formulate and formally adopt written policies and procedures concerning decisional capacity assessment for facility residents. These institutional protocols should address, at a minimum (1) when a psychiatric consultation must/should be ordered, (2) under what circumstances the facility's institutional ethics committee should be involved in decision making for a cognitively impaired resident, (3) in what situations judicial involvement to definitively resolve questions about a resident's decisional capacity ought to be involved, and (4) the decision-making process for actual (de facto) but not judicially declared (de jure) incapacitated residents with and without formal advance directives. These institutional protocols should be woven into the facility's overall risk-management program (Kapp, 1987).

Although courts now are, and ought to be, approached only rarely for de jure declarations concerning a resident's competence (the legal determination of decision-making capacity), apprehension has been expressed by nursing facility providers and resident advocates that the emphasis of OBRA 1987's residents' rights guarantees of resident participation in decisions may exert the paradoxical effect of motivating more providers to resort to the judiciary for formal clarification of decision-making authority for decisionally questionable residents. Such a development and its impact on resident care and facility operation would have to be monitored closely.

Advance Medical Directives

Recent legal developments encouraging the use of advance medical directives are intended to facilitate medical decision making for individuals, including nursing facility residents, who no longer have the ability to make and express their own autonomous treatment choices. The availability of these legal devices, however, raises several additional implications for clinicians who deal with cognitively compromised residents.

Federal and State Legislation

In the wake of the U.S. Supreme Court's lone "right to die" decision in *Cruzan v. Director, Missouri Department of Health*, 110 S.Ct. 2841 (1990) (Emanuel, 1992), Congress enacted the federal Patient Self-Determination Act (PSDA) in November 1990 as §§4206 and 4751 of that year's OBRA (Public Law 101-508). The PSDA was not intended to create new substantive rights for individuals but rather to impose certain process requirements on health care providers to facilitate and encourage patients in the exercise of their existing medical decision-making rights (McCloskey, 1991). The PSDA requirements encompass all nursing facilities (in addition to hospitals, home health agencies, hospices, health mainte-nance organizations, and preferred provider organizations) that participate in the Medicare and Medicaid programs. Implementing regulations were promulgated by DHHS in 1992 (42 Code of Federal Regulations §489.102).

Specifically, nursing facilities are mandated by the PSDA to take several actions. First, they must develop and provide to incoming residents or, for resi-dents who are cognitively incapacitated to their proxies, a formal policy statement regarding the facility's handling of advance medical directives. This statement may not conflict with applicable state law. Next, the nursing facility must inquire whether the entering resident has previously written any kind of advance directive. If the reply to this inquiry is in the negative, a presently decisionally capable resident must be informed of his or her rights under pertinent state law to execute such a directive. Last, the nursing facility is expected under the law to sponsor educational opportunities on this subject for its staff, residents, and more gen-eral communities.

In the midst of the *Cruzan* decision, congressional action on the PSDA, and a large amount of accompanying publicity surrounding the dilemma of medical decision making near the end of life, virtually every state legislature in the early 1990s revisited and amended existing state law on the subject. Those few states that had not previously enacted legislation in this realm got on the bandwagon.

These state statutes vary somewhat in their specifics, particularly concerning their purported limitations of and checks on personal autonomy in the name of protecting vulnerable persons from abuse or neglect. Many of these legislatively enacted limitations raise serious constitutional as well as public policy questions. Putting those problems to one side and emphasizing the need to carefully consult the precise legislation in one's own jurisdiction, it is possible to generically describe the three chief components present in most of these state statutes.

First, all of these statutes authorize a device for mentally capable adults to execute an instruction-type directive, usually called a living will or declaration. This formal advance directive offers residents the opportunity to document the types of medical interventions they would wish to have or refuse in the event of future critical illness accompanied by an incapacity at the time to make and express autonomous choices. Interesting questions have been suggested concern-ing the ability of people to foresee accurately their future preferences concerning life-sustaining medical treatments, when those predictions are made now in a hypothetical context (Cantor, 1992). Nonetheless, the instruction directive repre-sents the best attempt at an educated guess about resident wishes when contempo-raneous discussion with the resident is impossible because of intervening incapac-ity. Some have suggested that the reliability of such inferences may be improved by encouraging residents to document broad "values histories" instead of more particular, intervention-oriented instruction directives (Lambert et al., 1990).

Values histories can also help in comprehending and applying instruction directive provisions whose interpretation often ends up being quite ambiguous in actual treatment contexts.

A second aspect of most modern state life-sustaining medical treatment (LSMT) statutes aims at overcoming some of the limitations of instruction directives. This component authorizes currently able persons to execute a written proxy directive for health care purposes (New York Task Force, 1992). A proxy directive, usually taking the form of a durable power of attorney (Annas, 1991), enables presently capable adults to designate others to act as their medical decision-making agents in the future if the residents are no longer capable of deciding or speaking independently. Legally empowering a proxy gives the resident an actual advocate, with whom the resident should have earlier discussed personal treatment values and preferences, to speak on the resident's behalf during a time of total dependence. At the same time, the availability of an authorized proxy offers the nursing facility and its staff a chance to consult with someone presumably knowledgeable about the resident's desires.

A third point covered by statute explicitly in approximately half of the country is decision making for a currently incapacitated person who has not previously executed an advance instruction or proxy directive. Family consent statutes designate relatives, in a stated priority order, as agents with authority to make certain kinds of medical decisions on behalf of people in this category provided that specific procedural safeguards have been satisfied. In essence, family consent statutes codify or legitimate the long-standing medical practice of turning to "next of kin" for advice and decisions when the resident is decisionally unavailable.

Clinical Implications

By emphasizing the large role of resident autonomy in LSMT decisions, the PSDA and state advance directive legislation is likely to have a substantial impact on the role of clinicians who are involved with mental health issues in the nursing facility. Some of the clinician's tasks here will be familiar but with different, challenging twists, while other professional and public expectations will be relatively novel.

Evaluating Decisional Capacity

As has already been noted, developing valid and reliable protocols and techniques for assessing decisional capacity is important regarding informed consent and medical decision making generally. It is likely that the PSDA and state advance directive legislation will raise the importance and complexity of resident capacity evaluations to a new level. A proactive approach to compliance with statutory obligations suggests that nursing facilities should delineate a clear framework, reflected in written policies and procedures, for assessing and documenting every resident's ability to understand the nature and consequences of advance directives and to execute them if desired. For some residents in a gray zone of cognitive ability, a greater degree of explicit psychiatric input than ordinary and more elaborate documentation may be indicated.

Clinicians are used to conducting assessments of decisional capacity based on "real time"—that is, which evaluate an individual's ability to make medical decisions around the same time the assessment is conducted. Under the PSDA, clinicians may be asked to conduct more retrospective and prospective rather than just concurrent assessments.

For persons who are admitted to a Medicare or Medicaid-participating nursing facility, retrospective evaluation of decisional capacity may be called for in two kinds of circumstances. For people who enter a facility with a previously executed advance medical directive, a question may be posed about the validity of that advance directive based on uncertainty concerning the decisional capacity of the resident at the earlier time that directive execution took place. For the new resident who desires at the time of admission to execute an advance directive for the first time or to revise an existing one, decisional capacity may be questionable and in need of formal assessment. In both of these situations, a psychiatrist may be requested to conduct a capacity assessment, ordinarily at some time after the resident's admission, aimed at advising the attending physician or a court about the resident's previous mental ability.

Additionally, when a person of questionable capacity indicates a wish to execute or revise a medical directive at the point of admission to a nursing facility, the clinician will have to conduct an evaluation of that individual's ability to make medical choices today that will not become effective until some future time. Further, since advance directives ordinarily are executed by decisionally capable people with the proviso that they spring into effectiveness only upon the individual's subsequent incapacity, the clinician will be called upon to determine at what moment an advance directive should become operative. In the absence of an advance directive, evaluation of the resident's decisional capacity may be indicated in more situations to help figure out when the health care team ought to rely upon its jurisdiction's family consent statute in turning to next of kin. (See Chapter 17 for a complete discussion of advance directives.)

Facilitating Decision Making

Beyond its decisional capacity assessment ramifications, the PSDA also will probably enhance the role of clinicians involved in mental health care in many cases as facilitators of prospective and concurrent medical decision making. For a start in this regard, the nursing facility should incorporate mental health perspectives and expertise into the ongoing process of development and revision of the written institutional policies and procedures that are mandated by the PSDA. For nursing facilities with institutional ethics committees, mental health representation on (or at least consultation to) this body should be prominent.

Even many residents who are capable and desirous of exercising autonomy may need counseling assistance to sufficiently understand their alternatives and to make and express a choice among competing courses. Mental health skills will often be especially valuable in providing this sort of guidance and support. For the dying resident, the mental health professional can convey comfort and assurance that the resident will not be abandoned regardless of the treatment (or non-treatment) regime selected.

Advance directives may be useful for nondying residents also, such as chronically ill individuals who are likely to need extensive mental health services in the future but whose decisional capacity may wax and wane. One unintended but legitimate consequence of the PSDA may be to encourage clinicians to try to persuade presently capable residents to execute forms of a ''psychiatric will'' that would consent in advance to mental health treatment in the event of subsequent need but decisional incapacity (Appelbaum, 1991).

Where a treatable medical problem, such as depression, interferes with a resident's ability to rationally arrive at treatment decisions (including the decision to execute an advance directive), mental health professionals may contribute to promoting individual autonomy—and the relief of suffering that may be coloring the resident's ostensible choices—by providing effective treatment for the underlying cognitive impairment. For the resident who is admitted in the midst of a temporary decisional incapacity brought about by intercurrent physical or mental illness, the mental health professional can assist in determining when the resident has regained sufficient lucidity to be approached about advance directives and other facets of medical decision making.

For decisionally capable and incapacitated residents alike, both nursing home admission and critical illness are times of great stress for families. The emphasis of the PSDA on decisional autonomy for residents and their families will probably strain fragile family dynamics even further in many situations. Mental health professionals should be expected to play an even more significant part than at present in guiding medically, morally, and emotionally perplexed families through the difficult decision-making processes accompanying nursing facility admission and critical illness (Orr et al., 1991).

Finally, the function of the mental health care team by no means ends once a decision to forego certain components of LSMT has been made and recorded. On the contrary, there is a strong ethical as well as legal imperative against abandoning the resident and family at this time. It is precisely at this point that emotional support to residents and their families for their stress and bereavement is most essential. This role must not be forgotten or sacrificed in the rush to impress governmental surveyors by complying with the formal documentation mandates of the PSDA.

Physical Restraints and Psychotropic Drugs

The use of both physical or mechanical restraints and psychotropic drugs in nursing facilities is a subject that is addressed extensively in the OBRA 1987 legislation and implementing regulations. Current legal provisions quite clearly convey congressional and regulatory intentions to reduce markedly the unnecessary and inappropriate utilization of these behavior control modalities. These legal provisions have substantial implications for professionals concerned with the care of mentally compromised nursing facility residents.

Physical Restraints

Defined in the HCFA *Interpretative Guidelines for Surveyors* as "any manual method or physical or mechanical device, material, or equipment attached or adjacent to the resident's body that the individual cannot remove easily which restricts freedom of movement or normal access to one's body," physical restraints have been a regular part of the institutional long term care scene in the United States for hundreds of years (Evans and Strumpf, 1989). The growing professional and public perception that the use of physical restraints in nursing facilities in many instances is unnecessary, improper, and even abusive has culminated in detailed federal and state regulation.

The present federal rule, published February 5, 1992, provides that "the resident has the right to be free from any physical restraints imposed or psychoactive drug administered for purposes of discipline or convenience, and not required to treat the resident's medical symptoms," 42 Code of Federal Regulations §483.13[a]. The OBRA 1987 statute itself goes even further:

> Restraints may only be imposed to ensure the physical safety of the resident or other residents, and only upon the written order of a physician that specifies the duration and the circumstances under which the restraints are to be used (except in emergency circumstances which are to be specified by the secretary [of DHHS] until such an order could reasonably be obtained), Public Law No. 100-203, §§4201(c)(1)(A)(ii) (Medicare) and 4211(c)(1)(A)(ii) (Medicaid).

The HCFA is encouraging state surveyors to take an aggressive stance in enforcing the new statutory and regulatory requirements concerning the use of physical restraints. This stance is consciously intended to be consistent with the resident outcome orientation characterizing the nursing home survey process under OBRA 1987, as exemplified by the requirements that all nursing facilities administer a comprehensive assessment for each resident based on a nationally uniform minimum data set (MDS) and "[t]hat each resident must receive and the facility must provide the necessary care and services to attain and maintain the highest practicable physical or mental and psychosocial well-being in accordance with the comprehensive assessment and plan of care." In addition to federal regulation by HCFA tied to a nursing facility's participation in Medicare and Medicaid, providers should also be aware of potential liability connected to regulation by the federal Food and Drug Administration (FDA) of physical restraints as medical "devices."

Additionally, virtually every state guarantees nursing home residents the right to be free from excessive physical restraints as part of that state's resident bill of rights. These state provisions are in accord with both the spirit and letter of the current federal requirements.

Contrary to popular belief in some provider circles, these governmental provisions limiting the permissible use of physical restraints do not unduly increase the potential negligence or malpractice exposure of nursing facilities based on resident falls or wandering. In fact, the exact opposite is true (Johnson, 1990). Cases holding providers liable in the absence of restraints are far eclipsed in number and amount of damages by legal judgments and settlements made on the basis of inappropriate ordering of restraints, failure to monitor and correct their adverse effects on the resident, or errors in the mechanical application of the restraint.

The question of physical restraint reduction in nursing facilities is no longer a matter for debate but only for implementation. Nursing facilities must develop and carry out policies and procedures to comply with all applicable legal requirements in this regard. Less restrictive alternatives to the use of restraints, including both environmental and administrative changes in the facility, must be explored fully and explained to staff, residents, and families (Libow and Starer, 1989).

Psychotropic Drugs

Psychotropic drugs have been prescribed profusely, and often improperly, in American nursing homes (Waxman et al., 1985; Avorn et al., 1989; Sternberg et al., 1990; Beers et al., 1991; Garrard et al., 1991; Svarstad and Mount, 1991). Prescriptions for them frequently have been issued in the absence of any specific psychiatric diagnosis for the resident, let alone a comprehensive treatment plan explaining the rationale for the drugs. Instead of being prescribed on the basis of medical indications, psychotropics have sometimes been used for environmental control or to appease the strenuous demands of families or staff.

The OBRA of 1987 and its implementing regulations, as well as corresponding resident rights laws in every state, aim at major changes from the previously prevailing situation where psychotropic drugs were sometimes used for nonpsychiatric treatment purposes (Burke, 1991; Jencks and Clauser, 1991; Senate Special Committee on Aging, 1991). As noted previously, 42 Code of Federal Regulations §483.13(a) assures each nursing facility resident "the right to be free from any . . . psychoactive drug administered for the purposes of discipline or convenience, and not required to treat the resident's medical symptoms." Additionally, 42 Code of Federal Regulations §483.25(1)(1) states that each resident's drug regimen must be free from unnecessary drugs, and 42 Code of Federal Regulations §483.25(1)(2) requires that a resident for whom antipsychotics have not been used previously may be given them only to treat a specific condition. Residents getting antipsychotic drugs must receive gradual dose reductions or drug holidays. HCFA's *Interpretive Guidelines for Surveyors* should be consulted for guidance concerning criteria for unnecessary drugs, specific indications for permissible psychotropic drug prescription behaviors that should not be considered an indication for psychotropic drug use, and drug discontinuation methodologies (Burke, 1991).

Beyond governmental regulations, a current standard of the Joint Commission on Accreditation of Healthcare Organizations (JCAHO) speaks clearly about the need for medications, specifically antipsychotic drugs. The 1994 *Accreditation Manual for Long-Term Care* states that "antipsychotic drug therapy [may only be] used to treat a specific condition," and that a resident has a right to freedom from chemical and physical restraints, except as authorized in writing by a physician for a specified time period and when necessary to protect the resident from self-injury or from injuring others.

The OBRA statute and regulations, plus the JCAHO standards, recognize the professional consensus (Board of Directors, 1992) that there may often be quite legitimate therapeutic indications for the prescription of psychotropics. Legal standards to which providers are held obviously assume that prescribers will keep abreast of the current professional literature in this sphere (Beers et al., 1991). Even when prescribed for the correct reasons, however, possible drug toxicities may be underestimated. It is important, therefore, for facility staff to carefully monitor residents on psychotropics for timely indications of negative side effects. Liability may be imposed for negligence in monitoring and response even where the resident assessment and the prescription itself were initially defensible. Further, when a resident is taken off a particular medication, adequate monitoring for untoward reactions is an expected part of the standard of care.

Federal regulations require within each nursing facility a regular pharmacist-conducted drug regimen review (DRR). This should be incorporated into the facility's more comprehensive drug utilization review (DUR) program, with which medical and nursing staff should cooperate completely and in an ongoing manner.

Conclusion

Psychiatric care in the nursing home entails many interesting legal considerations. The picture has been made considerably more complicated over the last several years by the enactment of statutes, regulations, and voluntary standards on the federal and state levels designed to improve the quality of care—long deficient—available to mentally disordered nursing home residents and to promote the principles of individual self-determination and least intrusive alternative as much as possible. Understanding and dealing creatively and positively with these legal requirements may make the role of clinician in a nursing facility more difficult than before, but no doubt also more satisfying and fulfilling.

References

Annas GJ. The health care proxy and the living will. *N Engl J Med* 324:1210–1213, 1991.

Appelbaum PS. Advance directives for psychiatric treatment. *Hosp Commun Psychiatry* 42:983–984, 1991.

Avorn J, Dreyer P, Connelly K, Soumerai SB. Use of psychoactive medication and the quality of care in rest homes. *N Engl J Med* 320:227–232, 1989.

Beers M, Avorn J, Soumerai S, et al. Psychoactive medication use in intermediate-care facility residents. *JAMA* 260:3016–3020, 1988.

Beers MH, Ouslander JG, Rollingher I, et al. Explicit criteria for determining inappropriate medication use in nursing home residents. *Arch Intern Med* 151:1825–1832, 1991.

Board of Directors of the American Association for Geriatric Psychiatry, Clinical Practice Committee of the American Geriatrics Society, and Committee on Long-term Care and Treatment for the Elderly of the American Psychiatric Association. Psychotherapeutic medications in the nursing home. *J Am Geriatr Soc* 40:946–949, 1992.

Burke WJ, Neuroleptic drug use in the nursing home: The impact of OBRA. *Am Fam Physician* 43:2125–2130, 1991.

Burns BJ, Wagner HR, Taube JE, et al. Mental health service use by the elderly in nursing homes. *Am J Public Health* 83:331–337, 1993.

Cantor NL. Prospective autonomy: On the limits of shaping one's postcompetence medical fate. *J Contemp Health Law Policy* 8:13–48, 1992.

Eichmann MA, Griffin BP, Lyons JS, et al. An estimation of the impact of OBRA-87 on nursing home care in the United States. *Hosp Commun Psychiatry* 43:781–789, 1992.

Emanuel EJ. Securing patients' right to refuse medical care: In praise of the Cruzan decision. *Am J Med* 92:307–312, 1992.

Evans LK, Strumpf NE. Tying down the elderly: A review of the literature on physical restraint. *J Am Geriatr Soc* 37:65–74, 1989.

Freedman M, Stuss DT, Gordon M. Assessment of competency: The role of neurobehavioral deficits. *Ann Intern Med* 115:203–208, 1991.

Freiman MP, Arons BS, Goldman HH, Burns BJ. Nursing home reform and the mentally ill. *Health Affairs* 9:47–60, 1990.

Galen KD. Assessing psychiatric patients' competency to agree to treatment plans: *Hosp Community Psychiatry* 44:361–364, 1993.

Garrard J, Makris L, Dunham T, et al. Evaluation of neuroleptic drug use by nursing home elderly under proposed medicare and medicaid regulations. *JAMA* 265:463–467, 1991.

Grof GN. *From Asylum to Community: Mental Health Policy in Modern America.* Princeton NJ: Princeton University Press, 1991.

Jencks SF, Clauser SB. Managing behavior problems in nursing homes. *JAMA* 265:502–503, 1991.

Johnson SH. The fear of liability and the use of restraints in nursing homes. *Law Med Health Care* 18:263–273, 1990.

Kanter AS. Abandoned but not forgotten: The illegal confinement of elderly people in state psychiatric institutions. *NYU Rev Law Social Change* 19:273–307, 1991–92.

Kapp MB. *Preventing Malpractice in Long-term Care: Strategies for Risk Management:* New York: Springer, 1987.

Knight JA. Judging competence: When the psychiatrist need, or need not, be involved. In: Cutter MA, Shelp ES, eds. *Competency.* The Netherlands: Kluwer, 1991.

Lambert P, Gibson JM, Nathanson P. The values history: An innovation in surrogate medical decision-making. *Law Med Health Care* 18:202–212, 1990.

Libow LS, Starer P. Care of the nursing home patient. *N Engl J Med* 321:93–93, 1989.

McCloskey E. Between isolation and intrusion: The patient self-determination act. *Law Med Health Care* 19:80–82, 1991.

Mental Health Law Project. Making choices: Challenges for advocates and elderly nursing home residents with mental illness. *Mental Disability Law and the Elderly.* Issue Paper #2. Washington, DC: Bazelon Mental Health Law Center, 1991.

New York State Task Force on Life and the Law. *When Others Must Choose: Deciding for Patients Without Capacity.* New York: New York State Task Force on Life and the Law, 1992.

Orr RD, Paris JJ, Siegler M. Caring for the terminally ill: Resolving conflicting objectives between patient, physician, family, and institution. *J Fam Pract* 33:500–504, 1991.

Ouslander JG, Osterweil D, Morley J. *Medical Care in the Nursing Home.* New York: McGraw-Hill, 1991.

Post SG. Values in geriatric psychiatry. *J Geriatr Psychiatry* 25:125–137, 1992.

Searight HR. Assessing patient competence for medical decision making. *Am Fam Physician* 45:751–759, 1992.

Senate Special Committee on Aging. *Reducing the Use of Chemical Restraints in Nursing Homes.* (S. Hrg., 102-554, Serial No. 102-6). Washington, DC: U.S. Government Printing Office, 1991.

Sternberg J, Spector WD, Drugovich ML, et al. Use of psychoactive drugs in nursing homes: Prevalence and residents' characteristics. *J Geriatr Drug Ther* 4:47–60, 1990.

Smyer MA. Aging and decision-making capacity. *Generations* 17:51–56, 1993.

Svarstad BL, Mount JK. Nursing home resources and tranquilizer use among the institutionalized elderly. *J Am Geriatr Soc* 39:869–875, 1991.

Waxman HM, Klein M, Carner EA. Drug misuse in nursing homes: An institutional addiction? *Hosp Commun Psychiatry* 36:886–292, 1985.

Index